Caregiving Contexts

Maximiliane E. Szinovacz, PhD, is professor and director of the Gerontology Institute at the University of Massachusetts Boston. She received her doctorate from the University of Vienna, Austria. She has coauthored or edited four books—most recently the *Handbook of Grandparenthood*—and has published over 70 articles and book chapters. She is a fellow of the Gerontological Society of America and of the National Council on Family Relations. Her research interests focus on retirement, intergenerational relationships and caregiving, and grandparenthood.

Adam Davey, PhD, is an associate professor in the College of Health Professions at Temple University. Dr. Davey is a developmental psychologist with training in human development and family studies from the Pennsylvania State University. Previously, he was senior research scientist at the Polisher Research Institute and an associate professor at the University of Georgia. Dr. Davey's research addresses issues of marital and intergenerational relationships, family caregiving, and comparative analysis of the interface between formal and informal care networks, particularly in the United States, Great Britain, and Sweden. Currently, Dr. Davey is examining regional variability in how families have responded to changes over a 6-year period in the availability of formal services across Sweden. He has published more than 60 articles and book chapters.

Caregiving Contexts

Cultural, Familial, and Societal Implications

Edited by

Maximiliane E. Szinovacz, PhD

and

Adam Davey, PhD

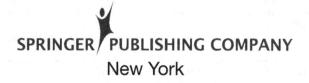

SPRINGER PUBLISHING COMPANY
New York

Springer Publishing Company, LLC
11 West 42nd Street
New York, NY 10036
www.springerpub.com

Acquisitions Editor: Sheri W. Sussman
Managing Editor: Mary Ann McLaughlin
Project Manager: Carol Cain
Cover design: Joanne E. Honigman
Composition: Apex Publishing, LLC

08 09 10/ 5 4 3 2 1

Library of Congress Cataloging-in-Publication Data

Caregiving contexts : cultural, familial, and societal implications / Maximiliane E. Szinovacz, Adam Davey.
    p. cm.
  Includes bibliographical references and index.
  ISBN-13: 978-0-8261-0287-4 (alk. paper)
  ISBN-10: 0-8261-0287-5 (alk. paper)
  1. Older people—Care—Cross-cultural studies. 2. Older people—Home care—Cross-cultural studies. 3. Older people—Family relationships—Cross-cultural studies. 4. Caregivers—Cross-cultural studies. 5. Older people—Government policy—Cross-cultural studies. I. Szinovácz, Maximiliane. II. Davey, Adam.
  HV1451.C325 2008
  362.6—dc22   2007020081

Printed in the United States of America by Maple-Vail.

Contents

List of Contributors

Élena del Barrio, MA
IMSERSO (Instituto de Migraciones y
Servicios Sociales)
Madrid, Spain

Penélope Castejon, MA
IMSERSO
Madrid, Spain

Mayte Sancho Castiello, MA
IMSERSO
Madrid, Spain

Michelle Cheuk, MA
Department of Sociology
University of North Carolina at Chapel Hill
Chapel Hill, NC

Stephen Conroy, PhD
University of San Diego
San Diego, CA

Amanda Cott, BA
Carolina Population Center
University of North Carolina at Chapel Hill
Chapel Hill, NC

Daphna Gans, PhD
University of Southern California
Los Angeles, CA

Nurit Gur-Yaish, PhD
Center for Research and Study of Aging
Faculty of Social Welfare and Health Studies
University of Haifa
Haifa, Israel

Kathryn A. Henderson, PhD
Department of Sociology
Indiana University
Bloomington, IN

Lennarth Johansson, PhD
National Board of Health and Welfare
Stockholm, Sweden

Richard W. Johnson, PhD
Income and Benefits Policy Center
Urban Institute
Washington, DC

Ruth Katz, PhD
Department of Human Services
Center for Research and Study of Aging
Faculty of Social Welfare and Health Studies
University of Haifa
Haifa, Israel

Ariela Lowenstein, PhD
Department of Masters in Gerontology
Center for Research and Study of Aging
Faculty of Social Welfare and
Health Studies
University of Haifa
Haifa, Israel

Bo Malmberg, PhD
Institute of Gerontology
Jönköping, Sweden

Casey Schroeder Miklowski, MA
Department of Sociology
Case Western Reserve University
Cleveland, OH

Eliza K. Pavalko, PhD
Department of Sociology
Indiana University
Bloomington, IN

Merril Silverstein, PhD
University of Southern California
Los Angeles, CA

Eleanor Palo Stoller, PhD
Department of Sociology
Wake Forest University
Winston-Salem, NC

Gerdt Sundström, PhD
Institute of Gerontology
Jönköping, Sweden

Maria Angeles Tortosa, PhD
Department of Economics
University of Valencia
Valencia, Spain

Peter Uhlenberg, PhD
Department of Sociology
University of North Carolina at Chapel Hill
Carolina Population Center
Chapel Hill, NC

Steven K. Wisensale, PhD
Department of Family Studies
College of Liberal Arts
University of Connecticut Storrs, CT

Steven H. Zarit, PhD
Department of Human Development and Family Studies
Pennsylvania State University
University Park, PA

Foreword

The study of care by families to older adults is a relatively recent focus in the social and behavioral sciences. Until the late 1970s, only a handful of articles had addressed the family's role in assisting elders. Family gerontology had instead been concerned with a different issue: the withering of traditional support for older generations. It was widely believed that older people would be left alone and lonely, living in age-segregated communities or institutional settings. Much of the research at that time sought to establish whether there was still any contact between elders and their families (e.g., Shanas, 1968). While academics were pondering these questions, ordinary people found themselves increasingly concerned about and engaged in the care of their parents and spouses. Their worries worked their way into the media, and finally to the research community (Neugarten, 1979).

Although families have always provided care, the emerging public awareness in the last 30 years reflects a substantial change in the conditions of care. In the past, caring for elders within the family was the norm, but care was rare, since most people did not live to old age, and the period of decline at the end of life was typically brief. Now, of course, life expectancy is longer and most people live to ages when it is likely that they will develop chronic illnesses and disabilities that require ongoing care. Furthermore, the same improvements in medicine and public health that have promoted long life have also extended life after the onset of disease and disability (Cassel, Rudberg, & Olshansky, 1992). As a result, more older people need care than ever before and for longer periods of time.

In light of these changes, the resilience of families is remarkable. Despite the fractures in family life caused by divorce and other problems and the declining economic resources of many working- and middle-class families, family ties to their elders have largely remained strong and they remain the main source of care, even in countries with well-developed public support programs (Shea et al., 2003).

It is not surprising, given the pressures on families, that much of the research on caregiving has been preoccupied with questions of stress and burden. This has been an important focus because of the public health implications associated with chronic stress and the need to develop reasonable systems of support to help families provide care. It was also an important step in establishing family care as a legitimate field of study and for the practical goal of obtaining research funding.

An unintended side effect of this emphasis, however, has been to decontextualize family care. The focus has been almost exclusively on a single caregiver, who has been viewed from within a relatively narrow, albeit important, frame: how stress affects health and well-being. Despite this focus, the most consistent and enduring finding in the caregiving literature from the earliest to the most current research is the heterogeneity among caregivers, caregiving families, and the stresses and outcomes they experience. There is surprisingly little attention paid to the sources of this variability, particularly how the social connections between the caregiver and his or her family, community, and the wider social milieu affect the care process and outcomes.

This volume represents a major step forward in the literature by placing its focus squarely on the caregiving context, its dimensions and how it shapes the process and outcomes of family care. The chapters locate care within the family, rather than a single individual. A husband, wife, daughter, or other family member may take on the lion's share of responsibility, but other kin and nonkin are usually involved in giving help and support on a regular basis, and the transactions and negotiations among them are a critical dimension of the care process. The family, in turn, is embedded within a larger cultural, community, and social context. Cultural expectations affect decisions about who becomes a caregiver, who else might provide help, the meanings attributed to disability and care, willingness to make personal sacrifices in providing care, openness to outside services and support, and a variety of other issues. The community and its ecology can facilitate or hinder care through such factors as ease of access to everyday services such as groceries or health care, as well as acceptance and support. The larger social and policy context has an obvious effect on whether and in what ways caregivers and disabled elders might be supported.

These explorations of context will give us a broader view of how caregiving occurs. It will help us improve our theories about care and about the family's role in contemporary society. An understanding of the variability in family care also can lead to development of more effective ways of supporting families. Rather than a one-size-fits-all approach, which has largely characterized social programs and public policy, we need to devise strategies that complement the heterogeneity of families. These approaches can grow out of an understanding of the conditions under which families manage the multiple challenges of care and how some families learn to manage more effectively.

We also need to recognize that families have limited resources and ability to provide care, especially as disabilities of the person they care for become more severe. Rather than viewing the institution as the end of the process, however, the reality is that families continue to be involved. We need more thoughtful plans for incorporating families into the life of a residential setting.

Care of our elders is an enduring and yet evolving part of life. The focus on context will help us understand, support, and learn from the ways that families meet the challenges involved.

Steven H. Zarit, PhD
Professor and Head
Department of Human Development and Family Studies
Pennsylvania State University

REFERENCES

Cassel, C. K., Rudberg, M. A., & Olshansky, S. J. (1992). The price of success: Health care in an aging society. *Health Affairs, 11*, 87–99.

Neugarten, B. L. (1979). The middle generations. In P. K. Ragan (Ed.), *Aging parents*. Los Angeles: University of Southern California Press.

Shanas, E., and others. (1968). *Old people in three industrial societies*. New York: Atherton Press.

Shea, D. G., Davey, A., Femia, E. E., Zarit, S. H., Sundstrom, G., Berg, S., & Smyer, M. A. (2003). Exploring assistance in Sweden and the United States. *Gerontologist, 43*, 712–721.

Caregiving Contexts

CHAPTER ONE

Introduction: Caregiving in Context[1]

Adam Davey and Maximiliane E. Szinovacz

Although contexts are rarely considered, the majority of issues associated with aging of individuals and societies are socially and culturally bound. Most of the key issues—such as household structure and living arrangements; work, leisure, and retirement; and health and social policies—vary considerably from one sociocultural context to another. There is also considerable heterogeneity within contexts that has not received a great deal of attention in previous research. This volume attempts to increase our understanding of caregiving through a wide variety of contextual frameworks, as opposed to the more common disciplinary perspective.

As the baby boom cohorts move from mid-life toward old age, demand for caregivers will increase significantly, and issues surrounding caregiving will reach even greater societal significance than they already have today. Much of the existing caregiving literature has focused on the caregiver or care recipient, their relationship, and caregivers' burdens and stress. However, fuller understanding of caregiving issues requires a broader, contextual perspective. Such a perspective is particularly important to prepare caregiving-related programs and policies for the challenges of the aging baby boom cohorts.

The objective of this volume is to present a contextual perspective on caregiving. We focus on three interrelated contexts: the sociocultural, familial, and sociopolitical. This perspective is pursued in a dual manner. First, each chapter addresses a specific caregiving context. Second, the individual chapters pay attention to contexts other than those of specific

1

focus in the chapter. For example, all chapters consider selected relevant subcultural variations (race and ethnicity, gender differences, regional variations, etc.). In addition, individual chapters demonstrate linkages between different contexts, such as between cultural and familial contexts. Insights pertaining to the familial contexts of care (e.g., the familial support network) could be linked to societal-level family structural change or to cultural variations in norms about filial obligations to provide care.

As a result, the content of this book is structured somewhat differently from many other edited volumes. Each chapter begins with an introduction to the topic and a thorough review of the relevant literature. Each chapter then continues to present new data or a novel conceptualization relevant to the contexts of care. Each chapter, then, represents a unique contribution to our knowledge base that can stand on its own. Each chapter, however, also provides a contrast or counterpoint to the other contributions in this volume to illustrate the same topic from multiple vantage points, or in divergent contexts. In this way, it becomes possible to begin unpacking the various assumptions and presuppositions that guide our work or that of the dominant paradigm.

The first section addresses the sociocultural contexts of care. Uhlenberg and Cheuk use data from the Second Longitudinal Study on Aging to address the question of how the availability of caregivers is projected to change in the future, relative to today's levels. Their analyses expand on questions of how society will be fundamentally altered by the aging of this demographically large cohort. Adding to our concerns about what will happen to programs such as Social Security and Medicare, Uhlenberg and Cheuk consider the solvency of informal care. To the extent that their assumptions and projections reflect reality, the implications of their research for the largest single source of support—informal caregivers—are sobering. The breadth of data sources they bring to bear on addressing this topic speaks volumes about the extent to which the study of aging requires an interdisciplinary perspective. Given the societal significance of the baby boom cohorts thus far, it would be surprising if they failed to exert lasting changes on formal and informal care as well.

Johnson builds on these demographic trends by considering the factors affecting decisions individuals make regarding the choice of long-term care services—including home care, nursing home care, and informal care from children and other sources—using data from the 2002 wave of the Health and Retirement Study. This chapter and the data it presents have important implications given the considerable changes in women's labor force participation. This chapter illustrates the extent to which economic perspectives on care have been elaborated to consider a wider range of individual, family, and social variables than would have been common a decade ago. It reminds us, as well, that the costs (both real and opportunity) of care, and factors associated with variations in them, are an important and often overlooked aspect of old-age care.

Taking a slightly different approach, Silverstein, Conroy, and Gans adopt a focus that blends social psychological and economic perspectives to understand what leads one child to step forward and provide care for a mother in light of expectations about what one's siblings will provide. The resulting analyses of data from the Longitudinal Study of Generations (LSOG) demonstrate the intricate relationships between norms and costs on each sibling's care decisions. The central issue is that the care decisions made by one sibling have important implications for the other siblings. This should remind us that it is nearly impossible under most conditions to consider the perspective of a single actor without also considering the family context. It reminds us, as well, that some constellations of support are likely to be more satisfactory than others. As these authors demonstrate, formalized models of care can be quite useful in considering important conditions and dimensions along which care decisions vary within a single family.

The issues of population aging are truly global in their implications. In a significant extension of their previous research, Lowenstein, Katz, and Gur-Yaish examine cross-national variability in elder care using the rich data from the Old Age and Autonomy: The Role of Service Systems and Intergenerational Family Solidarity (OASIS) study. Their chapter considers both the expectations for assistance from formal and informal sources and their associations with quality of life in four European nations and Israel. Cross-national research is difficult to do well, and researchers must often rely on comparisons of data from diverse samples and measures collected with different purposes in mind. Thus, the use of OASIS data provides a good way to make cross-national comparisons directly and reliably. Their findings underscore the fact that high levels of state-provided services do not appear to deter support from informal sources. Rather, older adults receive more assistance, or at least assistance from a wider range of sources, in nations with more extensive services for older adults. Given the high observed levels of unmet need in the United States, this has important implications for aging populations.

What these chapters have in common is that they display the central role played by family in support and assistance to older adults. With this in mind, the second section of this book is devoted exclusively to considering the role of family as perhaps the most proximal context from which care emerges. It is interesting to note that, while each chapter in this section focuses on care within a single type of family relationship, the questions each seeks to address, the assumptions each brings to bear, and the methodology employed varies widely across chapters. Rather than presenting contradictory perspectives on similar issues, the diversity of approaches highlights both the complexity of the family as a context as well as the unique perspective on family contexts that multiple methods can provide.

The chapter by Stoller and Miklowski addresses assistance provided by spouses, the most common type of helpers for married older adults. Many changes over the past 60 years have affected the institution of marriage and how couples reach old age together, but the centrality of marriage remains strong. As with so many other aspects of marriage, the implications of care are different for husbands than wives. Stoller and Miklowski are sensitive not just to gender differences, but also to how gender plays out through the multiple contexts in which individuals and couples are likely to be embedded. They carry forward the differences identified by the literature to consider a range of practical implications and recommendations that are likely to be useful when working with spouse caregivers.

Addressing a different set of relationships and their interplay, Davey and Szinovacz consider the ways in which adult children divide assistance to older parents. Using data from the Health and Retirement Study (HRS), they parse these ties in two different ways that integrate the information from the two preceding chapters. One section of the chapter addresses the issue of how siblings divide assistance to a specific parent. They examine the extent of change within these care networks over time, as well as factors associated with these changes. Considerable evidence emerges for flexibility and fluidity in these adult child care networks, and this change is not limited to children participating in a peripheral caregiver role. Another section of this chapter considers how couples divide assistance to parents (and parents-in-law). Here again, the modal situation is one in which assistance to parents is shared between husbands and wives, with lineage being the primary dimension along which responsibilities are divided; gender is an important but secondary dimension. A final section extends these analyses to consider some potential implications of changes in the care network for individual well-being. In this way, then, we can extend our understanding of filial obligation to in-law relationships as well as one's own parents, but care must be paid to social structural and demographic differences associated with one's "risk" of having a parent in need of assistance.

The implications of care for an older parent extend beyond one's siblings and spouse. Szinovacz uses a conceptual framework derived from the stress process model to organize and synthesize the diverse and disparate literature on how care affects children within the family, both directly in terms of their involvement with care and indirectly with regard to parents' involvement in care. One of the unique elements of this chapter is that it integrates first-person accounts from a qualitative study conducted with children in caregiving families. The chapter is just as illustrative in pointing out where the considerable knowledge gaps are as it is with regard to highlighting the implications of care across three generations.

A final section of this book expands the focus to the sociopolitical contexts in which care is embedded. Chapters in this section can be seen as bridging the content and contexts of the two earlier sections, and each of the chapters either directly or indirectly addresses an aspect of the implications of social policies for caregiving. Not surprisingly, these chapters cover a wide range of content.

Whereas Johnson's contribution in the first section of this book directs attention toward the costs for individuals of providing care directly versus indirectly via paid services or other care arrangements, Pavalko, Henderson, and Cott consider the nature of policies that can support caregivers within the workforce. Workplace elder care policies and associated benefits have generally lagged behind those for child care, and the United States has lagged behind many other industrialized nations. The authors use an ambitious scope of data resources, including the National Compensation Survey, the Current Population Survey, and the National Longitudinal Studies to provide a more comprehensive portrait of workplace policies as they pertain to caregiving. Their charting of changes in workplace policies that can support caregivers shows both progress and erosion in selected policies over time.

Broadening the consideration of policies affecting caregivers, Wisensale picks up where Pavalko and colleagues leave off. He extends the discussion to consider family care within the broader network of relevant policies in the United States such as the National Family Caregiver Support program and the Family Medical Leave Act. He also provides some comparative cross-national perspectives and concludes with the presentation of an integrative framework to unify the discussion of policy issues. There are also connections with Johnson's chapter as Wisensale provides more detail about the nature and extent of home- and community-based services in the United States, with additional information regarding how they are financed. His chapter also points to the wide regional variations in services, as federal programs pass through state-level systems and are implemented at the local levels. Just how contextual these policies are stands out in stark relief when they are contrasted with family care policies from France, Germany, and Italy.

With all of this information as ground work, Sundström, Malmberg, Castiello, del Barrio, Castejon, Tortosa, and Johansson remind us that there is often at least as much variation in the nature and extent of services for old-age care within countries as between them. These authors present in-depth information about home- and community-based services across a wide variety of European nations, organized into three broad categories along geographical and ideological-political dimensions. What emerges is a sense of the rich array of services—some directed toward older adults, others directed toward supporting family members, and still others nascent or nonexistent. Going beyond a simple survey of policies and services, the authors proceed to a more in-depth comparison of two contrasting nations: Sweden and Spain. The rich set of analyses they present draw from a wide variety of data sources within countries (such as the Levels of Living survey in Sweden), and across nations (such as the SHARE study, designed to mirror the HRS in the United States, and the EUROFAMCARE project). One of the most striking features of their in-depth comparisons is that policies emerge out of specific family contexts as much as families respond to the policies that are available. Formal services rarely appear to supplant support by families, but at their best they can encourage and sustain the help that families do provide. In every nation considered, families were the primary source of support for older adults, although they need not do so on their own. That services begin to strain under the rapidly aging population in the Nordic countries can be readily seen in the changing mix of formal and informal support to older adults.

In preparing a volume such as this one, it was never our aim to be comprehensive. We hope instead that we have succeeded in presenting views on caregiving for older adults from as wide a range as possible. It is not until we begin to shift figure and ground in dialectic fashion that the centrality, yet tremendous variability, in the contexts from which care emerges can be fully appreciated. Our consideration of the three inter-related contexts of culture, family, and society can help to broaden perspectives on caregiving and to lay a solid foundation for the next generation of dialogue on policy, research, and practice of caregiving.

NOTE

1. Preparation of this chapter was funded in part by a grant from the National Institute on Aging, R01 024045, Maximiliane E. Szinovacz, PI.

SECTION I

Sociocultural Contexts

CHAPTER TWO

Demographic Change and the Future of Informal Caregiving

Peter Uhlenberg and Michelle Cheuk

In recent years, a great deal of attention has focused on issues related to the rapid aging of the U.S. population that is anticipated as the baby boom cohorts enter old age. Journalists, aging researchers, and policymakers are interested in the social, economic, political, and health implications associated with the expected doubling of the size of the older population between 2010 and 2040. So far, the greatest attention has been paid to the challenges associated with funding the Social Security program. The key issue here involves the changing ratio of the working population to the retired population receiving old-age pensions. Obviously, changes will be required in the pay-as-you-go Social Security program as the ratio of workers (those paying the Social Security tax) to beneficiaries drops from 3.3 in 2005 to 2.0 in 2040. The challenge of funding the existing Medicare program in the face of population aging is even greater. The issue for Medicare involves not only the same change in the ratio of workers paying taxes to retirees receiving benefits, but also the anticipated continuing inflation in per capita health care costs. Recent projections show that, by 2028, Medicare will cost more than Social Security (Palmer & Saving, 2005).

Still another issue related to population aging, and the focus of this chapter, involves providing care for older people who cannot function independently. Despite receiving less attention, the challenges of caring for the dependent older population in coming decades are no less formidable than those facing the Social Security and Medicare programs. The challenges of

9

caring for the frail elderly population in the future involve not only funding for long-term care but also the supply of caregivers. Most of the care that older people currently receive comes from unpaid caregivers—family members and other informal caregivers (Knickman & Snell, 2002; Rein & Salzman, 1995; Stone, 2000). For example, 65% of older people receiving help with activities of daily living who live in the community rely exclusively on informal care, and an additional 30% rely in part on informal care. In other words, about 95% of older people outside of institutions who rely on others for daily assistance are receiving that care, wholly or in part, from unpaid sources (Knickman & Snell, 2002). Should we assume that this high level of informal caregiving will be available for the future population of dependent older people?

The future supply of informal caregivers is an important issue because of its economic implications and its relationship to quality of care. The economic significance of informal care can be seen from estimates of the economic value of the informal caregiving that occurs in the United States—$196 billion in 1997. By comparison, national spending for nursing home care was $83 billion in that year, and spending on paid home health care was $32 billion. (Arno, Levine, & Memmott, 1999). Even without any change in the frequency of care being provided by unpaid sources, the cost of long-term care would be expected to increase rapidly because of population aging. If, in addition, there is a shift away from using informal care toward using formal care, we could experience even greater growth in public and/or out-of-pocket expenditures for long-term care. Currently, about 60% of formal long-term care is paid for by public sources, and 40% is paid for out of pocket (Knickman & Snell, 2002).

In addition to the economic concern, a decline in the availability of informal caregivers could have a negative effect on the quality of care received. First, unavailability of informal care increases the risk of institutionalization (Lo Sasso & Johnson, 2002). Most people strongly feel that quality of life is enhanced by living at home rather than in an institution, and physical and mental health outcomes tend to be better for those receiving care outside of institutions (Uhlenberg, 1997). Moreover, there are widespread concerns that the quality of care provided by home health aides tends to be inferior to that provided by family members (Wiener & Hanley, 1992).

This chapter explores how the supply of informal caregivers for the disabled older population may change as the population ages over coming decades. We first review what is known about informal caregiving and how recent changes in the older population may affect the future need for caregivers. Then we examine what currently predicts whether an older disabled person receives formal versus informal long-term care. Finally, we look at how projected changes in the sociodemographic character-istics of both the older and the younger populations may challenge the existing caregiving arrangements that rely so heavily on informal care.

BACKGROUND

How Many Need Assistance?

Because the prevalence of frailty and disability increases in later life, a substantial proportion of the older population must depend on others for daily care. Several large, national surveys over the past 20 years provide information about the number and characteristics of both the users and the providers of long-term care for disabled older persons. For example, the National Long-Term Care Survey (NLTCS) has col-lected information from about 17,000 older people. In this survey, a user of long-term care is defined as anyone receiving help for activi-ties of daily living (ADLs) or instrumental activities of daily living (IADLs) due to a disability or health problem lasting at least 3 months (Spillman, 2004). The ADLs in this definition were bathing, dressing, eating, walking, transferring, and toileting; the IADLs were preparing meals, telephoning, shopping, and managing money. The NLTCS found that about 16% of the population over age 65 in 1999 was receiving long-term care (Spillman, 2004). Among the 5.5 million older people receiving long-term care in 1999, 30% were in institutions, and 70% were community residents.

The probability of an older person receiving long-term care varies a great deal depending on the person's age. The age pattern of receiv-ing long-term care is shown in Table 2.1. Among the young-old (aged 65–74), about 7% were receiving long-term care in 1999, and most of those (84%) were community residents. But among those over age 90, the need for daily assistance is very different—63% are users of long-term care, and only slightly more than half of these are still living out-side of institutions. The strong relationship of disability with age has led some to suggest that caregiving research should focus on the popula-tion over age 80. However, the situation looks quite different when we examine the age distribution of all long-term care users. Because the total number of people in each age category declines steeply with age, it turns out that 42% of all older long-term care users are less than 80 years of age. Because a significant proportion of long-term care users are in the young-old category and because these individuals are the most likely to be receiving care from informal caregivers, we include all persons over age 65 in this study.

Changing Age Composition and the Ratio of Potential Caregivers to Older Care Receivers

A number of factors will influence the future demand for care by older persons and the supply of people available to provide that care. Perhaps the most obvious factor that will affect the ratio of potential caregivers to care receivers is the shifting age composition of the population. This does not mean that demography is destiny (Friedland & Summer, 1999), but it recognizes that population aging should not be ignored in discussions of how to meet caregiving needs in the future. A simple way of seeing the implications of the changing age composition is to calculate the ratio of potential caregivers to care receivers, assuming that the age-specific rates of care receiving do not change. As discussed below, this assumption may not be realistic. However, showing the results of projections using this assumption demonstrates the relevance of population age composition for future caregiving needs.

To calculate the ratio of potential caregivers to older people in need of care, one must estimate both the numerator and the denominator. Although caregivers can be any age, the population aged 35–64 can be used as an approximation of the potential supply of caregivers. Spillman and Pezzin (2000) estimate that about 75% of potential family caregivers were in this age category in 1994, and most formal caregivers are in this age category. The projected size of the population aged 35–64 at future dates comes from the middle-range projections provided by the U.S. Census Bureau (2000). The projected number of older people in need of care is obtained by applying the age-specific rates of receiving long-term care given in Table 2.1 to the projected size of the population in each age category.

The results of this exercise in calculating the ratio of potential caregivers to long-term care receivers are shown in Table 2.2. If current patterns of disability persist, the number of persons aged 35–64 per older disabled person will fall from 18.8 in 2000 to 8.6 in 2040. This striking change occurs because the proportion of the total population in the 35–64 age category declines (from 39% in 2000 to 34% in 2040), the proportion of the total population in the 65 and over category increases (from 13% to 20%), and the proportion of the older population over age 85 increases (from 12% to 19%). Other things being equal, population aging would greatly increase the need for caregivers. If the availability of family members to provide unpaid care should decline, there could be a tremendous increase in the demand for geriatric health care workers. Before discussing potential changes in the availability of informal caregivers, we consider the possibility that the demand for care might decline.

TABLE 2.1 Persons Aged 65 and Older Receiving Long-Term Care, 1999 National Long-Term Care Survey

Age	Population (in thousands)	Percent receiving long-term care[a]	Percent receiving long-term care in community[b]	Percent receiving long-term care in institutions[c]
65–69	9,443	5.7	5.0	0.7
70–74	8,785	8.8	7.2	1.7
75–79	7,305	13.6	10.1	3.5
80–84	4,797	24.8	17.3	7.4
85–89	2,601	39.8	24.8	15.0
90–94	1,133	59.8	33.7	26.1
95 and older	396	72.1	35.7	36.4
Total	34,459	15.9	11.1	4.8

[a] Receipt of long-term care is defined as receiving human assistance or standby help with at least one of six activities of daily living (ADLs) or being unable to perform at least one of eight instrumental activities of daily living (IADLs) without help. The ADLs included are eating, transferring, toileting, getting around inside, dressing, and bathing. The IADLs are meal preparation, grocery shopping, light housework, laundry, financial management, taking medication, telephoning, and getting around inside.

[b] This does not include about 1.3 million persons with disabilities who do not receive chronic help but who use special equipment to manage their disabilities.

[c] This includes about 1.5 million persons in nursing homes and slightly more than 150,000 persons in other care facilities.

Source. Table B-15 U.S. House of Representatives (2004).

TABLE 2.2 Projection of Potential Caregivers and Long-Term Care Receivers

Year	Caregivers (population aged 35 to 64)	Long-term care receivers aged 65 and older	Ratio
2000	106,061,000	5,642,000	18.8 to 1
2020	121,657,000	8,448,000	14.4 to 1
2040	129,665,000	15,077,000	8.6 to 1

Source. Calculated from Table 2.1 and U.S. Census Bureau (2000).

Trends in Demand for Care

An assumption of no change in rates of using long-term care in coming decades could be wrong. If age-specific disability rates decline, then the number of old people needing assistance would not increase as rapidly as projected above. Greater use of assistive technology and higher education levels could reduce the need for caregivers for the population with disabilities. A starting place for considering these possibilities is an examination of recent trends.

The trend in age-specific use of long-term care is clear. Data from the NLTCS show that the proportion of older people receiving care has declined in recent years, from 14.6% in 1984 to 12.8% in 1989, 11.6% in 1994, and 10.7% in 1999. This downward trend occurred despite some aging of the older population, which, other things being equal, would have increased the use of long-term care. The next question that researchers ask, of course, is why these data show such a large decline in the use of long-term care.

Part of the answer to why the need for caregivers declined is straightforward—there was a notable decline in disability rates from 1982 to 2005. Although a number of studies have examined this issue, there is not full agreement over how much improvement there was in underlying capacity. Generally, disability studies report that rates of IADL disability have declined (Freedman et al., 2004), and these declines appear to be driven by increased levels of education, greater use of assistive technology, and changes in environmental accommodations (Freedman & Martin, 1999; Spillman, 2004). Findings on changes of rates of ADL disability are mixed; several studies show no significant change in ADL disability rates, but two studies show declines (Freedman et al., 2004; Manton, Gu, & Lamb, 2006). Thus, in recent years, IADL disability rates have declined and ADL disability rates may have as well.

As noted already, one factor contributing to the decline in IADL disability rates is the rising levels of education in the older population from 1984 to 1999. The other major factor is an increase in the use of assistive technology during this time. The NLTCS found that the percentage of disabled people using "assistive devices only" increased from 13.4% in 1984 to 25.8% in 1999 (Federal Interagency Forum on Aging-Related Statistics, 2004), and the National Health Interview Survey on Disability found a substantial age-adjusted increase in the use of assistive devices (e.g., wheelchairs, walkers, leg braces, and canes) during this time as well (Russell, Hendershot, LeClere, Howie, & Adler, 1997). The use of assistive technology not only allows some people to avoid dependency, but also is associated with a decline in hours of personal care (Hoenig, Taylor, & Sloan, 2003), time and difficulty in performing tasks

(Mann, Ottenbacher, Frass, Tomita, & Granger, 1999), and residual disability (Agree, 1999; Verbrugge, Rennert, & Madans, 1997). Given that many people still do not use assistive technology (Mann, Hurren, & Tomita, 1993) and have unmet needs (Edwards & Jones, 1998), it is possible that use of assistive technology will continue to increase and thereby further reduce the demand for personal care.

Because educational attainment and assistive technology are likely to increase in the future, the demand for IADL caregiving is likely to decrease. However, recent trends suggest that demand for the more intensive ADL care is likely to continue at its current level unless ADL disability rates begin to drop (Spillman, 2004).

Looking ahead, some researchers argue that disability rates might increase as new cohorts enter old age in coming decades. The reason for this gloomy forecast is the much-publicized increasing rates of obesity among younger adults after 1980. The proportion of adults under age 75 who were obese doubled, from 15% to 30%, in the period from 1976–1980 to 1999–2002 (National Center for Health Statistics, 2005). Because of the strong relationship between obesity and disability (Gregg et al., 2005; Strum, Ringel, & Andreyeva, 2004), there is concern that increasing obesity rates among cohorts entering old age in the years ahead could lead to increasing rates of disability (Reynolds, Saito, & Crimmins, 2005; Strum et al., 2004). It is not clear that rising levels of obesity at younger ages will translate into greater prevalence of disability at older ages (Gregg et al., 2005; Preston, 2005; Williamson, 2003). However, it is noteworthy that, while disability rates were falling for older people between 1984 and 1996, they were increasing for the adult population under age 60—that is, for those cohorts that were experiencing large increases in rates of obesity (Lakdawalla, Bhattacharya, & Goldman, 2004). As these cohorts enter old age in coming decades, one cannot assume that they will have lower rates of chronic disability than those who preceded them.

Who Provides Care?

Who currently provides care for the millions of older long-term care users? A useful way to approach this question is to distinguish four types of long-term care users. The most studied category consists of those who receive paid care because they reside in long-term care institutions. In 1999, 30% of all elderly long-term care users were living in institutions, and 70% were residing in the community (Spillman, 2004). Elderly long-term care users residing in the community can be divided into three categories: those who rely on formal (paid) care, those who rely on informal (unpaid family and friends) care, and those who use a combination of formal and informal care. A majority of those living in the community relies solely on informal caregivers, and another large proportion relies on a combination of informal and formal caregivers. Only 5% of all long-term care users live in the community and rely exclusively on formal care providers (Spillman & Pezzin, 2000). Thus, the distribution of all long-term care users by type of caregiver is as follows: 35% rely wholly on formal care (30% in institutions and 5% in the community), 25% use both formal and informal care, and 40% depend wholly on informal care. This means that almost two-thirds of all disabled older people in the population are receiving all or part of their caregiving from informal sources in the community. Clearly, these informal caregivers—unpaid relatives and friends—play an enormously significant role in meeting the needs of older people who are no longer able to function independently.

In the United States there exists a hierarchy in preferences for who should provide informal care, with spouses and children being called upon for help before other relatives, friends, or neighbors (Cantor, 1980). By far the most important sources of informal caregivers are the spouses and children of older disabled people (Stoller & Martin, 2002; Stone, Cafferata, & Sangl, 1987; Wolff & Kasper, 2006). Furthermore, in recent years the proportion of all informal caregivers who are spouses and children has increased. Therefore, the discussion of informal caregiving in this chapter will focus on the children and spouses of older people.

How has the distribution across types of caregivers been changing? The proportion of people using "formal care only" has increased slightly since the 1980s. Although the proportion of older people living in nursing homes declined from 5.4 to 4.3% between 1985 and 1999, the proportion living in the community who used formal care exclusively increased from 5.1 to 8.5% (Federal Interagency Forum on Aging-Related Statistics, 2004). However, over this time period, there was no clear trend in the use of "informal care only." The proportion of older people in the community using informal care alone declined from 68.9% in 1984 to 57.1% in 1994 but then increased to 65.5% by 1999 (Federal Interagency Forum on Aging-Related Statistics, 2004). The proportion using both formal and informal care followed the reverse pattern, increasing and then decreasing.

During these years, the changes in use or nonuse of formal care to supplement informal care are likely related to changes in Medicare coverage of home health care. In the late 1980s, several court decisions expanded Medicare's home health care coverage. People who were receiving home health care visits received more visits, and people who did not have home health care visits began to have them. The increase in home health care likely accounts for the reduction in reliance on only informal care observed from 1984 to 1994, as more people utilized the home health care visits covered by Medicare. The increased use of Medicare-funded home health care in this period resulted in a massive upsurge in Medicare costs. Subsequently, steps were taken to curtail the use of home health care. In 1997, the Balanced Budget Act limited Medicare coverage of home health care, and this change explains both the decline in home health care visits after 1997 and the increase in informal care use only by 1999 (Federal Interagency Forum on Aging-Related Statistics, 2004; Health Care Financing Administration, 1999; Scanlon, 1997).

The point to be emphasized here is that informal caregiving continues to be extremely important in meeting the needs of disabled older people. But we can anticipate that demographic forces will challenge the existing arrangements. Substantial changes in the size and composition of cohorts of both care users and care providers are on the horizon. Before examining these demographic changes, we carefully examine the factors other than policy that promote informal versus formal caregiving for disabled persons.

PREDICTING USE OF FORMAL VERSUS INFORMAL CARE

As mentioned previously, the availability of informal caregivers has important implications for those receiving care and for the public cost of providing care to older people. In anticipating how the supply of informal caregivers might change in coming decades, it is useful to know what characteristics of older dependent people are related to their use of paid versus unpaid caregivers. We briefly summarize the findings of previous research on this subject. Then we present findings from our multivariate analysis of data from the second Longitudinal Study on Aging (LSOA II). This analysis will provide more detail on the differences in the use of unpaid care across individuals with different characteristics.

Past Studies

A recent analysis of data from the 2002 Health and Retirement Survey by Johnson and Wiener (2006) provides information on the bivariate relationship between selected characteristics of care receivers and their use of paid versus unpaid care. The results are unsurprising, if one assumes that the probability of using informal care is related to the degree of disability and to the resources available to the dependent person. As severity of the disability requiring assistance increases, measured as number of ADLs, the reliance on informal care decreases. An important resource for an older person can be family members, such as a spouse and adult children. As expected, among older disabled people, the unmarried are more likely than the married to rely on paid care, and the childless are more likely than those who have children to use paid caregivers. Economic resources to purchase help might also be expected to influence whether a person makes use of formal caregiving. Using education as a proxy for economic resources, the Johnson and Wiener study shows that those with a college education are more likely than those with less education to use formal caregiving. However, the relationship between income and use of paid care is curvilinear. Those in or near poverty and those in the highest income category are more likely than those in the middle income category to use paid caregivers. This income pattern probably exists because low-income older people have access to paid home health care services through Medicaid, and high income older people have adequate resources to purchase care, but those in the middle lack adequate resources to purchase care.

Other studies report findings consistent with those described above. For example, being unmarried and/or having fewer children increases the risk of an older disabled person receiving care in an institution (Crystal, 1982; Freedman, 1999). Childless older people have been shown to rely more on formal care (Boaz & Muller, 1994; Crimmins & Saito, 1993; Zimmer & Kwong, 2003).

Further Analysis

To extend our understanding of the determinants of using informal care, we use a simple model (shown in Table 2.3) to predict the use of paid caregiving by dependent older persons living in the community. First, consistent with findings reported above, we expect formal care to be used more often when the level of care required is greater. The logic of this argument is that informal caregivers may be less able or willing to provide care that requires special skills and/or is more physically demanding. Second, based on economic reasoning, we expect that the likelihood of purchasing care increases as the resources needed to purchase care increase. Third, again consistent with previous findings, we expect that use of formal care increases as the supply of kin (spouse, children, and siblings) decreases. Finally, several standard control variables (sex, age, race/ethnicity) are included in the model, although we do not hypothesize what effects they might have. Using this multivariate model, we examine the effect of each variable controlling for other related variables, and we can address questions regarding how much difference particular variables make.

Data

The data used in this analysis come from the first wave of the second Longitudinal Study on Aging, conducted in conjunction with the 1994

TABLE 2.3   Odds Ratios for Logistic Regression of Use of Paid
Caregiving by Dependent Older People on Independent Variables
(N = 2,884)

Independent variable	Odds ratio		
		Predictor	Block
Age	1.00		
Number of activities of daily living	1.13	**	
Number of instrumental activities of daily living	0.99		**
Female	1.20		
Black	0.97		
Hispanic	0.40	***	**
Asian	0.42	*	
Other race	0.92		
Less than high school	0.60	***	***
College	1.44	*	
Missing education	0.85		
Married, spouse present	0.41	***	
Married, spouse not present	1.19		***
Missing marital status	0.66		
0 children	1.72	**	***
2 children	0.85		
3 children	1.10		
4 or more children	0.76		
Number of siblings	0.93	*	

Source. Authors' calculation from 1994–1995 second Longitudinal Study on Aging
(LSOA II).
* $p < .05$. ** $p < .01$. *** $p < .001$.

National Health Interview. The sample for the study was obtained
through a stratified multistage sample design and is representative of the
civilian noninstitutionalized population, age 70 and older, in the United
States in 1994–1995. A total of 9,447 respondents had face-to-face interviews. Information on disability, type of health care, demographic characteristics, family structure, and living arrangements were collected in the
interviews. Our analysis is based on the 2,884 respondents who reported
that they were receiving help with activities of daily living (ADLs or
IADLs) and for whom crucial information was not missing (347 cases
were dropped because of missing information).

The dependent variable in the analysis is dichotomous—whether
the older person's primary caregiver was a paid caregiver or an informal

caregiver. One-fourth of the weighted sample (25.6%) had a paid caregiver, while three-fourths (74.4%) had an informal caregiver. With this outcome variable, we use logistic regression and report odds ratios in Table 2.3. The independent and control variables in the regression equation are coded as follows:

> *Age:* A continuous variable from 70 to 99 and over. The last category is coded as 99. The mean age of the weighted sample is 79.4.
>
> *Level of disability:* The sum of ADL and IADL disabilities. The means of the weighted sample are 0.5 ADLs and 1.4 IADLs.
>
> *Sex:* A dummy variable, with 1 being female. Seventy % of the weighted sample is female.
>
> *Race/ethnicity:* A nominal variable with mutually exclusive categories of White, Black, Hispanic, Asian, and other race. Eighty-two percent of the weighted sample is White, 9% is Black, 4% is Hispanic, 1.7% is Asian, and 2.6% is other race.
>
> *Education:* Coded as less than high school, high school but not college, college, or missing information. The mean level of education for the weighted sample is 10.5 years.
>
> *Marital status:* The four categories are not married, married and the spouse is present in the household, married but the spouse is not present in the household, and missing marital status. In the weighted sample, 59% is not married, 39% is married and the spouse is present in the household, 1% is married but the spouse is not present in the household, and 1% is missing marital status.
>
> *Children:* Number of living children are coded as 0, 1, 2, 3, 4+. Twelve % of the weighted sample has no child, 19% has one child, 23 percent has two children, 18% has three children, and 28% has four or more children.
>
> *Siblings:* Number of living siblings. The mean of the weighted sample is 1.9 siblings.

Results

The results of the logistic regression analysis are shown in Table 2.3. After briefly describing these results, we examine the magnitude of selected differences. First, the control variables age and sex do not have a significant effect on using paid versus informal care, net of the other variables in the model. Regarding race/ethnicity, there is no difference between Blacks and Whites, but Hispanics and Asians were more likely than Whites to rely on informal caregivers. As expected, people with more ADLs are more likely than people with fewer ADLs to use paid care.

Of greater interest for our purposes are the effects of resources possessed by older people. Net of other variables, older people who receive care are more likely to use paid care when they have more education rather than less education. This finding fits with our expectation that those with more economic resources (indicated by higher levels of education) are more likely to pay for care. The variables we are most interested in are related to the supply of potential kin caregivers: marital status, number of children, and number of siblings. All three of these variables have a significant effect on informal caregiving. Those who are not married, and hence do not have a spouse who can provide care, are more likely to use paid care than those who are married. People with no children are more likely to rely on paid care than those who have at least one child. People with one child are more likely to pay for care than those who have four or more children. However, those with two or three children were not more likely than those with only one child to use only informal caregiving. This suggests that greater attention should be given to childlessness than to number of children when discussing implications of demographic change for supply of informal caregiving. Finally, people with fewer siblings are more likely than those with many siblings to pay for care. Thus, each aspect of family structure is a significant predictor, in the direction expected, of whether a disabled older person receives care from paid sources.

We next looked more closely at married people to see if there are differences between those who are remarried and those who are in their first marriage (analysis not shown). Compared to those who are in their first marriage, remarried people are more likely to have a spouse caregiver. This is especially true for men. One possible explanation is that men who remarry, compared to those in first marriages, may be more likely to have spouses who are younger and healthier than they are. On the other hand, compared to people in their first marriage, those who are remarried are less likely to have a child as their caregiver. Overall, the differences between these groups in spousal and in child caregiving roughly balance out, so that remarried long-term care users were about as likely as those in first marriages to have a spouse or a child as caregivers.

In addition to knowing that marital status and number of children have a significant effect on the probability of using paid care, we also want to know how much of a difference these particular variables make. To get a sense of the magnitude of the effects, we take a typical respondent (average values for age, race/ethnicity, education, disability level, and number of siblings), vary the marital status and number of children, and calculate predicted probabilities of using paid versus unpaid care for men and women. Figure 2.1 shows the results of this exercise. First, having children has a large impact on using paid care, especially for women. For example, married women with no children are twice as likely as those with four or more children to use paid care (28% versus 12%). Similarly, the fewer children that unmarried women have, the more likely they are to rely on paid care. Forty-six percent of unmarried women without children used paid care compared to 24% of unmarried women with four or more children. In contrast to women, the number of children has relatively little impact on the probability of men using paid versus unpaid care.

The second finding highlighted in Figure 2.1 is the critical influence of marital status for both men and women. Controlling for number of children, marital status has a significant effect on the likelihood that an older long-term care user receives help from a paid caregiver. As one might expect, the impact of being married is greater for men than women. For example, among childless people, being unmarried increases the likelihood of using paid care by 2.5 times for men, compared to 1.3 times for women. Similarly, for those who have one child, being unmarried increases the likelihood of using paid care by 2.5 times for men, compared to 1.8 times for women.

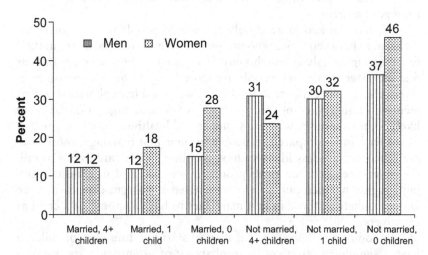

FIGURE 2.1   Percent of long-term care users predicted to use a paid caregiver, by sex, marital status, and number of children, with control variables held constant at their means.

Source: Authors' calculation from 1994–1995 second Longitudinal Study on Aging (LSOA II).

To summarize the key findings from our analysis, older people are more likely to use formal care than informal care when they

- have higher education,
- are not married,
- are childless,
- have few children compared to many, and
- have few siblings.

DEMOGRAPHIC CHANGE

The characteristics of the older population change as new cohorts enter old age and replace the cohorts who previously occupied the older age categories. Assuming that the individual-level characteristics that predict use of formal versus informal caregivers persist, these changing characteristics of the older population could alter the extent to which older people in the future will rely on family and kin as caregivers. How will the characteristics that affect the use of informal care by older people—education, marital status, and number of children—change in coming decades? To answer this question we will focus on expected change among older White women between 2000 and 2040, recognizing that subsequent analyses should complete the projections for other segments of the future older population.

Data

To illustrate changes in the older population in coming decades, we focus on three age categories (70–74, 80–84, and 90–94) in the years 2000, 2020, and 2040. To estimate the distribution of older White women in these years by education, marital history, and number of children, we begin with data from around 2000 provided by the U.S. Census Bureau. For example, among White women aged 70–74 in 2000 (survivors of the birth cohort of 1926–1930), 15% were college graduates, 4% were never married, and 11% were childless (see Figures 2.2, 2.3, and 2.4). In 2020, this cohort born in 1926–1930 will have aged into the 90–94 age category, and we assume that these characteristics of the cohort will not have changed. That is, the characteristics of women aged 90–94 in 2020 is projected to be the same as for women aged 70–74 in 2000. The assumption of no change in the distribution across characteristics as a cohort ages is not entirely plausible because there is likely to be differential survival by these characteristics. For example, we should expect survival to be positively related to educational achievement, so the proportion with low education should decline with time and the proportion with high education should increase. Nevertheless, this approach of assuming no change in cohort characteristics as they age in later life provides a reasonable approximation to what can be anticipated.

To project the characteristics of younger age categories in 2020 and 2040, we start with data from 2000 for the appropriate cohort. For example, women who will be 80–84 years old in 2040 are in the birth cohort of 1956–1960, which was aged 40–44 in 2000. By assuming that women have completed their education and childbearing by age 40, we project that these characteristics of this cohort will not change as it ages. In projecting its marital history in 2020 and 2040, we assume that age-specific transition rates will resemble those existing around 2000. For Census Bureau data on education for various cohorts of White women around 2000, see Day and Bauman (2000); for data on marital history, see Kreider (2002); and for data on fertility, see National Center for Health Statistics (2003).

Educational Change

As shown in Figure 2.2, we anticipate a substantial increase in the educational levels of older women, reflecting the very different school experiences in earlier life of the cohorts that will replace the contemporary older population. In 2000, four times as many women aged 80–84 had less than a high school education than had a college education. By 2040, this ratio will be reversed, because five times as many will be college- educated as will have less than a high school education. Assuming that educational differences in use of paid care persist, other things being equal, the coming large increase in the educational levels of the older population should significantly increase the future demand for paid caregivers. Because education is associated with lower rates of disability, there could be a lower demand for caregiving among individuals in an age category. Nonetheless, more people who become disabled will have high education levels and therefore will be more likely to demand paid care.

Marital Status Changes

The proportion of older people who have never married is expected to slightly increase over the next 40 years, as shown in Figure 2.3. The effect of this change, of course, will be to decrease the supply of potential spouse caregivers. However, the expected increase in the proportion of older White women who never marry (for example, an increase from 5% of women aged 80–84 in 2000 to 7% in 2040), is too small to have much impact on the overall supply of informal caregivers.

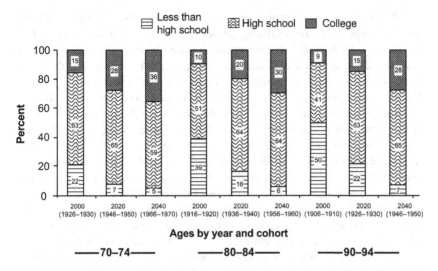

FIGURE 2.2   Educational attainment of White women by age: 2000, 2020, 2040.
Source: Day and Bauman (2000).   [AuQ1]

In contrast to the experience of White women, the retreat from marriage in recent decades by younger Black women has been dramatic—a third of all Black women aged 40 in 2000 may never marry (Blau, 2007). This racial contrast suggests that discussions of future spouse caregiving need to carefully consider racial/ethnic differences.

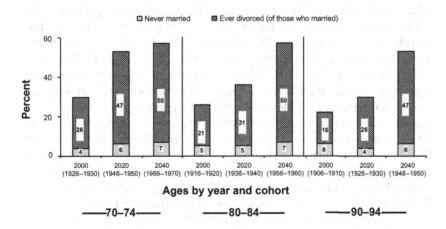

FIGURE 2.3   Marital status of White women by age: 2000, 2020, 2040.
Source: Kreider (2002).

Probably a more important factor affecting the future supply of spouse caregivers is the declining gender gap in age at marriage and in life expectancy. Gender differences in median age at first marriage declined over the 20th century, and the gender gap in life expectancy declined since 1970 (Federal Interagency Forum on Aging-Related Statistics, 2004). Consequently, married couples who enter old age in the future can anticipate spending fewer years widowed, which implies an increase in the supply of potential spouse caregivers. These changes are reflected in the increase between 1990 and 2000 in the proportion of older women who were married (Kreider & Simmons, 2003) and in the forecast by the Social Security Administration that the proportion of married persons over age 85 will increase in coming years (Siegel, 1996).

Potentially the most important change in marital patterns affecting future informal caregiving, however, is neither the increase in percent who never marry nor the decrease in length of widowhood. It is the expected dramatic increase in the proportion of women who have their first marriage end in divorce that could most alter current caregiving arrangements (Uhlenberg, Cooney, & Boyd, 1990). In 2000, about 20% of ever-married women aged 80–84 had experienced divorce; in 2040 it will be nearly 50%. The crucial question is what effect divorce in earlier life has on availability of informal caregivers in later life.

The impact of divorce on availability of children to provide care seems clear. Compared to married people, divorced people are more likely to use paid care and less likely to rely on children for care when they are disabled. The negative effect of divorce on children as caregivers is true for both men and women, but especially for men (Cooney & Uhlenberg, 1990; Hagestad, 1986; Marks, 1991). The decreased strength of father-child relationships in later life resulting from divorce (Uhlenberg, 1993) reflects the consequences of fathers not coresiding with their children during childhood (Furstenberg, 1990; Seltzer & Bianchi, 1988). Theoretically, those who remarry after divorce could expand their supply of child care-givers by adding stepchildren (Wachter, 1997). However, findings from our analysis (discussed above) replicate results from other studies that show that remarried people are less likely than people in first marriages to use any child caregivers (Marks, 1991). Remarried people may be more likely than divorced people to receive care from children, but they are less likely to receive such care than people in first marriages (Knickman & Snell, 2002). Thus, the increasing prevalence of divorce among cohorts that will occupy the older ages after 2020 or 2030 is a major demographic force working to decrease the supply of child caregivers in the future.

In addition to decreasing the availability of children to provide care, divorce can also decrease availability of spouses to provide care. Clearly this is the case for those who divorce and do not remarry. However, as shown above, people who remarry are somewhat more likely than people who stay in first marriages to rely on a spouse caregiver. This is especially true for men. Thus, remarriage can moderate the negative impact of increasing divorce on the availability of informal caregivers. However, the rate of remarriage has been decreasing steadily since 1960 (Bramlett & Mosher, 2002). The persistent high rate of divorce in recent decades, when combined with a decreasing rate of remarriage, produces an expected large increase in the proportion of people whose marital status in old age will be divorced. Thus, the overall effect of changing marital patterns on the use of informal caregivers in coming decades will almost certainly be negative.

Changes in Number of Children

The significant decline in the number of children that baby boomers had compared to the cohorts that precede them will produce a large change in the number of living adult children available to provide long-term care for older parents in the future. The total fertility rate of cohorts that produced the baby boom was over 3.0, compared to about 2.0 for the baby boom cohorts (National Center for Health Statistics, 2003). As shown in Figure 2.4, when the mothers of the baby boom are in greatest need of caregiving (i.e., when they are over age 80 around 2020), more than a fourth of them will have at least four children. However, 20 years later when baby boomers are over age 80, only 10 percent of them will have four or more children. There will also be an increase in the proportion of those over age 70 who are childless between 2020 and 2040. This change in family size is significant because older people with fewer living children tend to use paid care more often, as indicated in Figure 2.1. Also, women with fewer children are more likely to be cared for in institutions (Crystal, 1982; Freedman, 1999). Thus, the decrease in the number of children per capita among older long-term care users can be expected to increase the demand for paid caregivers in coming decades.

However, the effect of declining fertility on the use of child caregivers by older adults should not be exaggerated. The most important contrast in availability of having a child caregiver is between the childless and those with at least one child. Those who have one child are less likely than those with two children to have a child who provides care, but the difference is less than that between the childless and the mothers with one child (Uhlenberg, 1993; Zimmer & Kwong, 2003). At higher parities, there are diminishing returns associated with having more children, so that differences between those with four or more compared to those with two or three are small. As shown in Figure 2.4, the proportion of women over age 80 who are childless is not expected to increase—it will be lower in 2020 than it was in 2000 and will be about the same in 2040 as in 2000. The big change in family size will be the decrease in the proportion of women

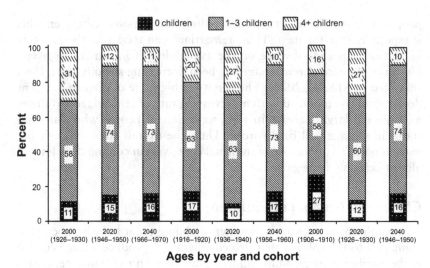

FIGURE 2.4   Number of living children by age of White mothers:
2000, 2020, 2040.
Source: National Center for Health Statistics (2003).

with large families, but, as noted above, those with four or more children
rely on paid caregivers only slightly less often than those who have one or
two children. It is a significant advantage to have a daughter if one wants
to receive long-term care from a child (Rein & Salzman, 1995; Stone,
2000), and the odds of having a daughter increase with the number of
children born.

In conclusion, the smaller average family size for women who
will occupy the oldest age categories by 2040 will reduce the supply of
informal caregivers for dependent older persons, but not dramatically.
In addition, decline in fertility across cohorts will result in older people
in the future having fewer siblings, nephews, nieces, and grandchildren
available for caregiving. Although these other kin constitute a relatively
smaller proportion of family caregivers than spouses and children, their
shrinking numbers will have some additional impact on the supply of
informal caregivers.

Changes in Characteristics of Younger Cohorts

The future availability of informal caregivers depends not only on changing
characteristics of the older population but also on changing characteristics

of the cohorts that will comprise the younger population. High rates of divorce and declining rates of remarriage among these cohorts may decrease the availability of adult children to provide care (Uhlenberg, 1994) because divorced women who maintain separate households tend to have less time and money to invest in caregiving. Also, increasingly, the daughters of older people are in the labor force, which decreases the time and energy that they have for caregiving (Doty, Jackson, & Crown, 1998; Pavalko & Artis, 1997). Research has shown that when daughters provide care in addition to being employed, their parent tends to receive less informal care and more formal care (Doty et al., 1998). In addition, longer life expectancy and later age at childbearing mean that more parents in need of care in the future will have adult children who also are old. Adult children who are themselves old may be less able or willing to care for their parents who are very old than are middle-aged children with old parents. On the other hand, adult children who are old will also more likely be retired, and therefore they may be more available to provide care than their younger, working counterparts.

CONCLUSION

Population aging over the next several decades will challenge existing social institutions in a number of ways. As long as growing old is associated with withdrawal from the labor force, increasing health problems, and growing risks of disability, the challenges of dealing with Social Security, Medicare, and long-term care issues will all occur at about the same time. There is no reason to expect that social institutions cannot adapt to meet these challenges, but substantial changes will need to begin soon. The ratio of older people to working-age people will occur abruptly after 2010 as the baby boom cohorts arrive at old age with very different educational and family experiences than those of the contemporary older population.

This chapter has explored the challenges ahead to the current arrangement of relying on kin for almost two-thirds of the long-term care received by older disabled people. Some disabled people rely on paid care more than on informal care by family members. Individuals are at higher risk of using paid care when they have high disability levels, have resources to pay for care, and/or lack family members to provide informal care. Those most able to pay for care either have high incomes or receive Medicaid benefits because of low income. People who are divorced, unmarried, childless, and/or have a small extended family are more likely to rely on paid care because they have fewer family members available for assistance. Cohorts of Black women entering old age have a high proportion who are unmarried and are therefore more likely to rely on paid care. Hispanics and Asians, on the other hand, are less likely to rely on paid care and are more likely to rely on informal care.

As fewer people arrive at old age with stable marriages and large families, the availability of informal caregivers will shrink. Further, as educational levels among older people increase, we can expect the demand for formal care to increase, although this may be offset by the fact that people with higher educational levels are less likely to become disabled in the first place. But the forces that point to an increase in demand for paid care relative to informal care will occur at the same time as the overall ratio of older retired persons to workers is increasing. In this context, several important questions will need to be answered. How much growth in the geriatric workforce will be needed to meet the demands of the future disabled older population? How will the nation's resources be allocated to pay for geriatric care? And who will pay for the increase in formal care?

REFERENCES

Agree, E. (1999). The influence of personal care and assistive devices on the measurement of disability. *Social Science & Medicine, 48,* 427–443.

Arno, P. S., Levine, C., & Memmott, M. M. (1999). The economic value of informal caregiving. *Health Affairs, 18,* 182–188.

Blau, D. M. (2007). Some thoughts on aging, marriage, and well-being in later life. In K. W. Schaie & P. Uhlenberg (Eds.), *Social structures: Demographic changes and the well-being of older persons* (pp. 230–238). New York: Springer.

Boaz, R. F., & Muller, C. F. (1994). Predicting the risk of permanent nursing-home residence: The role of community help as indicated by family helpers and prior living arrangements. *Health Services Research, 29,* 391–414.

Bramlett, M. D., & Mosher, W. D. (2002). Cohabitation, marriage, divorce, and remarriage in the United States. *Vital and Health Statistics, 23*(22). National Center for Health Statistics, Hyattsville, MD.

Cantor, M. (1980). The informal support network, its relevance in the lives of the elderly. In E. Borgotta & N. McCluskey (Eds.), *Aging and society* (pp. 111–146). Beverly Hills, CA: Sage.

Cooney, T., & Uhlenberg, P. (1990). The role of divorce in men's relations with their adult children after midlife. *Journal of Marriage and the Family, 52,* 677–688.

Crimmins, E. M., & Saito, Y. (1993). Getting better and getting worse: Transitions in functional status among older Americans. *Journal of Aging and Health, 5,* 3–36.

Crystal, S. (1982). *America's old age crisis.* New York: Basic Books.

Day, J. C., & Bauman, K. J. (2000). *Have we reached the top? Educational attainment projections of the U.S. population.* Working Paper Series No. 43, Population Division, U.S. Census Bureau, Washington, DC.

Doty, P., Jackson, M. E., & Crown, W. (1998). The impact of female caregivers' employment status on patterns of formal and informal eldercare. *The Gerontologist, 38,* 331–341.

Edwards, N. I., & Jones, D. A. (1998). Ownership and use of assistive devices amongst older people in the community. *Age and Ageing, 27,* 462–469.

Federal Interagency Forum on Aging-Related Statistics. (2004). *Older Americans 2004: Key indicators of well-being*. Washington, DC: Author.

Freedman, V. A. (1999). Family structure and the risk of nursing home admission. *Journal of Gerontology: Social Sciences, 51B*, S61–S69.

Freedman, V. A., Crimmins, E., Schoeni, R. F., Spillman, B. C., Aykan, H., Kramarow, E., et al. (2004). Resolving inconsistencies in trends in old-age disability: Report from a technical working group. *Demography, 41*, 417–441.

Freedman, V. A., & Martin, L. G. (1999). The role of education in explaining and forecasting trends in functional limitations among older Americans. *Demography, 36*, 461–473.

Friedland, R. B., & Summer, L. (1999). *Demography is not destiny*. Washington, DC: National Academy on an Aging Society.

Furstenberg, F. F. (1990). Divorce and the American family. *Annual Review of Sociology, 16*, 379–403.

Gregg, E. W., Cheng, Y. J., Caldwell, B. L., Imperatore, G., Williams, D. E., Flegal, K. M., et al. (2005). Secular trends in cardiovascular disease risk factors according to body mass index in US adults. *Journal of the American Medical Association, 293*, 1868–1874.

Hagestad, G. O. (1986). The aging society as a context for family life. *Daedalus, 115*, 119–139.

Health Care Financing Administration. (1999). *A profile of Medicare home health: Chart book*. Washington, DC: Author.

Hoenig, H., Taylor, D. H., & Sloan, F. A. (2003). Does assistive technology substitute for personal assistance among the disabled elderly? *American Journal of Public Health, 93*, 330–337.

Johnson, R. W., & Wiener, J. M. (2006). A profile of frail older Americans and their caregivers. *Occasional Paper Number 8: The Retirement Project*. Washington, DC: Urban Institute.

Knickman, J. R., & Snell, E. K. (2002). The 2030 problem: Caring for aging baby boomers. *Health Services Research, 37*, 849.

Kreider, R. M. (2002). Number, timing, and duration of marriages and divorces: 2001. *Current Population Reports*, P70-97.

Kreider, R. M., & Simmons, T. (2003). *Marital status: 2000*. Washington, DC: U.S. Census Bureau.

Lakdawalla, D., Bhattacharya, J., & Goldman, D. P. (2004). Are the young becoming more disabled? Rates of disability appear to be on the rise among people ages eighteen to fifty-nine, fueled by a growing obesity epidemic. *Health Affairs, 23*, 168–176.

Lo Sasso, A. T., & Johnson, R. W. (2002). Does informal care from adult children reduce nursing home admissions for the elderly? *Inquiry, 39*, 279–297.

Mann, W. C., Hurren, D., & Tomita, M. (1993). Comparison of assistive device use and needs of home-based older persons with different impairments. *American Journal of Occupational Therapy, 47*, 980–987.

Mann, W. C., Ottenbacher, K. J., Frass, L., Tomita, M., & Granger, C. V. (1999). Effectiveness of assistive technology and environmental interventions in maintaining independence and reducing home care costs for the frail elderly: A randomized controlled trial. *Archives of Family Medicine, 8*, 210–217.

Manton, K. G., Gu, X., & Lamb, V. L. (2006). Change in chronic disability from 1982 to 2004/2005 as measured by long-term changes in function and health in the U.S. elderly population. *Proceedings of the National Academy of Sciences, 103*, 18374–18379.

Marks, N. F. (1991). *Remarried and single parents in middle adulthood: Differences in psychological well-being and relationships with adult children*. National Survey of Families and Households Working Paper No. 47. Madison: University of Wisconsin.

National Center for Health Statistics. (2003). *Cumulative birth rates by live-birth order.* Retrieved June 6, 2003, from http://www.cdc.gov/nchs/data/statab/t991x31.pdf

National Center for Health Statistics. (2005). *Health, United States, 2005.* Washington, DC: U.S. Government Printing Office.

Palmer, J. L., & Saving, T. R. (2005). *Status of the Social Security and Medicare programs* (Vol. 2006). Baltimore, MD: Social Security Administration, Office of the Chief Actuary.

Pavalko, E. K., & Artis, J. E. (1997). Women's caregiving and paid work: Causal relationships in late life. *Journals of Gerontology Series B-Psychological Sciences and Social Sciences, 52B,* 170–179.

Preston, S. H. (2005). Deadweight? The influence of obesity on longevity. *New England Journal of Medicine, 352,* 1135–1137.

Rein, M., & Salzman, H. (1995). Social integration, participation and exchange in five industrialized countries. In S. Bass (Ed.), *Older and active* (pp. 238–263). New Haven, CT: Yale University Press.

Reynolds, S. L., Saito, Y., & Crimmins, E. M. (2005). The impact of obesity on active life expectancy in older American men and women. *The Gerontologist, 45,* 438–444.

Russell, J. N., Hendershot, G. E., LeClere, F., Howie, J., & Adler, M. (1997). *Trends and differential use of assistive technology devices: United States, 1994.* Hyattsville, MD: National Center for Health Statistics.

Scanlon, W. J. (1997). Medicare home health care: Success of Balanced Budget Act cost controls depends on effective and timely implementation. In *Subcommittee on Oversight and Investigations, Committee on Commerce, House of Representatives.* Washington, DC: United States General Accounting Office.

Seltzer, J. A., & Bianchi, S. M. (1988). Children's contact with absent parents. *Journal of Marriage and the Family, 50,* 663–677.

Siegel, J. S. (1996). *Aging into the 21st century.* Washington, DC: National Aging Information Center, Administration on Aging.

Spillman, B. C. (2004). Changes in elderly disability rates and the implications for health care utilization and cost. *Milbank Quarterly, 82,* 157–194.

Spillman, B. C., & Pezzin, L. E. (2000). Potential and active family caregivers: Changing networks and the "sandwich generation". *Milbank Quarterly, 78,* 347–374.

Stoller, E. P., & Martin, L. (2002). Informal caregiving. In D. J. Ekerdt (Ed.), *Encyclopedia of aging* (pp. 185–190). New York: Macmillan.

Stone, R. I. (2000). *Long-term care for the elderly with disabilities: Current policy, emerging trends, and implications for the twenty-first century.* Farmington Hills, MI: Milbank Memorial Fund.

Stone, R. I., Cafferata, G., & Sangl, J. (1987). Caregivers for the frail elderly: A national profile. *The Gerontologist, 20,* 616–627.

Strum, R., Ringel, J. S., & Andreyeva, T. (2004). Increasing obesity rates and disability trends. *Health Affairs, 23,* 199–205.

Uhlenberg, P. (1993). Demographic change and kin relationships in later life. *Annual Review of Gerontology and Geriatrics, 13,* 219–238.

Uhlenberg, P. (1994). Implications of being divorced in later life. In United Nations (Ed.), *Ageing and the family* (pp. 121–127). New York: Author.

Uhlenberg, P. (1997). Replacing the nursing home. *Public Interest, 128,* 73–84.

Uhlenberg, P., Cooney, T., & Boyd, R. (1990). Divorce for women after midlife. *Journals of Gerontology Series B-Psychological Sciences and Social Sciences, 44,* 3–11.

U.S. Census Bureau. (2000). *Annual projections of the resident population by age, sex, race, and Hispanic origin: 1999 to 2100.* Retrieved September 14, 2006, from http://www.census.gov/population/www/projections/natdet-D1A.html

U.S. House of Representatives, Committee on Ways and Means. (2004). *House Ways and Means Committee Prints: 108-6, 2004 Green Book.* U.S. Government Printing Office, http://www.gpoaccess.gov/wmprints/green/2004.html

Verbrugge, L. M., Rennert, C., & Madans, J. H. (1997). The great efficacy of personal and equipment assistance in reducing disability. *American Journal of Public Health, 87,* 384–392.

Wachter, K. W. (1997). Kinship resources for the elderly. *Philosophical Transactions of the Royal Society of London, Series B Biological Sciences, 352,* 1811–1817.

Wiener, J. M., & Hanley, R. J. (1992). Caring for the disabled elderly: There's no place like home. In S. M. Shortell & U. Reinhart (Eds.), *Improving health policy and management* (pp. 75–109). Ann Arbor, MI: Health Administration Press.

Williamson, J. D. (2003). Forecasting health service needs for older adults: Some sun, some clouds. *Medical Care, 41,* 25–27.

Wolff, J. L., & Kasper, J. D. (2006). Caregivers of frail elders: Updating a national profile. *The Gerontologist, 46,* 344–356.

Zimmer, Z., & Kwong, J. (2003). Family size and support of older adults in urban and rural China: Current effects and future implications. *Demography, 40,* 23–44.

CHAPTER THREE

Choosing Between Paid Elder Care and Unpaid Help From Adult Children: The Role of Relative Prices in the Care Decision[1]

Richard W. Johnson

INTRODUCTION

Providing long-term care services to frail older adults is a critical challenge for U.S. families. About 10 million adults ages 65 and older needed long-term care services in 2002 (Johnson & Wiener, 2006; Spillman & Black, 2005a), and the number is projected to rise in the future as the population continues to age (Knickman & Snell, 2002). Much of the long-term care received by frail elders is provided informally by the family at home, with adult daughters often assuming primary responsibility for the care of their parents, especially when the parent is widowed or divorced (Arno, Levine, & Memmott, 1999). Care activities are often physically exhausting and emotionally draining. Many caregivers report high stress levels, depression, and physical health problems (Yee & Schulz, 2000). Burdens are often particularly intense for employed caregivers, who must balance caregiving duties with their employment responsibilities. Many workers are forced to reduce their hours of employment when caring for their aging parents, or drop out of the labor force altogether (Johnson & Lo Sasso, 2006).

However, social and demographic changes may soon transform the delivery of long-term care services. Women may be less able or willing to fulfill their traditional care responsibilities in the future as they become increasingly attached to the labor market, and falling fertility rates will further limit the future availability of family caregivers. The impact of these social and demographic pressures will intensify once the baby boomers—people born between 1946 and 1964—reach their 70s and 80s and many develop long-term care needs. (See also the chapter by Uhlenberg & Cheuk in this volume.)

How families respond to these pressures will have important consequences for older adults, younger family members, and the cost of public programs. If family members respond by providing less informal care in coming years, many older adults may turn to paid services, such as formal home care or nursing home care. Such a trend may worsen the financial outlook for Medicare and especially Medicaid, which already devotes much of its budget to long-term care services (Georgetown University Long-Term Care Financing Project, 2007). This trend also could raise the financial burden of long-term care for those who do not qualify for public benefits, especially since only about 9% of Americans ages 55 and older currently hold private long-term care insurance (Johnson & Uccello, 2005). Alternatively, families could respond by working harder to provide informal care, with women juggling their schedules to accommodate both their employment and care responsibilities and men accepting more care duties. Better information is needed about how families currently provide care for elderly adults to understand how the future demand for long-term care services will likely evolve.

This chapter examines how families with frail elders choose between long-term care services from paid providers and unpaid family members. The analysis modeled the receipt of paid home care, nursing home care, unpaid care provided by adult children, and unpaid care from other sources as functions of disability, income, demographics, and the price of each type of service. The price of unpaid care from children—the opportunity cost to children of helping their frail parents—equaled the hourly wage that the elder's child with the lowest potential earnings could receive in the labor market. Data came from the 2002 Health and Retirement Study (HRS), a nationally representative survey of older Americans that collects detailed information on disability, long-term care services, and family characteristics. The results show that frail older people with high-earning adult children received less unpaid care from their offspring and more care from paid sources than frail older adults whose children had worse labor market prospects. These findings imply that the demand for paid services will likely rise in the future as the opportunity cost of care from adult children, especially daughters, grows.

BACKGROUND AND SIGNIFICANCE

Most frail older Americans rely on informal help from family and friends. In 2002, about 57% of community-dwelling adults ages 65 and older with functional limitations received unpaid help with basic personal care or household chores during a month-long period (Johnson & Wiener, 2006). Only about 14% received paid home care (excluding medical services provided at home). Among more severely disabled older adults— those reporting difficulty with three or more activities of daily living (ADLs), such as bathing, dressing, or transferring—about four of five living at home received unpaid help and more than one in three received paid services. Most paid home care recipients also obtained unpaid help from family and friends. Only about one-quarter of older adults who received paid home care in 2002 did not also obtain unpaid help (Johnson & Wiener, 2006).

About 34 million adults provided care in 2004 to frail Americans ages 50 and older (National Alliance for Caregiving and AARP, 2004). Although the number of men providing care has increased rapidly in recent years (Spillman & Pezzin, 2000), women still make up the majority of caregivers. For example, 64% of primary caregivers in a recent survey were women (Donelan et al., 2002). And women devote about 50% more time to care activities than men (U.S. Department of Health and Human Services, 1998). Most people caring for adults are middle-aged, although about one in eight is age 65 or older (National Alliance for Caregiving and AARP, 2004).

Spouses and adult children (especially daughters) provide much of the unpaid care received by frail older adults. Nine in 10 older care recipients living at home receive help from their spouses (Johnson & Wiener, 2006), who account for about two-thirds of all of their unpaid helpers (McGarry, 1998). However, only about 4 in 10 at-home frail older adults are married and living with their spouses (Johnson & Wiener, 2006). Children play the dominant caregiving role for older people who are not married. About three-fourths of unmarried older care recipients receive help from their children, with more than one-half receiving help from daughters and slightly more than one-quarter receiving help from sons (Johnson & Wiener, 2006). However, children are more likely to provide help with errands and household chores than basic personal care (McGarry, 1998). Although most care is provided by a single caregiver, many older people obtain assistance from a network of helpers.

For example, nearly one-quarter of frail older care recipients with two or more children receive help from more than one child (Checkovich & Stern, 2002).

Some previous research has examined the factors influencing which child in the family provides care to the frail parent. It is well known, for example, that daughters are much more likely than sons to serve as caregivers (e.g., Dwyer & Coward, 1991). Children who coreside with their parents or live nearby are more likely than other children to provide care, although the coresidence decision is not fully understood (McGarry, 1998; Pezzin, Pollak, & Schone, 2004). Children who received financial help from their parents in the past are more likely to provide care when their parents become ill (Henretta, Hill, Li, Soldo, & Wolf, 1997). Emotional closeness between a parent and child also appears to play an important role in caregiver selection (Pillemer & Suitor, 2006). The number of siblings reduces the odds that a given child helps his or her parents (Wolf, Freedman, & Soldo, 1997), but it increases the chances that the elder receives help from any child. Some studies have found that schooling decreases the likelihood that an adult child provides care (Henretta et al., 1997; Johnson, Lo Sasso, & Lurie 2004), but other studies have failed to find a significant effect of education on caregiving (McGarry, 1998). (See also the chapter by Davey & Szinovacz in this volume.)

Caregiver Burden

Caregiving responsibilities often involve long hours of arduous work that leaves caregivers feeling overwhelmed. On average, caregivers for frail adults spend 4.3 years providing care (National Alliance for Caregiving and AARP, 2004). Those caring for older people average about 150 hours per month helping, and primary ADL caregivers average 260 hours per month (Johnson & Wiener, 2006). Most caregivers are ill-prepared for their role and provide care with little or no support (Alzheimer's Association and National Alliance for Caregiving, 2004). Their care responsibilities often leave them feeling frustrated, angry, drained, guilty, or helpless (Center on an Aging Society, 2005).

These burdens take emotional, physical, and financial tolls on caregivers. They exhibit higher levels of depressive symptoms and mental health problems than their peers who do not provide care (Marks, Lambert, & Choi, 2002; Pinquart & Sorensen, 2003; Schulz, O'Brien, Bookwals, & Fleissner, 1995). Caregiver depression intensifies as the care recipient's functional status declines. For example, between 30 and 40 percent of dementia caregivers suffer from depression and emotional stress (Alzheimer's Association and National Alliance for Caregiving, 2004; Covinsky, Newcomer, Dan, Sands, & Yaffe, 2003). Caregiving responsibilities also appear to impair physical health. Caregivers are more likely to develop serious illness than noncaregivers (Shaw et al., 1997) and are less likely to engage in preventive health behaviors (Schulz et al., 1997). Stressed elderly spousal caregivers exhibit higher mortality rates than people of the same age who do not provide care (Schulz & Beach, 1999). Caregiving responsibilities also impose financial costs. About 6 in 10 caregivers of disabled adults are employed (National Alliance for Caregiving and AARP, 2004), and many middle-aged women participate less in the labor force when they spend time helping their frail parents (Johnson & Lo Sasso, 2006).

Social and demographic changes will likely intensify caregiver burdens in coming years. Balancing employment and care responsibilities is becoming more challenging as more women join the labor force. Between 1980 and 2004, the labor force participation rate of married women ages 45 to 64 increased from 47% to 67% (U.S. Census Bureau, 2006). Falling fertility rates will also limit the future availability of family caregivers, potentially increasing the burdens on those who provide care. Women born between 1956 and 1960 had only 1.9 children on average, compared with 3.2 children for women born between 1931 and 1935 (Redfoot & Pandya, 2002), while the share of women ages 40 to 44 without any children almost doubled (to 19%) between 1980 and 1998 (Bachu & O'Connell, 2001).

Alternatives to Family Care

Families may respond to the rising burdens of informal care by turning to paid helpers. The use of paid home care increased during the 1980s and early 1990s. Between 1982 and 1994, the share of older community-dwelling care recipients who relied solely on informal family help fell from 74% to 64%, while the share who received some assistance at home from paid helpers increased from 26% to 36% (Liu, Manton, & Aragon, 2000). The growth in paid help may have resulted partly from expansions in Medicare and Medicaid financing of home care services (Feder, Komisar, & Niefeld, 2000) as well as from the rising employment of women. In addition, advances in technology now allow complex illnesses, once treated only in hospitals, to be treated at home. However, the share of frail older adults receiving paid home care fell between 1994 and 1999, partly because of new restrictions in Medicare reimbursement for home health care (Spillman & Black, 2005b).

Assisted living and other congregate settings are another fast-growing housing and service option for adults with disabilities. Although they encompass a wide range of housing options and thus are difficult to define, they typically offer frail older adults basic services and round-the-clock oversight in settings that are less institutional than nursing homes. Most offer group meals, housekeeping services, medication reminders, and help with personal activities (Hawes, Rose, & Phillips, 1999). As many as 800,000 older people in the United States live in assisted living settings (National Center for Assisted Living, 2000).

About 1.4 million Americans lived in nursing homes in December 2006 (American Health Care Association, 2006), which primarily serve those with severe medical conditions and disabilities. The share of older adults in nursing homes has steadily declined over the past two decades, falling from 4.5% in 1985 to 3.6% in 2004 (Bishop, 1999; Lewin Group, 2006). Nursing home rates fell most dramatically among adults ages 85 and older, declining from 21% to 14% between 1985 and 2004 (Lewin Group, 2006). At the same time, the nursing home population has grown older and more frail. For example, 86% of residents needed help with three or more ADLs in 2004, up from 72% in 1987 (Lewin Group, 2006; Rhoades & Krauss, 1999).

Research on the interactions between formal home care, nursing home care, and informal family care is limited and inconclusive. Most studies conclude that home care benefits do not significantly reduce the use of nursing home services, perhaps because the study population was not at high risk of institutionalization (Hughes, 1985; Kemper, Applebaum, & Harrigan, 1987; Weissert, Cready, & Pawelak, 1988). Greene and his colleagues (Greene, Lovely, & Ondrich, 1993; Greene, Lovely, Ondrich, & Miller, 1995; Greene, Ondrich, & Laditka, 1998), however, found that certain home care services can reduce nursing home admissions for carefully targeted populations. The cash and counseling demonstration project found that Medicaid beneficiaries in Arkansas who were given consumer-directed allowances for paid home care services used more home care than those not offered the allowances but were less likely to enter nursing homes (Dale, Brown, Phillips, Schore, & Carlson, 2003). Other evidence suggests that home care benefits lead to only small declines in unpaid family care (Pezzin, Kemper, & Reschovsky, 1996). Studies based on nonexperimental data have not generally found that home care services significantly reduce nursing home admissions, although these studies do not fully account for the endogeneity of home care (Hanley, Alecxih, Wiener, & Kennell, 1990; Jette, Tennstedt, & Crawford 1995). Family care does, however, appear to reduce nursing home admissions (Freedman, 1996; LoSasso & Johnson, 2002).

Relative prices are also likely to play important roles in long-term care decisions. Couch, Daly and Wolf (1999) found that low-wage sons and unmarried daughters were more likely to spend time helping their parents than high-wage children, for whom the opportunity cost of caregiving activities is high. The price of informal care likely also affects the demand for all other types of services. For example, the parents of high-wage children may be more likely to receive formal home care or other types of market substitutes to offset the shortfall in family care, but there is no empirical evidence on this important issue. Better information is needed on how families choose long-term care arrangements so we can better assess how they may respond to the rising cost of providing informal care.

MODEL AND HYPOTHESES

We examined how families choose among alternative long-term care services by modeling paid home care, nursing home care, unpaid help from adult children, and unpaid help from other sources for a sample of frail older adults. The analysis was grounded in a theoretical framework that assumes family members make rational decisions about long-term care arrangements so as to maximize their well-being subject to financial and time constraints (Becker, 1991). The approach posits that family members value their own health, leisure, and consumption. Additionally, children and parents value each other's health, leisure, and consumption. Adult children bargain with their parents and siblings over the amount and type of care to provide to frail parents (Pezzin & Schone, 1999a). Children and parents have altruistic feelings toward each other, although family members may differ somewhat in how they value each other's welfare.

Hypotheses

The framework of our model implies that children and parents weigh relative costs and benefits when making long-term care arrangements. We predicted that the use of a particular service mode would rise as its price decreased and the price of other substitutable services increased. The effective price of unpaid care from adult children is the opportunity cost of their time, equal to the value of output from their most productive activities if they were not spending their time providing care to parents. We hypothesized, then, that frail older adults in families facing high prices for children's time and relatively low prices for paid home care and nursing home care would be less likely to receive unpaid care from children and more likely to receive paid services. Conversely, the framework predicted that frail older adults would be more likely to receive unpaid help from children and less likely to receive paid services as the value of the children's time declined and the price of home care and nursing home care increased. Children with high opportunity costs, such as those in high-paying jobs, may elect to help finance paid long-term care services for their parents instead of reducing their paid work hours to provide the care themselves. We also hypothesized that the likelihood of receiving unpaid care from nonchild sources would rise as the price of paid services and the value of children's time increased.

The framework suggests a role for other economic and demographic factors in long-term care arrangements. We expected that paid services would rise and unpaid care would fall as the frail elder's income and wealth increased, holding other factors constant (including price), because frail parents with many financial resources can generally afford to purchase long-term care without substantially reducing their consumption of other goods and services. However, this relationship may be difficult to detect because Medicaid subsidies reduce the effective price of paid long-term care services for people with little income and wealth. We expected all types of long-term care services to increase with age and disability, reflecting higher levels of need. Another hypothesis predicted that additional adult children would reduce the use of paid services and raise the use of unpaid care from children, holding prices constant, by better enabling siblings to share care responsibilities. We expected that married frail adults, who can generally rely on their spouses for help, would be less likely than unmarried adults to receive both paid care and unpaid care from children. However, the effect would likely be smaller if the spouse was also disabled and thus less able to offer assistance. Paid home care would likely be less common in rural areas, where home care agencies are generally more difficult to find.

Different approaches to family behavior generate different predictions about the relationship between parent and child characteristics and long-term care arrangements. Cultural norms may compel certain family members to provide care to others (Hamon & Blieszner, 1990; Lee, Netzer, & Coward, 1994). Daughters, for example, may feel obligated to serve as primary caregivers for their frail parents even if they earn high wages and paid home care would be more efficient. Other theories contend that children may tend to help their parents to improve their chances of receiving bequests, not out of feelings of love and affection (Bernheim, Shleifer, & Summers, 1985). In that case, high-income parents with more money to bequeath may be more likely than low-income parents to receive care from their children.

METHODS

The data came primarily from the 2002 HRS, a nationally representative survey of older Americans conducted by the University of Michigan with primary funding from the National Institute on Aging. Respondents, who entered the survey in 1992, 1993, or 1998, were followed over time, as were their spouses.[2] In 2002, the HRS sample consisted of 22,831 respondents age 55 or older or married to a spouse age 55 or older. All respondents were living in the community at baseline but were followed into nursing homes as necessary. Proxies provided information for respondents who were unable or unwilling to answer. The survey oversampled African Americans, Hispanics, and Florida residents but included sampling weights that we used to adjust our estimates so that they reflected the underlying population.

The HRS is uniquely well suited to a study of how families choose among different types of long-term care services. It collects detailed information on a wide range of topics, including demographics, health and disability, family structure, income, assets, and the receipt of care. At each wave, the survey asked respondents whether they had any difficulty because of physical, mental, emotional, or memory problems with each of the following ADLs: dressing (including putting on shoes or socks), walking across a room, bathing or showering, eating (including cutting up food), getting into or out of bed, and using the toilet (including sitting down or standing up). The questionnaire instructed respondents to exclude difficulties that they did not expect to last for at least 3 months. Additionally, the survey asked respondents whether they had any difficulty with any of the following instrumental activities of daily living (IADLs) because of health or memory problems: preparing hot meals, shopping for groceries, making phone calls, taking medications, and managing money (such as paying bills and tracking expenses).[3]

The HRS collected detailed information on children's characteristics and help received with ADLs and IADLs. Respondents reported how they were related to each of their helpers, the number of days and hours per day each helper provided assistance during the last month, and whether helpers were paid. The survey also identified respondents living in nursing homes at the time of the interview. Additionally, the HRS collected information about each respondent's offspring, including their age, gender, marital status, and education. The restricted-access version of the data that we used identified each respondent's state of residence, which we used to impute prices for long-term care services, as described below.

We restricted our sample to frail adults ages 65 and older with at least one surviving biological child. The analysis classified respondents as frail if they reported difficulty with at least one ADL or IADL. Because care arrangements may differ by disability level and marital status, we also examined outcomes among unmarried frail adults (who cannot turn to spouses for help) and severely disabled older adults, defined as those who reported any difficulty with three or more ADLs. After we eliminated 80 cases that lacked complete information on children, our final samples consisted of 2,714 frail older adults, 772 severely disabled older adults, and 1,489 frail unmarried adults.

Model Specification

The analysis estimated logit equations of the receipt of any unpaid help from biological children over the past month, any unpaid help from other sources over the past month, any paid home care over the month, and nursing home care at the time of the survey interview. We also estimated tobit equations of the number of hours of unpaid help received from children and from other sources over the past month, and the number of paid home care hours. To test whether price, income, and other factors affect the likelihood that frail older adults receive different combinations of services, we then estimated a multinomial logit model of three different long-term care arrangements: paid help but no unpaid help from children, paid help and unpaid help from children, and neither paid help nor unpaid help from children. The omitted reference category consisted of frail older adults who received unpaid help from children but no paid help.

The equations were estimated as functions of prices, income, disability, education, demographic characteristics, and urbanicity. Demographic characteristics consisted of the potential care recipient's gender, age, race and ethnicity, marital status, number of adult daughters, and number of adult sons. Disability level was measured by the number of ADL limitations and the number of IADL limitations. To account for differences in consumption needs by family size, we measured income as the ratio of household income to the federal poverty level. The analysis used the U.S. Department of Agriculture's rural-urban continuum code to classify the care recipient's place of residence as the central county of a metropolitan area with a population of 1 million or more, a suburb of a major metropolitan area, or an exurb or rural area.

Effective prices that families face for long-term care services are difficult to estimate because they depend on a number of different factors. The price of unpaid care from adult children depends on how much the children could earn in the labor market if they chose to work. The HRS did not ask respondents about their children's wages, so we could not use actual wages in the model. However, we would not use actual wages even if they were available, because they likely reflect caregiving activities. Instead, we imputed earnings from ordinary least squares regressions of the natural logarithm of hourly wages for a sample of workers in the 2002 Current Population Survey, a nationally representative monthly household survey conducted by the U.S. Census Bureau. We pooled data from the June, July, August, and September waves. The regressions were estimated separately for men and women as functions of age and its square, race and ethnicity, education, and marital status.[4] We excluded other variables from the specification because these variables were the only child characteristics available in the HRS. The analysis used the regression results to impute an hourly wage to every adult child of each frail older adult in the sample, including those children who were not actually employed, because some nonworking caregivers might have elected to work for pay if they were not providing care.

For frail older adults with more than one adult child, we set the price of unpaid care from children equal to the imputed hourly earnings of the child with the lowest imputed wage. Although other possible approaches exist, such as setting the price equal to the average potential wage across all adult children in the family, our approach is consistent with the notion that families choose care options that minimize total costs. The analysis focused on help from biological children and grouped assistance from stepchildren and children-in-law with unpaid help from all other sources, because biological children provide much more elder care than stepchildren or children-in-law (Ganong & Coleman, 2006; Pezzin & Schone, 1999b).[5]

We based prices for paid home care and nursing home care on average costs that prevailed in the respondent's state of residence. The average daily pay rate for nursing home care (excluding therapy, rehabilitation, and medication costs) came from a national survey by the long-term care division of GE Financial (AARP, 2002). Home health care costs equaled the hourly price charged by an agency for a home health aide, based on a survey of 521 agencies (MetLife, 2002).

Medicaid Eligibility

Some users of formal home care and nursing home care qualify for Medicaid benefits, reducing the price they pay for these services. Medicaid pays for nursing home and home care services for disabled older adults with limited income and virtually no assets. We estimated Medicaid eligibility by combining income and asset data with eligibility rules.

Eligibility rules are complex and vary by state. In most states, older adults who are eligible for Supplemental Security Income (SSI) also qualify for Medicaid. Thirty-one states allow people with incomes up to 300% of the federal SSI benefit (or $1,635 per month for single adults and $2,451 for couples in 2002) to receive Medicaid-funded nursing home care (Bruen, Wiener, & Thomas, 2003). Other states allow people to exclude medical and long-term care expenses from income when determining Medicaid eligibility. However, the income thresholds in medically needy cases are lower than the SSI income thresholds. In states without medically needy programs, people with incomes exceeding eligibility standards can qualify for Medicaid benefits by assigning their incomes to special trusts, called Miller trusts.

The wealth threshold in most states is $2,000 in countable assets for individuals and $3,000 for couples. Countable assets exclude the value of the primary residence and assets reserved for spouses living in the community. People with more wealth can qualify once they have spent nearly all of their assets on long-term care and other allowable expenses.

Long-term care users with incomes above the SSI benefit level who receive Medicaid-funded services must contribute to the cost of their care. Aside from income they may protect for a community-dwelling spouse, Medicaid long-term care users may keep only a small monthly allowance. These monthly allowances vary by state, ranging from $30 to $90 for nursing home residents and from 100% to 300% of the SSI benefit amount for home care users. Spousal allowances also vary by state but in 2002 could not exceed $2,232 in monthly income or $89,324 in assets.

RESULTS

About two-thirds of older adults with ADL or IADL limitations and with surviving adult children received unpaid help from family and friends, paid home care, or nursing home care in 2002. Table 3.1 shows the breakdown by type of service. About 6 in 10 frail older adults with adult children obtained unpaid help, with 36% receiving help from their children and 37% receiving unpaid help from other sources (primarily their spouses). About 23% received paid home care, and another 12% resided in nursing homes.

Most older people receiving assistance with ADLs or IADLs obtained help from multiple sources.[6] For example, two-thirds of older adults receiving help from unpaid children obtained assistance from other people. More than three-quarters of paid home care users and nursing home residents also received unpaid help.

Unmarried frail older adults were about as likely as married people to receive long-term care services, but the types of services differed by marital status. Unmarried people were more likely to receive unpaid help from adult children but less likely to receive unpaid help from other sources because they did not receive spousal help. Additionally, they were more likely than married people to obtain paid home help or nursing home care.

More than 9 in 10 severely disabled older adults (with three or more ADL limitations) received long-term care services in 2002. About 83% received unpaid help from any source, 55% received paid home care,

TABLE 3.1   Percentage of Frail Older Adults Receiving Long-Term Care Services

	All frail older adults	Unmarried frail older adults	Adults with severe disabilities
Help from any source	66.4	68.4	92.9
Unpaid help	61.0	60.2	83.4
Unpaid help from adult children	35.9	51.0	54.2
Unpaid help from other sources	37.2	22.2	48.7
Paid home care	22.5	30.1	54.8
Nursing home care	11.8	17.0	30.8
Only unpaid help	42.6	36.4	38.0
Only unpaid help from adult children	13.1	21.0	8.9
Only unpaid help from other sources	20.2	5.8	16.9
Only paid home care	2.9	4.0	4.3
Only nursing home care	2.6	5.4	4.3
Unpaid help from adult children and other sources	12.3	13.1	19.7
Unpaid help and paid home care	17.5	22.4	45.2
Unpaid help from adult children and paid home care	12.9	19.3	33.0
Unpaid help from other sources and paid home care	7.6	6.4	19.7
Unpaid help and nursing home care	9.2	12.7	25.4
Unpaid help from adult children and nursing home care	7.1	11.3	19.0
Unpaid help from other sources and nursing home care	2.9	2.5	8.7
Number of observations	2,714	1,489	772

Note. The sample was restricted to adults ages 65 and older with at least one limitation with an activity of daily living (ADL) or instrumental activity of daily living (IADL) and with surviving biological children. Help received at home was measured during the month preceding the survey interview, and nursing home care was measured at the time of the interview. Respondents were classified as having severe disabilities if they reported three or more ADLs. Help from children included only assistance from biological children. Data are from the author's computations from the 2002 Health and Retirement Study (HRS).

and 31 percent resided in nursing homes. Help from multiple sources was especially common. For example, about five out of six recipients of unpaid help from children also obtained assistance from paid helpers (at home or in nursing homes) or other unpaid helpers. About the same fraction of paid home care users also received unpaid help.

Care Differences Across Groups

Table 3.2 reports how the receipt of long-term care services by frail older adults in 2002 varied by personal characteristics. The proportion receiving services increased rapidly with age and level of disability. For example, about 81% of frail older adults ages 85 and older received some type of care, compared with only 52% of those ages 65 to 69. Only about 41% of older adults with exactly one ADL limitation received any care, compared with 93% of those with three or more ADL limitations. Interestingly, however, older people with IADL limitations but no ADL limitations were more likely to receive long-term care services than people with only one or two ADL limitations, perhaps because many people with IADL limitations but no ADL limitations had memory problems. The prevalence of unpaid help from adult children, paid home care, and nursing home care all increased steadily with age and—for people with at least one ADL limitation—disability levels. However, the oldest old were significantly less likely than younger people to receive unpaid help from sources other than their children, because they were less likely to be married and receive spousal help.

The use of long-term care services declined sharply with income. About four in five frail older adults with household incomes below the federal poverty level received care, compared with about one-half of those with incomes exceeding four times the poverty level.[7] Care from adult children, paid at-home providers, and paid providers in nursing homes all fell with income, although the declines were most rapid for unpaid help from children. Income-related differences in nursing home care were evident only between those with incomes below twice the poverty level and those with more income. Unpaid help from friends, spouses, and other family members except children did not vary systematically with the frail adult's income.

Frail older college graduates were significantly less likely than those with no more than a high school diploma to receive unpaid help from their children, but there were no significant educational differences in the receipt of paid home care or nursing home care. Those who never attended high school were more likely to receive help from any source and unpaid help from nonchild sources than those with more education.

Long-term care varied by gender and race and ethnicity. African Americans and Hispanics were significantly more likely than non-Hispanic Whites to receive any services. African Americans were less likely to receive nursing home care than Whites and more likely to receive unpaid help from children. Frail older women were more likely than men to receive paid home care, nursing home care, and unpaid help from children. However, they were less likely than men to receive unpaid help from other sources, because they were more likely to be widowed and thus lack access to spousal care. There were no significant gender differences in the receipt of long-term care services overall.

TABLE 3.2   Percentage of Frail Older Adults Receiving Long-Term Care Services, by Personal Characteristics

	Any services	Unpaid help from biological children	Unpaid help from other sources	Paid home care	Nursing home care
All	66.4	35.9	37.2	22.5	11.8
Gender					
Male	64.0	21.9*	48.3*	15.8*	8.2*
Female	67.7	43.5	31.2	26.2	13.8
Age					
65–69	51.5*	21.1*	38.6*	8.1*	5.0*
70–74	59.9*	25.7*	42.1*	13.1*	6.6*
75–79	65.9*	31.0*	41.7*	18.4*	9.6*
80–84	68.3*	40.9*	34.3	23.7*	12.1*
85 and older	81.1	55.1	30.5	43.5	22.9
Marital status					
Widowed	72.7*	53.1*	21.9*	31.5*	18.1*
Divorced or separated	61.1	41.5*	21.7*	22.8*	12.4*
Never married	75.5	33.8	49.7	30.4	0.0*
Currently married	65.2	15.5	57.6	12.3	4.9
Race and ethnicity					
African American	72.8*	47.0*	39.4	20.6	8.3*
Hispanic	74.8*	37.0	40.7	23.3	7.8
Non-Hispanic White and other	65.0	34.5	36.7	22.7	12.5
Education					
Did not attend high school	79.5*	47.3*	43.5*	25.6	13.2
High school dropout	65.5	37.7*	35.4	21.9	12.1
High school graduate	63.7	34.5*	35.6	20.8	10.9
Some college	68.7	28.0	34.3	21.4	12.6
Four or more years of college	59.5	25.1	36.1	24.0	10.8
Ratio of income to federal poverty level					
Less than 1	80.2*	57.9*	30.7	29.5*	16.0*
1 to 1.24	68.7*	44.8*	33.8	28.9*	14.1
1.25 to 1.99	71.8*	41.3*	38.0	25.1*	14.7*
2 to 4	61.7*	27.4*	41.9*	17.3	8.3
More than 4	52.9	17.6	36.0	17.9	9.0
Number of ADL limitations					
None	72.8*	36.6*	40.5*	8.7*	4.1*
One	40.9*	21.7*	23.4*	7.9*	3.6*

Continued

TABLE 3.2   Percentage of Frail Older Adults Receiving Long-Term Care Services, by Personal Characteristics *(Continued)*

	Any services	Unpaid help from biological children	Unpaid help from other sources	Paid home care	Nursing home care
Two	64.0*	32.4*	41.3*	14.6*	5.8*
Three or more	92.9	54.2	48.7	54.8	30.8
Number of Children					
One	67.5	34.1*	36.8	28.6*	16.5*
Two	67.8	35.3*	41.0*	23.7*	11.8
Three	61.7*	33.9*	34.0	20.8	11.1
Four	66.1	31.3*	39.9	23.6*	11.4
Five or more	68.7	43.7	33.8	16.8	9.1
Number of daughters					
Zero	64.2	24.9*	41.9*	25.4	15.6*
One	66.5	36.4	37.9	23.2	12.4
Two	66.2	39.2	34.6	21.1	9.3
Three or more	68.2	40.9	34.7	20.5	10.4
Number of sons					
Zero	69.3	41.5	34.4	24.4*	14.0*
One	66.3	34.4	37.5	26.2*	12.3
Two	65.7	32.7	39.9	19.2	11.7
Three or more	64.7	37.4	35.8	18.0	9.2

Note. The sample was restricted to 2,714 adults ages 65 and older with at least one limitation with an activity of daily living (ADL) or instrumental activity of daily living (IADL) and with surviving biological children. Help received at home was measured during the month preceding the survey interview, and nursing home care was measured at the time of the interview. Help from children included only assistance from biological children. An asterisk indicates a significant difference ($p < .05$) in the portion receiving help between the given group and the last group in the category. Data are from the author's computations from the 2002 Health and Retirement Study (HRS).

Unmarried frail older adults were more than twice as likely to receive paid home care, nursing home care, and unpaid help from adult children as their married counterparts, who generally received assistance from their spouses. For example, about 53% of frail older widows and widowers received help from their adult children, compared with only 16% of married frail older adults. However, married people with long-term care needs were more than twice as likely as widows and widowers to receive unpaid help from other sources. Widowed frail older adults were more than three times as likely as married frail older adults to reside in nursing homes, and about two and a half times as likely to receive paid home care. Frail older adults with five or more children were also more likely to receive help from children and less likely to receive paid home care and nursing home care than those with fewer children.

Differences in long-term care use by income, education, and race and ethnicity appear to arise from differences across groups in disability levels. Table 3.3 shows the share of frail older adults receiving long-term care services by personal characteristics for the subset with severe disabilities. The likelihood of any long-term care use among severely disabled older adults did not vary significantly by income, education, or race and ethnicity. Additionally, nursing home care did not vary significantly by income or gender among severely disabled older adults, and paid home care did not vary significantly by income. Other differences, however, persisted. For example, high-income adults with severe disabilities were significantly less likely than their lower-income counterparts to receive unpaid care from children and more likely to receive unpaid help from other sources. Older women and unmarried adults with severe disabilities were especially likely to receive paid home care and unpaid care from children but unlikely to receive unpaid help from other sources. Rates of long-term care use increased with age among severely disabled older adults. And White non-Hispanics were significantly more likely than African Americans and Hispanics to receive nursing home care.

Model Estimates of the Receipt of Long-Term Care

To disentangle the effects of these various factors on long-term care services, Table 3.4 shows estimates from our models of any unpaid help from adult children, any unpaid help from other sources, any paid home care, and any nursing home care. The table reports odds ratios, with asterisks identifying those that differ significantly from one and daggers denoting marginally significant differences. Odds ratios significantly greater than one indicate that the associated factor was positively correlated with the outcome, and those less than one indicate negative correlations. The appendix table reports sample means and standard deviations.

The price of children's time, measured as the imputed hourly wage that could be earned by the frail elder's lowest-paid child, significantly reduced the likelihood that frail older adults received any unpaid help from their adult children and increased the likelihood that they received paid home care and nursing home care. The price of children's time had relatively small effects on the probability of help from children but had larger effects on paid services. A one-dollar increase in the hourly price of children's time reduced the probability of unpaid help by 3% increased the probability of paid home care by 8% and increased the probability of nursing home residence by 10%. The value of children's time did not significantly affect the likelihood of unpaid help from other sources.

The price elasticity, defined as 100 times the percent change in the outcome induced by a 1% change in own price or the price of some other good or service, is a common way of measuring how outcomes respond

TABLE 3.3　Percentage of Older Adults With Severe Disabilities Receiving Long-Term Care Services, by Personal Characteristics

	Any services	Unpaid help from biological children	Unpaid help from other sources	Paid home care	Nursing home care
All	92.9	54.2	48.7	54.8	37.9
Gender					
Male	93.6	41.9*	62.3*	48.6*	26.0
Female	92.6	59.7	42.6	57.6	33.0
Age					
65-69	86.4*	39.7*	61.7*	32.1*	17.3*
70-74	90.2*	43.6*	57.4*	39.7*	20.9*
75-79	94.0	48.1*	58.7*	43.9*	21.4*
80-84	92.4	55.0*	43.4	61.8*	38.0
85 and older	96.3	68.2	36.3	73.5	42.5
Marital status					
Widowed	93.1	69.2*	29.0*	66.1*	39.9*
Divorced or separated	90.1	63.3*	26.2*	54.8*	32.8*
Never married	100.0*	47.0	44.6	60.6	0.0*
Currently married	93.3	30.0	83.4	38.4	17.5
Race and ethnicity					
African American	87.2	58.2	44.2	46.8	18.2*
Hispanic	95.7	46.3	54.9	45.6	12.4*
Non-Hispanic White and other	93.4	54.4	48.7	56.7	34.2
Education					
Did not attend high school	95.9	55.2*	52.8	54.9	26.5
High school dropout	91.2	59.9*	44.1	53.2	31.9
High school graduate	89.6	52.3	45.1	50.8	29.7
Some college	95.3	62.1*	47.1	60.0	42.6
Four or more years of college	95.1	40.5	57.4	63.3	31.7
Ratio of income to federal poverty level					
Less than 1	95.5	68.8*	36.4*	64.4	29.6
1 to 1.24	95.6	60.2*	46.3*	65.6	38.1
1.25 to 1.99	92.0	56.5*	43.5*	49.2	30.0
2 to 4	93.0	48.6*	57.7	48.4	27.5
More than 4	88.0	32.7	61.7	56.0	34.6
Number of children					
One	90.1	51.4*	44.2	59.4*	39.2*
Two	94.1	53.8*	54.4	59.3*	31.7*

Continued

TABLE 3.3   Percentage of Older Adults With Severe Disabilities Receiving Long-Term Care Services, by Personal Characteristics *(Continued)*

	Any services	Unpaid help from biological children	Unpaid help from other sources	Paid home care	Nursing home care
Three	93.3	53.4*	47.8	53.4	33.2*
Four	93.2	47.6*	47.4	57.3*	28.2
Five or more	93.6	65.1	47.5	42.7	20.3
Number of daughters					
Zero	93.9	36.1*	58.5*	63.5	43.6*
One	93.4	55.6	48.9	53.3	29.9
Two	91.3	61.6	44.7	52.1	27.2
Three or more	92.9	57.9	44.8	53.8	26.7
Number of sons					
Zero	88.9	60.5	38.9	56.1	34.0
One	93.4	54.2	49.0	59.9*	32.4
Two	95.2	47.5	55.8	50.4	32.0
Three or more	93.7	55.2	50.4	48.5	22.9

Note. The sample was restricted to 772 adults ages 65 and older with three or more limitations with activities of daily living (ADL) and with surviving biological children. Help received at home was measured during the month preceding the survey interview, and nursing home care was measured at the time of the interview. Help from children included only assistance from biological children. An asterisk indicates a significant difference ($p < .05$) in the portion receiving help between the given group and the last group in the category. Data are from the author's computations from the 2002 Health and Retirement Study (HRS).

to prices. Elasticities of less than one in absolute value generally indicate that the outcome does not vary much in response to price changes. Economists describe these outcomes as being price inelastic. With children's time valued at a mean hourly price of $13.90, the results in Table 3.4 implied an own price elasticity of –0.42. The elasticity of paid home care with respect to the price of children's time was 1.11, and the elasticity of nursing home care was 1.39.

Out-of-pocket prices for nursing home care significantly reduced the likelihood of nursing home residence, although the effects were modest. The model predicted that a one-dollar increase in effective nursing home prices reduced care probabilities by 0.4 percent, implying an elasticity of –0.41 (given that the mean effective price was $103.59). Nursing home prices did not significantly affect the probability of unpaid help, but they decreased the probability of paid home care (although the effect was only marginally significant). We expected nursing home prices to raise the likelihood of paid home care use, holding home care prices constant, because home care may substitute for nursing home care when nursing

TABLE 3.4 Determinants of Long-Term Care Service Use

	Any unpaid help from children		Any unpaid help from other sources		Any paid home care		Any nursing home care	
	Odds ratio	SE	Odds ratio	SE	Odds ratio	SE	Odds ratio	SE
Prices								
Children's time	0.97*	0.01	1.01	0.01	1.08**	0.02	1.10**	0.03
Home care	1.02	0.01	0.99	0.01	0.99	0.01	1.01	0.02
Nursing home	1.00	0.001	1.00	0.001	0.998†	0.001	0.996*	0.002
Number of children								
Daughters	1.19**	0.05	0.87**	0.03	1.07	0.06	1.073	0.09
Sons	1.02	0.04	0.98	0.04	0.98	0.05	1.00	0.06
Age	1.02**	0.01	0.99	0.01	1.07**	0.01	1.03*	0.01
Number of ADL limitations	0.96	0.04	1.02	0.03	1.60**	0.07	1.46**	0.08
Number of IADL limitations	1.91**	0.08	1.66**	0.06	1.73**	0.08	1.65**	0.11
Male	0.51**	0.07	1.14	0.12	0.69*	0.11	0.91	0.20
Race and ethnicity								
African American	1.24	0.21	1.25	0.21	0.87	0.20	0.53*	0.17
Hispanic	0.69	0.17	1.14	0.24	1.12	0.36	0.59	0.30
[Ref: White or other]	—	—	—	—	—	—	—	—
Marital status								
[Ref: widowed]	—	—	—	—	—	—	—	—
Divorced or separated	0.78	0.14	1.13	0.23	1.16	0.30	1.08	0.38

Never married	0.45	0.29	4.41**	2.04	1.93	1.43	—	—
Currently married	0.15**	0.03	9.99**	1.43	0.28**	0.06	0.22**	0.06
Married to spouse with disabilities	2.78**	0.59	0.53**	0.08	2.52**	0.64	1.76†	0.57
Education								
Did not attend high school	1.13	0.18	1.48**	0.22	0.92	0.19	1.14	0.29
High school dropout	0.94	0.15	1.12	0.17	1.07	0.22	1.26	0.33
[Ref: high school graduate]	—	—	—	—	—	—	—	—
Some college	0.77	0.14	1.00	0.15	0.95	0.22	1.13	0.32
Four or more years of college	0.86	0.18	0.76	0.13	1.20	0.28	0.91	0.28
Ratio of income to poverty level	0.98	0.04	0.99	0.01	1.03**	0.01	1.03*	0.01
Urbanicity								
[Ref: urban]	—	—	—	—	—	—	—	—
Inner suburbs	0.91	0.12	1.17	0.14	0.84	0.14	1.05	0.21
Outer suburbs and rural	0.75*	0.10	1.19	0.14	0.85	0.15	1.29	0.28

Note. Estimates were from logit models of any unpaid help from adult biological children, any unpaid help from other sources, any paid home care, and any nursing home. Help received at home was measured during the month preceding the survey interview, and nursing home care was measured at the time of the interview. *SE* denotes the standard error of the odds ratio. The sample was restricted to 2,714 adults ages 65 and older with at least one limitation with an activity of daily living (ADL) or instrumental activity of daily living (IADL) and with surviving children. The price of children's time was set equal to the imputed hourly wage of the child with the lowest wage. Data are from the author's computations from the 2002 Health and Retirement Study (HRS).

† $.05 \leq p < .1.$ * $.01 \leq p < .05.$ ** $p < .01.$

homes are particularly expensive. However, effective home care prices and nursing home care prices were closely correlated ($r = 0.57$), because many people who qualify for Medicaid when using home care also qualify when in nursing homes. Thus, the estimated negative effect of nursing home prices may reflect a negative impact of home care prices on home care use. In fact, when we reestimated the model after dropping nursing home prices from the equation, home care prices exerted a negative and marginally significant effect on the likelihood of paid home care use.

Long-term care use generally increased with age and disability level. For example, the likelihood that frail older adults received paid home care increased by about 7% with each additional year of age, holding other factors constant. Each additional IADL limitation increased the probability of unpaid help from children by about 91% and the probability of paid home care by about 73%. However, additional ADL limitations did not significantly affect unpaid care from children or other sources. These findings suggest that severe disabilities may require help from professional caregivers and are consistent with other evidence that children primarily provide help with household chores and errands (McGarry, 1998).

Married frail older adults were much less likely than unmarried adults to receive unpaid help from children, paid home care, and nursing home care. For example, controlling for other factors, the model showed that married frail older adults were only 15% as likely as widowed adults to receive unpaid help from children. The estimated differences were much smaller, however, when spouses were disabled and unlikely to provide much help.

Controlling for other factors, including the value of children's time, the models indicated that the number of daughters significantly increased the likelihood that frail older adults received any help from children and reduced the chances of receiving unpaid help from other sources. However, the number of daughters did not significantly affect the likelihood of paid services (either at home or in nursing facilities), and the number of sons did not significantly affect the use of any types of services.

Income increased the likelihood that frail older adults used paid home care or nursing home care, although the effects were modest. For an unmarried adult, boosting income by about $8,600 (in 2002 dollars) would raise the likelihood of obtaining assistance from paid helpers either at home or in nursing homes by about 3%. Income did not significantly affect the chances of unpaid help. Frail older adults who never attended high school were significantly more likely than high school graduates to obtain unpaid help from sources other than their children. Education differences, controlling for other factors, were not evident in the receipt of other services.

Finally, gender, race and ethnicity, and urbanicity influenced the use of certain services. Men were significantly less likely than women to receive unpaid help from children and paid home care, even when the models controlled for marital status and access to help from spouses. Nursing home care did not, however, differ significantly by gender. African Americans were significantly less likely than non-Hispanic Whites to receive nursing home care, but there were no other significant racial differences in the use of long-term care services. Frail older adults living in outer suburbs and rural areas were significantly less likely than other people to receive help from adult children, perhaps because they were less likely to have children living nearby. However, paid home care was not significantly less prevalent in rural areas than in more urban locales.

Model Estimates of Care Hours

Table 3.5 shows results from tobit models of hours of monthly help received by frail older adults. The price of children's time significantly reduced monthly unpaid hours from children and significantly increased monthly paid help hours. The effects were substantial. A one-dollar increase in the hourly value of children's time reduced unpaid help from children by nearly 5 hours per month and increased paid home care by almost 7 hours per month. These estimates imply a price elasticity of unpaid help from children of –2.1 and an elasticity of paid home care with respect to the price of children's time of 4.6. Surprisingly, the value of children's time also reduced unpaid hours of assistance from nonchild helpers, although the effects were small and only marginally significant. Effective home care and nursing home prices did not generally affect the amount of help received. Home care prices modestly increased monthly unpaid help hours from children, consistent with economic theory, but the estimated effect was only marginally significant.

Other economic, social, and demographic factors found to influence the likelihood of long-term care services also affected monthly help hours. For example, help hours generally increased with disability level. However, the number of ADL limitations did not increase unpaid help hours received from children, perhaps because severely disabled adults generally turn to spouses or paid helpers for assistance. Frail married adults received fewer hours of assistance from children and paid helpers than widows, but more unpaid hours from sources (including spouses) other than their children. The number of daughters, but not sons, increased help hours from children and paid providers and reduced unpaid help hours from other sources. Women received more hours of unpaid help from children and paid home care than men. Income and education did not significantly increase help hours, except that college graduates received significantly more hours of paid home care than high school graduates. There were no significant differences by race and ethnicity or urbanicity in help hours.

TABLE 3.5 Determinants of Monthly Help Hours

	Unpaid help from children		Unpaid help from other sources		Paid home care	
	Coefficient	SE	Coefficient	SE	Coefficient	SE
Prices						
Children's time	-4.83**	1.53	-2.97†	1.78	6.66*	3.22
Home care	1.37†	0.83	-0.36	1.03	-0.82	1.89
Nursing home	-0.11	0.09	-0.19	0.12	0.002	0.21
Number of Children						
Daughters	16.88**	3.73	-15.75**	4.80	15.87†	8.87
Sons	-0.73	0.66	-5.68	4.68	-3.26	8.92
Age	0.49	0.72	-1.55†	0.90	4.66**	1.63
Number of ADL limitations	-0.61	3.00	11.05**	3.73	26.39**	6.65
Number of IADL limitations	59.74**	3.73	65.60**	4.50	83.03**	8.51
Male	-57.93**	12.34	19.45	13.72	-49.14†	27.85
Race and ethnicity						
African American	-17.05	16.99	-30.34	21.33	-62.47	40.66
Hispanic	-17.98	22.53	-13.82	28.57	39.71	50.20
[Ref: White or other]	—	—	—	—	—	—
Marital status						
[Ref: widowed]	—	—	—	—	—	—
Divorced or separated	-30.34†	17.51	-2.65	26.22	29.43	41.28
Never married	-136.69†	74.63	34.88	86.52	111.68	129.99
Currently married	-175.30**	15.82	267.89**	17.35	-165.26**	35.82

Married to spouse with disabilities	65.65**	20.24	-76.49**	18.66	129.39**	42.97
Education						
Did not attend high school	17.13	14.51	6.41	18.06	-31.14	34.28
High school dropout	3.06	14.86	-6.75	18.41	-4.41	34.72
[Ref: high school graduate]	—	—	—	—	—	—
Some college	-9.33	16.86	-14.95	19.90	-60.31	39.37
Four or more years of college	3.74	19.70	-14.95	22.16	83.82*	39.36
Ratio of income to poverty level	-1.11	1.68	-2.90†	1.73	4.17	2.79
Urbanicity						
[Ref: urban]	—	—	—	—	—	—
Inner suburbs	8.70	12.51	19.97	15.30	-45.60	28.91
Outer suburbs and rural	-16.29	12.34	18.43	15.04	-23.03	28.02
Intercept	-157.65*	65.46	-172.00*	79.56	-1046.33**	155.12

Note. Estimates were from tobit models of the number of at-home help hours received during the past month from adult biological children, other unpaid sources (including spouses), and paid helpers. *SE* denotes the standard error. The sample was restricted to 2,714 adults ages 65 and older with at least one limitation with an activity of daily living (ADL) or instrumental activity of daily living (IADL) and with surviving children. The price of children's time was set equal to the imputed hourly wage of the child with the lowest wage. Data are from the author's computations from the 2002 Health and Retirement Study (HRS).

† $.05 \leq p < .1.$ * $.01 \leq p < .05.$ ** $p < .01.$

Multinomial Logit Estimates of Care Arrangements

Table 3.6 reports odds ratios and standard errors from our multinomial logit model of long-term care arrangements. All parameters were estimated relative to frail older adults who received unpaid help from children but no paid services (either at home or in nursing homes). The price of children's time significantly increased the odds of receiving paid services and no unpaid help from children, relative to receiving unpaid help from children but no paid services. The effects were fairly large, with a one-dollar increase in the hourly price of children's time raising by 10% the probability that frail older adults received paid services but no unpaid help from children. However, the price of children's time also increased the chances that frail older adults received both paid services and unpaid help from children and, to a lesser extent, that they received neither paid services nor unpaid help from children. In many cases, then, children with high opportunity costs continued to provide some care to their frail parents but often supplemented their help with paid home care or nursing home care. The effective prices of home care and nursing home care did not significantly affect long-term care arrangements in the multinomial logit model.

Health and demographic factors significantly influenced long-term care arrangements. The odds of receiving paid services, both with and without unpaid help from children, increased with age and the number of ADL limitations. Age and the number of IADL limitations significantly reduced the chances of receiving neither paid services nor help from children. Men were more likely than women, and frail older adults living in outer suburbs were more likely than urban residents, to receive neither paid services nor help from children. Care may be difficult to obtain in rural areas because children often move to more urban areas when they leave home, and home care agencies may be less available outside of metropolitan areas. The number of daughters reduced the odds of receiving neither paid services nor help from children, but sons had no significant effects. There were no significant differences by income, race and ethnicity, or education in long-term care arrangements.

CONCLUSIONS

Our findings suggest that efficiency considerations play a role in how families choose to provide long-term care. Frail older adults received less unpaid help from their children and more help from paid sources, both at home and in nursing homes, when all of their offspring could earn relatively high wages in the labor market than when some had relatively poor labor market prospects. Children's earnings capacity had larger

TABLE 3.6 Multinomial Logit Estimates of Paid and Unpaid Services

	Some paid services, no unpaid help from children		Paid services and unpaid help from children		No paid services and no unpaid help from children	
	Odds ratio	SE	Odds ratio	SE	Odds ratio	SE
Prices						
Children's time	1.10**	0.03	1.09**	0.03	1.04*	0.02
Home care	0.98	0.02	1.03†	0.01	1.00	0.01
Nursing home	1.00	0.002	0.997†	0.002	1.00	0.001
Number of children						
Daughters	0.89	0.08	1.08	0.06	0.84**	0.04
Sons	0.95	0.06	0.98	0.06	0.99	0.05
Age	1.04**	0.01	1.05**	0.01	0.97**	0.01
Number of ADL limitations	1.48**	0.08	1.46**	0.08	0.96	0.05
Number of IADL limitations	0.98	0.06	1.62**	0.10	0.44**	0.03
Male	1.35	0.29	1.01	0.23	2.36**	0.38
Race and ethnicity						
African American	0.68	0.20	0.76	0.21	0.80	0.15
Hispanic	1.78	0.66	0.81	0.32	1.25	0.36
[Ref: White or other]	—		—		—	
Marital status						
[Ref: widowed]	—		—		—	
Divorced or separated	1.16	0.43	1.46	0.44	1.51*	0.31
Never married	2.83	2.28	0.37	0.43	1.13	0.64
Currently married	1.48	0.38	0.13**	0.05	7.66**	1.55
Married to spouse with disabilities	0.92	0.29	6.91**	3.13	0.42**	0.11

Continued

TABLE 3.6 Multinomial Logit Estimates of Paid and Unpaid Services (*Continued*)

	Some paid services, no unpaid help from children		Paid services and unpaid help from children		No paid services and no unpaid help from children	
	Odds ratio	SE	Odds ratio	SE	Odds ratio	SE
Education						
Did not attend high school	1.03	0.27	0.72	0.18	0.74	0.14
High school dropout	1.19	0.32	1.15	0.31	1.10	0.20
[Ref: high school graduate]	—	—	—	—	—	—
Some college	1.25	0.39	0.99	0.30	1.29	0.27
Four or more years of college	1.50	0.47	1.25	0.43	1.14	0.29
Ratio of income to poverty level	1.04	0.04	1.00	0.04	1.00	0.04
Urbanicity						
[Ref: urban]	—	—	—	—	—	—
Inner suburbs	0.88	0.18	0.82	0.17	1.11	0.17
Outer suburbs and rural	1.15	0.25	1.19	0.26	1.52**	0.24

Note. Estimates were from a multinomial logit model of no unpaid help from children but some paid help, both unpaid help from children and paid help, and neither unpaid help from children nor any paid help, relative to unpaid help from children but no paid help. Help received at home was measured during the month preceding the survey interview, and nursing home care was measured at the time of the interview. *SE* denotes the standard error. The sample was restricted to 2,714 adults ages 65 and older with at least one limitation with an activity of daily living (ADL) or instrumental activity of daily living (IADL) and with surviving children. The price of children's time was set equal to the imputed hourly wage of the child with the lowest wage. Data are from the author's computations from the 2002 Health and Retirement Study (HRS).

$\dagger$ $.05 \leq p < .1$. * $.01 \leq p < .05$. ** $p < .01$.

effects on the amount of unpaid help provided than on the receipt of any help. Frail older adults with well-educated children tend to receive paid home care that supplements unpaid family help but does not completely replace it. These findings are consistent with other evidence that most paid home care recipients also obtain unpaid family care (Johnson & Wiener, 2006; Spillman & Black, 2005b). Given the imprecision of our imputations of children's potential wages, our results likely underestimate the true impact of opportunity costs on long-term care arrangements.

Surprisingly, we did not uncover much evidence that effective prices for paid services affect their use. Accounting for Medicaid eligibility, we found that nursing home prices moderately reduced the likelihood that frail older adults became institutionalized, but home care prices did not significantly influence the receipt of at-home assistance from paid helpers or the amount of help they provided. Effective home care prices were marginally significant predictors of any paid home care when we dropped from the model nursing home prices (which are correlated with home care prices), but the impact was small. It seems likely that home care use would be more—not less—price responsive than the use of nursing homes, which most people avoid until they are physically unable to live at home (AARP, 2003). Measurement error in the effective price for paid services likely led us to underestimate its true impact on usage. For example, our underlying private-pay prices for home care and nursing home care varied across states but not within states, so our measures did not capture any urban-rural price differentials within a particular state. Rates charged by many home care agencies vary with the number of hours purchased. And our estimates of Medicaid eligibility were necessarily imprecise.

Many unanswered questions remain about how families make decisions about long-term care. Our results suggest that families strive to choose the low-cost option and consider the opportunity cost of the unpaid caregiver's time. The empirical findings are consistent with a model of family dynamics in which the sibling with little education or in a low-paying occupation provides care to the parent while the well-educated sibling helps finance paid services. Although we did not examine financial transfers between children and their parents, Couch, Daly, and Wolf (1999) found that high-wage children were, in fact, more likely than low-wage children to give money to their parents but less likely to spend time helping them. However, our results could instead reflect class differences in the willingness to turn to paid providers. For example, well-educated families may have more experience using paid helpers to assist with such activities as child care and household chores and thus may be more willing than less-educated families (even after controlling for income differences) to pay for help with elder care. Noneconomic factors, such as the emotional ties between parent and child, probably also play a role in caregiving decisions. Additional research would be valuable in sorting out these different motives.

Finally, our results imply that the demand for paid services will likely surge in coming years as the opportunity cost of care from adult children grows, especially for adult daughters. Women continue to work more and earn more in late mid-life (U.S. Census Bureau, 2006). Because many caregivers are forced to reduce their work hours or drop out of the labor force (Johnson & Lo Sasso, 2006), women's labor market gains raise the cost of informal care. Other trends are also likely to increase the future demand for paid services. For example, the rising prevalence of diabetes and obesity in the nonelderly population may eventually reverse the recent trend toward declining disability rates at older ages (Freedman, Martin, & Schoeni, 2002; Lakdawalla et al., 2003; Olshansky et al., 2005). Rising divorce rates, increasing childlessness, and declining family sizes could reduce the future availability of family caregivers (Bachu, 1999; Bachu & O'Connell, 2001; Teachman, Tedrow, & Crowder, 2000), although the narrowing of the gender gap in life expectancy could increase the supply of spousal caregivers (Lakdawalla & Philipson, 2002). Together, these trends have important consequences for older adults, their families, and the federal, state, and local governments.

APPENDIX TABLE Sample Means and Standard Deviations

	Mean	Standard deviation
Dependent variables		
Any unpaid help from children	0.36	0.48
Any unpaid help from other sources	0.37	0.48
Any paid home care	0.23	0.42
Any nursing home care	0.12	0.32
Monthly unpaid help hours from children	31.30	109.22
Monthly unpaid help hours from others	45.26	142.36
Monthly hours of paid home care	19.91	99.54
Prices		
Children's time	13.90	4.30
Home care	14.00	7.14
Nursing home	103.59	70.46
Number of children		
Daughters	1.67	1.46
Sons	1.61	1.38
Age	78.23	7.89
Number of ADL limitations	1.91	1.80
Number of IADL limitations	1.64	1.66

Continued

APPENDIX TABLE Sample Means and Standard Deviations (Continued)

	Mean	Standard deviation
Male	0.35	0.48
Race and ethnicity		
African American	0.10	0.30
Hispanic	0.06	0.24
Marital status		
Divorced or separated	0.10	0.30
Never married	0.01	0.07
Currently married	0.42	0.49
Married to spouse with disabilities	0.12	0.33
Education		
Did not attend high school	0.22	0.42
High school dropout	0.18	0.38
Some college	0.15	0.35
Four or more years of college	0.11	0.32
Ratio of income to poverty level	2.89	4.10
Urbanicity		
Inner suburbs	0.28	0.45
Outer suburbs and rural	0.34	0.47

Note. The sample was restricted to 2,714 adults ages 65 and older with at least one limitation with an activity of daily living (ADL) or instrumental activity of daily living (IADL) and with surviving children. Help received at home was measured during the month preceding the survey interview, and nursing home care was measured at the time of the interview. Help from children included only assistance from biological children. Data are from the author's computations from the 2002 Health and Retirement Study (HRS).

NOTES

1. Desmond Toohey provided outstanding research assistance. Stephen Conroy, Daphna Gans, Merrill Silverstein, Maximiliane Szinovacz, and Joshua Wiener provided valuable comments on an earlier draft. This study was prepared under grant number 049919 from the Robert Wood Johnson Foundation's Changes in Health Care Financing and Organization Initiative. The views expressed are those of the author and should not be attributed to the Urban Institute, its trustees, or its funders.
2. In 2004, the HRS added a cohort of respondents born between 1948 and 1953, but those data were not finalized when this study began.
3. The HRS also asked respondents whether they had any difficulty using a map, but we excluded that information from our measure of IADL limitations because we did not consider map reading to be an important component of independent living.
4. The regressions were based on a sample of 29,188 working men and 26,995 working women. They showed that earnings increased significantly with education and age (up to about age 50). Earnings were significantly higher for Whites than Blacks and Hispanics, and for married adults than unmarried adults. The r-squared statistics were 0.36 for men and 0.33 for women.

5. The HRS asked respondents whether they lived within 10 miles of each of their children. Although it may be impractical for children to provide regular care for their parents when they live far away, we did not restrict our analysis to nearby children, because the decision to live near parents likely reflects care expectations. To incorporate parent-child proximity into our equations would have required us to model the children's relative locations, which was beyond the scope of this study.
6. As reported in Table 3.1, 13.1% of all frail older adults received *only* unpaid help from adult children, and 35.9% of all frail older adults received unpaid help from adult children.
7. The federal poverty level for a single adult age 65 or older was $8,628 in 2002.

REFERENCES

AARP. (2002). *Across the states: Profiles of long-term care* (5th ed.). Washington, DC: Author.

AARP. (2003). *Beyond 50 2003: A report to the nation on independent living and disability.* Washington, DC: Author.

Alzheimer's Association and National Alliance for Caregiving. (2004). *Families care: Alzheimer's caregiving in the United States.* Chicago: Alzheimer's Association.

American Health Care Association. (2006). Nursing facility total, average and median number of patients per facility and ADL dependence. *CMS OSCAR Data Current Surveys, December.* Retrieved November 7, 2006, from http://www.ahca.org/research/oscar/rpt_average_ADL_200612.pdf

Arno, P. S., Levine, C., & Memmott, M. M. (1999). The economic value of informal caregiving. *Health Affairs, 18*(2), 182–188.

Bachu, A. (1999). Is childlessness among American women on the rise? *Population Division Working Paper No. 37.* Washington, DC: U.S. Census Bureau.

Bachu, A., & O'Connell, M. (2001). Fertility of American women: June 2000. *Current Population Reports.* Washington, DC: U.S. Census Bureau.

Becker, G. S. (1991). *A treatise on the family* (enlarged ed.). Cambridge, MA: Harvard University Press.

Bernheim, B. D., Shleifer, A., & Summers, L. (1985). The strategic bequest motive. *Journal of Political Economy, 93*(6), 1138–1159.

Bishop, C. E. (1999). Where are the missing elders? The decline in nursing home use, 1985 and 1996. *Health Affairs, 18*(4), 146–155.

Bruen, B. K., Wiener, J. M., & Thomas, S. (2003). Medicaid eligibility policy for aged, blind, and disabled beneficiaries. *AARP Public Policy Institute Report No. 2003-14.* Washington, DC: AARP.

Center on an Aging Society. (2005). *How do family caregivers fare: A closer look at their experiences.* Washington, DC: Georgetown University. Retrieved November 7, 2006, from http://ihcrp.georgetown.edu/agingsociety/pdfs/CAREGIVERS3.pdf

Checkovich, T. J., & Stern, S. (2002). Shared caregiving responsibilities of adult siblings with elderly parents. *Journal of Human Resources, 37*(3), 441–478.

Couch, K. A., Daly, M. C., & Wolf, D. A. (1999). Time? Money? Both? The allocation of resources to older parents. *Demography, 36*(2), 219–232.

Covinsky, K. E., Newcomer, R., Dane, C. K., Sands, L. P., & Yaffe, K. (2003). Patient and caregiver characteristics associated with depression in caregivers of patients and dementia. *Journal of General Internal Medicine, 18,* 1006–1014.

Dale, S., Brown, R., Phillips, B., Schore, J., & Carlson, B. L. (2003). The effects of cash and counseling on personal care services and Medicaid costs in Arkansas. *Health Affairs Web Exclusive, W3,* 566–575.

Donelan, K., Hill, C. A., Hoffman, C., Scoles, K., Feldman, P. H., Levine, C., et al. (2002). Challenged to care: Informal caregivers in a changing health system. *Health Affairs, 21*(4), 222–231.

Dwyer, J. W., & Coward, R. T. (1991). A multivariate comparison of the involvement of adult sons versus daughters in the care of impaired parents. *Journal of Gerontology: Social Sciences, 46*(5), S259–S269.

Feder, J., Komisar, H. L., & Niefeld, M. (2000). Long-term care in the United States: An overview. *Health Affairs, 19*(3), 40–56.

Freedman, V. A. (1996). Family structure and the risk of nursing home admission. *Journals of Gerontology: Social Sciences, 51B,* S61–S69.

Freedman, V. A., Martin, L. G., & Schoeni, R. F. (2002). Recent trends in disability and functioning among older adults in the United States. *Journal of the American Medical Association, 288*(24), 3137–3146.

Ganong, L., & Coleman, M. (2006). Obligations to stepparents acquired in later life: Relationship quality and acuity of needs. *Journals of Gerontology: Social Sciences, 61B*(2), S80–S88.

Georgetown University Long-Term Care Financing Project. (2007). Medicaid and long-term care. Retrieved November 7, 2006, from http://ltc.georgetown.edu/pdfs/medicaid2006 .pdf

Greene, V. L., Lovely, M., & Ondrich, J. (1993). The cost-effectiveness of community services in a frail elderly population. *The Gerontologist, 33,* 177–189.

Greene, V. L., Lovely, M., Ondrich, J., & Miller, M. (1995). Reducing nursing home use through community-based care: An optimization analysis. *Journals of Gerontology: Social Sciences, 50B,* 259–268.

Greene, V. L., Ondrich, J., & Laditka, S. (1998). Can home care services achieve cost savings in long-term care for older people? *Journals of Gerontology: Social Sciences, 53B*(4), S228–S238.

Hamon, R. R., & Blieszner, R. (1990). Filial responsibility expectations among adult child–older parent pairs. *Journals of Gerontology: Psychological Sciences, 45*(1), P110–P112.

Hanley, R. J., Alecxih, L. M. B., Wiener, J. M., & Kennell, D. L. (1990). Predicting elderly nursing home admissions: Results from the 1982–1984 National Long-Term Care Survey. *Research on Aging, 12*(2), 199–228.

Hawes, C., Rose, M., & Phillips, C. D. (1999). *A national study of assisted living for the frail elderly: Results of a national survey of facilities.* Office of Disability, Aging, and Long-Term Care Policy, Assistant Secretary of Planning and Evaluation, U.S. Department of Health and Human Services, Washington, DC.

Henretta, J. C., Hill, M. S., Li, W., Soldo, B. J., & Wolf, D. A. (1997). Selection of children to provide care: The effect of earlier parental transfers. *Journals of Gerontology, 52B,* 110–119.

Hughes, S. (1985). Apples and oranges? A review of community-based long-term care. *Health Services Research, 20,* 461–487.

Jette, A. M., Tennstedt, S., & Crawford, S. (1995). How does formal and informal community care affect nursing home use? *Journals of Gerontology: Social Sciences, 50B*(1), S4–S12.

Johnson, R. W., & Lo Sasso, A. T. (2006). The impact of elder care on women's labor supply at midlife. *Inquiry, 43*(3), 195–210.

Johnson, R. W., Lo Sasso, A. T., & Lurie, I. Z. (2004). *How do families allocate elder care responsibilities between siblings?* Paper presented at the HRS Older Families Research Conference, Santa Fe, NM.

Johnson, R. W., & Uccello, C. E. (2005). *Is private long-term care insurance the answer?* Issue in Brief No. 29. Chestnut Hill, MA: Center for Retirement Research at Boston College.

Johnson, R. W., & Wiener, J. M. (2006). *A profile of frail older Americans and their care-givers*. Washington, DC: Urban Institute.

Kemper, P., Applebaum, R. A., & Harrigan, M. (1987). Community care demonstrations: What have we learned? *Health Care Financing Review, 8*, 87–100.

Knickman, J. R., & Snell, E. K. (2002). The 2030 problem: Caring for aging baby boomers. *Health Services Research, 37*(4), 849–884.

Lakdawalla, D., Goldman, D. P., Bhattacharya, J., Hurd, M. D., Joyce, G. F., & Panis, C. W. A. (2003). Forecasting the nursing home population. *Medical Care, 41*(1), 8–20.

Lakdawalla, D., & Philipson, T. (2002). The rise in old-age longevity and the market for long-term care. *American Economic Review, 92*(1), 295–306.

Lee, G. R., Netzer, J. K., & Coward, R. T. (1994). Filial responsibility expectations and patterns of intergenerational assistance. *Journal of Marriage and the Family, 56*(3), 559–565.

Lewin Group. (2006). *Nursing home use by "oldest old" sharply declines.* Retrieved November 7, 2006, from http://www.lewin.com/NR/rdonlyres/9A0A92A2–4D76–4397-A0A2–04EB20700795/0/NursingHomeUseTrendsPaper.pdf

Liu, K., Manton, K. G., & Aragon, C. (2000). Changes in home care use by disabled elderly persons: 1982–1994. *Journals of Gerontology: Social Sciences, 55B*(4), S245–S253.

Lo Sasso, A. T., & Johnson, R. W. (2002). Does informal care from adult children reduce nursing home admissions for the elderly? *Inquiry, 39*(3), 279–297.

Marks, N., Lambert, J. D., & Choi, H. (2002). Transitions to caregiving, gender, and psychological well-being: A prospective U.S. national study. *Journal of Marriage and the Family, 64*, 657–667.

McGarry, K. (1998). Caring for the elderly: The role of adult children. In D. A. Wise (Ed.), *Frontiers in the economics of aging* (pp. 133–163). Chicago: University of Chicago Press.

MetLife. (2002). *The MetLife market survey of nursing home and home care costs.* Westport, CT: MetLife Mature Market.

National Alliance for Caregiving and AARP. (2004). *Caregiving in the U.S.* Retrieved November 7, 2006, from http://www.caregiving.org/data/04finalreport.pdf

National Center for Assisted Living. (2000). *NCAL survey of assisted living facilities.* Washington, DC: Author.

Olshansky, S. J., Passaro, D. J., Hershow, R. C., Layden, J., Carnes, B. A., Brody, J., et al. (2005). A potential decline in life expectancy in the United States in the 21st century. *New England Journal of Medicine, 352*(11), 1138–1145.

Pezzin, L. E., Kemper, P., & Reschovsky, J. (1996). Does publicly provided home care substitute for family care? Experimental evidence with endogenous living arrangements. *Journal of Human Resources, 31*(3), 650–676.

Pezzin, L., Pollak, R. A., & Schone, B. S. (2004). *Bargaining power and intergenerational coresidence: Adult children and their disabled elderly parents.* Paper presented at the HRS Older Families Research Conference, Santa Fe, NM.

Pezzin, L. E., & Schone, B. S. (1999a). Intergenerational household formation, female labor supply, and informal caregiving: A bargaining approach. *Journal of Human Resources, 34*(3), 475–503.

Pezzin, L. E., & Schone, B. S. (1999b). Parental marital disruption and intergenerational transfers: An analysis of lone elderly parents and their children. *Demography, 36*(3), 287–297.

Pillemer, K., & Suitor, J. J. (2006). Making choices: A within-family study of caregiver selection. *The Gerontologist, 46*(4), 439–448.

Pinquart, M., & Sorensen, S. (2003). Differences between caregivers and noncaregivers in psychological health and physical health: A meta-analysis. *Psychology and Aging, 18*(2), 250–267.

Redfoot, D. L., & Pandya, S. M. (2002). *Before the boom: Trends in long-term supportive services for older Americans with disabilities.* AARP Public Policy Institute Report No. 2002-15. Washington, DC: AARP.

Rhoades, J. A., and Krauss, N. A. (1999). *Nursing home trends, 1987 and 1996.* AHCPR Pub. No. 99-0032. Rockville, MD: Agency for Health Care Policy and Research.

Schulz, R., & Beach, S. R. (1999). Caregiving as a risk factor for mortality: The caregiver health effects study. *Journal of the American Medical Association, 282,* 2215–2219.

Schulz, R., Newson, J., Mittelmark, M., Burton, L., Hirsch, C., & Jackson, S. (1997). Health effects of caregiving: The caregiver health effects study. *Annals of Behavioral Medicine, 19,* 110–116.

Schulz, R., O'Brien, A. T., Bookwals, J., & Fleissner, K. (1995). Psychiatric and physical morbidity effects of dementia caregiving: Prevalence, correlates, and causes. *The Gerontologist, 35,* 771–791.

Shaw, W. S., Patterson, T. L., Semple, S. J., Ho, S., Irwin, M. R., Hauger, R. L., et al. (1997). Longitudinal analysis of multiple indicators of health decline among spousal caregivers. *Annals of Behavioral Medicine, 19,* 101–109.

Spillman, B. C., & Black, K. J. (2005a). *The size of the long-term care population in residential care: A review of estimates and methodology.* Washington, DC: Assistant Secretary for Planning and Evaluation, U.S. Department of Health and Human Services.

Spillman, B. C., & Black, K. J. (2005b). *Staying the course: Trends in family caregiving.* Washington, DC: AARP.

Spillman, B. C., & Pezzin, L. E. (2000). Potential and active caregivers: Changing networks and the "sandwich generation." *Milbank Quarterly, 78,* 347–374.

Teachman, J., Tedrow, L., & Crowder, K. (2000). The changing demography of America's families. *Journal of Marriage and the Family, 62,* 1234–1246.

U.S. Census Bureau. (2006). *Statistical abstract of the United States* (126th ed.). Washington, DC: U.S. Department of Commerce.

U.S. Department of Health and Human Services. (1998). *Informal caregiving: Compassion in action.* Retrieved November 7, 2006, from http://aspe.hhs.gov/daltcp/reports/care bro2.pdf

Weissert, W., Cready, C. M., & Pawelak, J. (1988). The past and future of home- and community-based long-term care. *Milbank Quarterly, 66,* 309–388.

Wolf, D. A., Freedman, V., & Soldo, B. J. (1997). The division of family labor: Care for elderly parents. *Journals of Gerontology, 52B,* 102–109.

Yee, J. L., & Schulz, R. (2000). Gender differences in psychiatric morbidity among family caregivers: A review and analysis. *The Gerontologist, 40*(2), 147–164.

CHAPTER FOUR

Commitment to Caring: Filial Responsibility and the Allocation of Support by Adult Children to Older Mothers

Merril Silverstein, Stephen J. Conroy, and Daphna Gans

INTRODUCTION

Concerns over the social implications of population aging have stimulated much consideration of the role of adult children as providers of care and support to their older parents. A great deal of this literature is centered on the prospect of increasing uncertainty about intergenerational support for elders who are enjoying increasingly longer lives but with fewer opportunities to receive help from children. Even well-intentioned children face challenges to providing care based on their geographic proximity, competing family and work demands, and coordination problems with (or lack of) siblings. At present, middle-aged children of aging parents—members of the baby boom cohort—have relatively many siblings with whom they can divide care duties. However, the next generation of potential caregivers will have fewer siblings, further increasing doubt about the viability of family support to elders (Himes, 1994).

Research shows that older parents expect to rely on their adult children for care, support, and attention (Blieszner & Mancini, 1987; Burr

71

& Mutchler, 1999; Cicirelli, 1993; Rossi & Rossi, 1990; Stein et al., 1998); whether those expectations are fulfilled will hinge on their children's filial values and barriers to providing care. In this investigation, we focus on the process by which filial responsibility becomes enacted in supportive behavior to older parents. We treat filial obligation as the expressed preference that adult children take responsibility for the needs of aging parents. Specifically, we investigate how elder support is allocated depending on (a) how preferences to engage in elder care are reconciled with time costs of travel, competing role alternatives, and opportunity costs; and (b) the availability of siblings willing and able to provide care.

Norm of Filial Responsibility

As a social norm, filial responsibility reflects the generalized expectation that children should support their older parents at times of need (Cicirelli, 1988, 1990). Although filial norms are predictive of support (Bromley & Blieszner, 1997; Peek, Coward, Peek, & Lee, 1998; Silverstein & Litwak, 1993), they represent an ideal and, as such, can be distinguished from what is actually achievable (Finley, Roberts, & Banahan, 1988; Stein et al., 1998). More than an expectation of one's own behavior, filial norms refer to the responsibilities that define the social role of adult children with respect to their aging parents. Consequently, even children who embrace filial responsibility as a desired goal do not necessarily plan to, or actually provide, support to their parents (Peek et al., 1998). Elder care norms are malleable and have been shown to fluctuate over biographical and historical time (Gans & Silverstein, 2006).

Indeed, Finch and Mason (1991) challenge the very existence of a consensus for what constitutes the appropriate response to relatives in need. Rather than considering normative orientations as inherently fixed, the authors provide evidence for their plasticity based on the context of the situation and the circumstances of the parties involved. Although we believe that this position may be overstated, we take a similar approach by suggesting that normative obligations as ideals are differentially expressed depending on the resources, constraints, and alternatives of the provider and the needs of the recipient.

We investigate children's support for aging parents as a function of norms and the time costs related to travel. Although adult children who live long distances from their older parents tend to express weaker filial responsibility than siblings living closer (Finley et al., 1988), this relationship is by no means deterministic; adults may have a strong sense of responsibility and live at a distance or have a weak sense of responsibility and live at close proximity. Internalized norms and structural barriers may be starting points for understanding how families function in practice, but they are not sufficient as explanations of behavior in contemporary families.

Sibling Negotiations in Care Decisions

Caregiving to elderly persons is a family affair. Yet the standard family decision model is based on Becker's (1991) proposition that family members share a common set of preferences administered by an altruistically motivated family head. Scholars have challenged Becker's altruistic-dictator model, citing its unsustainable assumption of common preferences, and paved the way for models that recognize the possibility of conflicting interests among family members (Pezzin & Schone, 1997; Pollack, 2000). The literature on intergenerational caregiving and support is replete with evidence for structured differentiation of siblings in their parent care activities (for examples, see Henretta, Hill, Li, Soldo, & Wolf, 1997; Neuharth & Stern, 2002; Pillemer & Suitor, 2006).

Family size and gender composition are key factors in coordinating care across siblings. Adult children in larger families tend to provide less support per capita than those in smaller families (Wolf, Freedman, & Soldo, 1997). These findings suggest that siblings resolve their division of labor by offsetting each other's efforts, signaling a coordinated response in a zero-sum game of care. In the United States, adult daughters provide more support than sons to aging parents (Aronson, 1992; Rossi & Rossi, 1990; Silverstein, Parrott, & Bengtson, 1995; Sörenson & Zarit, 1996). That the presence of adult daughters appears to suppress the contributions of sons suggests that sibling negotiations divide along gender lines (Wolf et al., 1997). The parent's gender is also a factor in attracting support, as studies generally show that older mothers receive more instrumental, financial, and emotional support from their children than do older fathers (Rossi & Rossi, 1990; Silverstein & Bengtson, 1997).

The process by which interdependent care decisions are made is more complex than that suggested by examining only behavioral outcomes. We suggest that the division of labor among siblings is predicated on the degree to which each sibling feels it is a child's duty to support older parents, as well as the costs that each sibling would incur if he or she became more involved as a caregiver. Curiously, most studies that examine the division of labor in caregiving do not consider the perspectives of those who actually divide and provide the care and, consequently, cannot directly consider the interpersonal dynamics that underlie negotiations among adult children. Viewed from the perspective of adult children, imbalances in siblings' contributions to parent care sometimes result in feelings of unfairness in the allocation of care duties and lead to resentment, particularly as the inequality in effort falls along gender lines (Hequembourg & Brailler,

2005). Such aggrieved children may ask their siblings to change their behaviors to achieve equity, or they may alter their perceptions in an attempt to justify why they provide more than their fair share of parent care and their siblings provide less (Ingersoll-Dayton, Neal, Ha, & Hammer, 2003). Implicit in these formulations is the notion that siblings use persuasion, guilt, and rationalization to achieve a stable division of labor, if not always an efficient distribution of effort.

As a result of relying on parents' perspectives on the care they receive from children, scant attention has been paid to the role that values, attitudes, and beliefs held by adult children play in motivating them to provide care. While it is reasonable to assume that siblings share somewhat similar attitudes toward filial duty as a result of having been reared in common home environments, it is also likely that siblings differ based on their unique experiences and social characteristics. Research shows that family members vary substantially in the strength with which they endorse norms obligating adult children to care for their aging parents (Gans & Silverstein, 2006).

Filial Responsibility and Sibling Bargaining

How do siblings negotiate the division of labor in elder care duties given their varied preferences and constraints? Rational choice theories propose that adult children will provide support to their parents when the incentives for doing so (e.g., fulfilling a moral duty, gaining emotional satisfaction, positioning for a bequest) outweigh the disincentives (e.g., losing time to alternative activities, travel costs, opportunity costs of forgone income). A bargaining framework relies on the principle of rational choice but also takes into account siblings' commitment and costs. In posing the question this way, we place filial responsibility in the context of a bargaining framework typically used by economists to explain family decision making when there are personal and collective interests at stake (Pollack, 1988; Stark & Falk, 1998). Thus, adult children make decisions about caring for an aged parent partially based on their anticipation that siblings would (or would not) be willing to commit to caregiving. Rather than rely on the *behavior* of adult children to represent their willingness to adopt caregiving roles, we tell a more complex story that includes their values toward elder care as an observable indicator of underlying levels of normative commitment.

Our investigation treats adult children as a set of actors weighing their commitment to parent care against its cost and in relation to siblings who make the same commitment-to-cost calculation. We consider attitudes toward filial responsibility as a strategic element in the allocation of care duties among siblings, such that those with stronger commitment will provide care for their parents at increasing marginal costs, thereby saving their less committed siblings from costs they have less incentive to incur. When viewed in terms of power relations among siblings, very strongly committed children risk being exploited by their committed counterparts, a process that can lead to gender imbalances in care work if the former tend to be women and the latter men (Arber & Ginn, 1995).

Using this framework and assuming that siblings are aware of each other's level of commitment and costs, we posit that more committed children—those who more strongly endorse elder care as a filial duty—will be more willing than their siblings to incur greater costs in providing care, thus raising the threshold beyond which caregiving becomes intolerable. Conversely, less dutiful children, even those for whom costs of care would be relatively low, may be reluctant to devote themselves to caregiving knowing that their more committed siblings will likely provide care (a variant of the free-rider problem discussed extensively in the economics literature; see McMillan, 1979).

This principle leads to a set of deductions that treat filial obligation as a strategic factor in the allocation of caregiving duties. For instance, if more filially obligated children are willing to incur greater costs related to caregiving than their less obligated siblings (e.g., willing to travel farther, forgo more income), the latter may provide less care even if they live closer to their parent. Alternatively, more strongly committed children who face insurmountable structural barriers to enacting the caregiving role may release these duties to siblings who are more reluctant but better positioned to provide care by virtue of having lower costs. An empirical question to be answered is how strong or weak does filial responsibility need to be before filial support is so delegated?

Normative Bargaining as a Game

To demonstrate how decisions would be made within a normative-bargaining framework, we present examples using a simultaneous one-shot game, with son (S) and daughter (D). S and D are adult siblings considering the decision to care for an older mother. The underlying premise is that the care outcome is formed by each child's expectations about what the other child might do. The game could easily be extended to an n-player game without loss of generality. The following discussion outlines several hypothetical scenarios to predict how siblings distribute their support to aging mothers under various conditions.

We make several assumptions in specifying the model: (a) The amount of support is associated with a cost proportional to the level of effort expended; (b) children who more strongly endorse filial responsibility derive greater satisfaction from knowing that their aging parent is being taken care of—regardless of which child provides the care; (c) siblings are aware, or can formulate a reasonable guess, of each other's level of filial responsibility; (d) use of alternative sources of support are not correlated with filial responsibility of children (we later address this issue with a methodological solution).

We begin by examining the extreme case where S and D feel that adult children have no obligation to care for their elderly mother. Since they receive no "satisfaction" benefit from knowing that a child cares for his or her mother, the only stake these children have is to minimize their costs. In this scenario, the mother receives no care from her children. Let us now assume S and D have positive and equal levels of commitment and cost. When S and D are cooperative, then the two children will likely split the difference. If they are noncooperative, then each child may adopt an optimal strategy of doing the inverse of what the other does: If one child does more, the other does less. However, as compared to the previous example, the older mother is now assured of being cared for by at least one of her two children.

Now consider the case in which the commitment of one child, say, D, is stronger than the commitment of the other. In the noncooperative scenario, D would realize that S has a dominant strategy to shirk, and D's optimal strategy would be to care for her mother (D > S). In this instance, S is a free rider on the efforts of his sister. Strategically, all S would have to do is sufficiently adjust D's perception of the probability that he will shirk in order to move the outcome toward D caring more.

Next, we expand our discussion to the more realistic scenario where siblings have differential travel costs and differential commitments. Let us assume that D lives farther than S from her mother. For small distance differentials, sibling inequalities in level of commitment would tend to drive care allocation toward the more committed. However, if the distance that must be traversed by D is sufficiently large relative to S, then D's optimal strategy may be to shirk. Knowing this, S, who lives much closer to his mother, would have an optimal strategy to provide most of the care. However, if D's commitment were sufficiently strong to overcome the costs imposed by distance, then the outcome could be reversed, with D becoming a long-distance caregiver. Under this condition, S, by virtue of having much less commitment than D, has power over his sister to hold out longer despite his more convenient location.

RESEARCH AIMS

We use the theoretical possibilities outlined above as a heuristic tool to develop the aims of our research. These are:

1. To examine the rewards and costs to children of providing support to older mothers, with particular attention to how filial

obligation conditions the tolerance of time costs imposed by geographic distance and other structural barriers.

2. To examine how intrafamily differences among siblings in their norms and opportunity costs affect their allocations of support to older mothers.

3. To examine the relative levels of filial obligation of "anomalous" siblings who are at the margins of distance and care, specifically: (a) children who live closer to mothers than their siblings but provide less support than expected, and (b) children who live farther away than their siblings but provide more support than expected.

METHOD

Sample

The study uses data from the Longitudinal Study of Generations (LSOG), a study of three- and four-generation families. The LSOG began in 1971 with an original sample of 2,044 respondents ages 16 to 91 deriving from 328 three-generation families whose grandfathers were selected via a multistage stratified random sampling procedure from a population of 840,000 individuals enrolled in southern California's first large health maintenance organization. All available grandparents (G1), parents (G2), and grandchildren 16 years of age or older (G3) in the selected families were eligible for the study. In 1985, the original sample members were surveyed again, and since then data have been collected at 3-year intervals up to 2000. Response rates over time are in the range of 70% to 80% and are comparable to most long-term longitudinal surveys (see Bengtson, Biblarz, & Roberts, 2002).

We use data from all G3s who had a surviving mother in 2000. These adult children were mostly in their 40s and 50s, and their parents were in their 70s and 80s. A rare feature of this data set—and one that is crucial for addressing our research questions—is that lateral family members are in the sampling frame, resulting in the recruitment of multiple siblings within the same families. The sample we analyze consists of 424 individuals who were nested within 283 nuclear families. The average participation rate per family is 1.5, less than half the average family size of 3.3, and represents a 45% capture rate given the universe of all children in these families. Nonparticipation of G3 siblings in 2000 was the result of nonresponse at baseline, sample attrition, and systematic exclusion of children born after 1955 (these children were deemed too young to participate and never joined the sample). A description of the operational sample is provided in Table 4.1.

TABLE 4.1   Analytic Variables and Descriptive Characteristics of G3 Adult Children (Observations = 424; Family Clusters = 283)

Variables	M	SD	Range
Female	.60	.49	0 to 1
Age	47.84	2.72	44 to 59
Education	5.49	1.36	1 to 8
Income	5.68	3.77	1 to 21
Married	.68	.47	0 to 1
Full-time employment	.69	.46	0 to 1
Has child age 16 or younger in household	.39	.49	0 to 1
Filial responsibility	15.74	3.63	0 to 24
Number of siblings	2.58	1.75	0 to 11
Geographic distance from mother	3.57	1.94	0 to 6
Functional impairment of mother	6.88	3.14	5 to 20
Mother is unmarried	.31	.46	0 to 1
Support provided to mother	4.92	5.06	0 to 35

Source: Longitudinal Study of Generations, 2000.

Dependent Variable

Support to mothers is operationalized as the number of days per week adult children engaged in five activities that require physical presence: household chores, transportation, care when sick, personal care, and visiting. While visiting is not formally a support task, much like instrumental services, it imposes travel and time costs, tends to be normatively regulated, and provides a benefit (usually emotional) to mothers. Respondents rated each item on an eight-point scale corresponding to the following categories and coding scheme: *not at all* (0), *once a year* (1), *several times a year* (2), *monthly* (3), *several times a month* (4), *weekly* (5), *several times a week* (6), and *daily* (7). The reliability of the nine items was $\alpha = 0.90$. Items were summed to form a support scale score, ranging from 0 to 35.

Independent Variables

Geographic distance from mothers, our key indicator of the time/opportunity costs of care, is measured on a seven-point ordinal scale ranging from *living together* (0) to *more than 500 miles away* (6). Filial obligations, our indicator of underlying preferences to provide support, is measured as the strength with which it is felt that adult children have the responsibility to provide support to their older parents in the following six areas: (a) companionship; (b) household chores, repairs, and transportation; (c) listening to problems and concerns; (d) personal and health care; (e) financial support; and (f) housing. For each item, the respondent assigned responsibility on a five-point Likert-type scale ranging from *none* to *total*. Responses were summed to create an additive scale with a potential range from 0 (*no filial responsibility*) to 24 (*total filial responsibility*). The reliability of the scale is $\alpha = 0.91$

Role competition is measured with three dichotomous variables to indicate whether adult children are married (vs. nonmarried), are working full-time in the paid labor force (vs. not working full-time), and are parents of a child 16 years old or younger living in the household (vs. not having such a child in the household). Personal income is rated on a 21-point ordinal scale ranging from *none* (1) to *more than $250,000* (21). Gender (0 = *male*; 1 = *female*), age (in years), and education (rated from 1 to 8 where 1 = *less than 8 years* and 8 = *postgraduate*) are also considered. We control for the total number of siblings of each respondent to adjust for variation in the opportunity to diffuse responsibility (whether one had sisters had no bearing on support provision).

We also consider several characteristics of older mothers that tend to be strongly associated with the demand for support: functional impairment and marital status. Functional impairment is measured as the inability to perform activities of daily living. Adult children answered five questions about their mothers' ability to (a) walk up and down stairs, (b) walk more than one block, (c) prepare meals, (d) do household chores, (e) take care of her own personal hygiene needs such as bathing and cutting toenails. Degree of difficulty was rated on a four-point scale: no difficulty (1), *can perform with difficulty* (2), *can perform with assistance* (3), and *unable to perform at all* (4). The items formed a reliable scale at $\alpha = 0.88$, and an additive scale score was calculated. Functional impairment scores ranged from 5 to 20, where 5 represented the ability to perform all tasks with no difficulty and 20 represented complete incapacity. To obtain a single impairment score for each mother, we averaged these scores across all siblings. Marital status of mothers was coded as a dichotomous variable (1 = *unmarried*; 0 = *married*). For 62 cases where information about marital histories was incomplete, we imputed marital status from children's reports of paternal death, a technique that produced an assignment error rate of 10% as judged by simulations with observed data. The majority of unmarried mothers were widowed.

Analytic Strategy

We adopt a three-pronged strategy to address our research questions. In our first analysis, we use the full sample of adult children to examine how personal costs, filial responsibility, and their interaction predict the amount of support children provide to their older mothers. Because ordinary least squares regression may produce downwardly biased standard errors in clustered designs, we use regression with robust standard errors to account for nonindependence of siblings nested within nuclear families (Stata, 2001). This approach is recommended when the primary interest is in explaining variation across individuals and when group characteristics are of secondary concern (Hu, Goldberg, Hedeker, Flay, & Pentz, 1998). Indeed, most (about 70%) of the variation in support provision occurred within nuclear family clusters, indicating that siblings are quite diverse. Because our interest lies more in explaining why some adult children provide more support than others (and less on why some mothers receive more support than others) this modeling strategy (also called population-averaged models) is better suited to the goals of the study than multilevel random effects models. In addition, it makes fewer distributional assumptions and allows more child-level predictors.

In our second analysis, we focus explicitly on how differences in the costs and benefits among siblings affect the way support is distributed among them. For this analysis, we select 241 adult children from the 106 families in which at least two siblings responded. We use a fixed-effects approach that transforms all variables into deviations from within-family means (Stata, 2001). The fixed-effects model takes the form

$$(y_{it} - y_i) = a + b(x_{it} - \bar{x}_t) + (e_{it} - \bar{e}_t),$$

where y_{it} represents support provided by each of T adult children to I parents, x stands for a predictor variable, b is the regression coefficient, and e_{it} is the remaining within-family residual for each sibling. Note that the three observed variables and the error term are each centered by their respective within-family mean. The intercept, a, represents the grand mean that is reintroduced to correctly estimate standard errors (Stata, 2001). There are two major benefits to using fixed effects in this study. First, observed and unobserved variables at the family level of analysis are conditioned out of the model because they are constrained to zero as a result of family-centering all variables. Consequently, variation in support based on the mother's characteristics (e.g., health, income, marital status, family size) and her reliance on sources of care other than her children (e.g., formal services, friends, other relatives) are rendered inconsequential in this modeling approach. Second, within-family deviation scores correspond well to bargaining as an intrafamilial process in which sibling differences form the basis for their division of labor.

To explore our third research question, we examine anomalous cases by comparing the filial commitment of children who provide unusually high or unusually low amounts of support given the distance they live from their mothers. Our interest here is in examining filial responsibility expressed by siblings who are at the margins of costs and care—those providing substantially more and substantially less than their expected share. This analysis is more descriptive than the previous two analyses for several reasons—one theoretical and the other practical. First, we are uncertain of the distance thresholds that define atypical amounts of support and are capable of detecting differences in levels of filial responsibility. Second, since family clusters are too small to efficiently estimate interaction terms, we turn to a more descriptive analysis of residuals from the fixed-effects model to determine whether filial beliefs of over- and underperforming siblings are different from each other.

Prior to conducting our analyses, we imputed for missing values using an expectation maximization (EM) algorithm. EM uses an iterative algorithm that imputes values from known associations among observed variables to produce optimal maximum likelihood estimates. This method of imputation has been shown to provide unbiased estimates under the assumption that data are missing at random and represents a substantial improvement over listwise deletion of data in terms of inferring to the population of interest (Little & Rubin, 1987).

RESULTS

Our first question addresses the influence of distance and competing roles on the amount of support provided to older mothers. Following Litwak and Kulis (1987), we expect the effect of distance to be nonlinear with a rapid initial decline that moderates at increasingly farther distances. Therefore, geographic distance is parameterized with linear and quadratic terms. We present estimates from these regression equations in Table 4.2. All significance tests are computed using robust standard errors that have been adjusted for family clustering. The results in the first equation demonstrate the expected nonlinear pattern, with a negative coefficient for the linear term and a positive coefficient for the quadratic term. In addition, the equation shows that daughters tend to provide significantly more support than sons. Children also provide more support to functionally disabled and unmarried mothers compared to healthier and married mothers, respectively. Neither filial responsibility nor any of the competing roles influence support provided.

In our next test, we examine the interaction between filial norms and geographic distance to test whether filial responsibility to provide support is more readily acted upon with greater proximity—when the costs of provision are lower. We note that interactions between filial norms and other possible barriers to providing support were not significant and, thus, are not presented in our equations. Indeed, employment and the presence of a spouse and child in the household may provide access

TABLE 4.2 Ordinary Least Squares Regression of Support Provided to Older Mothers Estimated With Robust Standard Errors (Observations = 424; Family Clusters = 283)

Predictors	Main effects		Main effects + interactions	
	Unstandardized estimates	SE	Unstandardized estimates	SE
Female	1.151**	.384	1.150**	.380
Age	.076	.086	.061	.082
Education	.052	.188	.016	.186
Income	-.050	.059	-.076	.061
Married	-.319	.533	-.218	.531
Full-time employment	.158	.460	.259	.461
Has child age 16 or younger in household	-.241	.445	-.250	.447
Filial responsibility	.101	.070	.812***	.217
Number of siblings	-.109	.160	-.132	.154
Functional impairment of mother	.444***	.110	.447***	.109
Mother is unmarried	1.128*	.529	.948†	.526
Geographic distance from mother	-2.599***	.724	9.398**	3.039
Geographic distance from mother squared	.196*	.095	-1.417**	.432
Filial responsibility × geographic distance	—	—	-.539***	.143
Filial responsibility × geographic distance squared	—	—	.073***	.020
Constant	1.536	4.892	-13.335**	5.545
R-square	.361		.383	

†$p < .10$. *$p < .05$. **$p < .01$. ***$p < .001$.

Source: Longitudinal Study of Generations, 2000.

to resources that assist the caregiver (see the chapter in this volume by Szinovacz) and cannot be considered a net cost as unambiguously as can geographic distance.

Interactions between norms of filial responsibility and distance, added to the second equation in Table 4.2, reveal a negative interaction with linear distance and a positive interaction with quadratic distance. To better interpret these interaction patterns, we present in Figure 4.1 the predicted relationship between norms and support for three specific geographic conditions: less than 50 miles, 50 to 100 miles, and more than 100 miles away. Children who are more proximate have a stronger positive relationship between their filial norms and their behavior in providing support. If fulfilling preferences is construed as an intrinsic reward to the committed provider, then the net benefit of providing support accrues most rapidly at closer distances when costs are low but begins to lose salience (at an accelerating rate) as distances increase. In other words, at close proximity, the low cost of providing support requires relatively little commitment, while at far distances, the high cost of providing support inhibits provisions even among those with the strongest commitment. One hour of time represents the threshold beyond which filial obligation ceases to be a strong enough motivator to overcome the costs of travel.

Our next model concerns the intrafamilial process by which support contributions are negotiated. We conjecture that the absolute strength of commitment may be less consequential in terms of motivating behavior than its *relative* strength within families. That is, even though siblings may share similar normative orientations, variation among them may

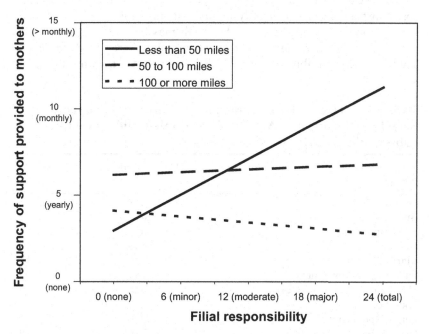

FIGURE 4.1 Predicted values from regression of support to mothers on filial responsibility, geographic distance, and their interaction (other covariates are held constant at their mean).

Source: Longitudinal Study of Generations, 2000.

determine the allocation of support roles. The same logic applies to the impact of competing roles and opportunity costs. Thus, we estimate a fixed-effects model that relies on within-family differencing, where each score is transformed into a deviation from the average family response. We estimate the model using the natural log of support as the dependent variable to capture the proportionate decline in support with increasing geographic distance. In choosing this type of nonlinear approach, we were cognizant of the fact that power terms have altered meanings in the fixed-effects approach because difference scores do not necessarily correspond with the original distance gradient, essentially losing their absolute quality. Taking the log of the dependent variable linearizes the nonmonotonic form of the relationship between distance and support and allows the use of linear predictors.

Estimates from the fixed-effects model are shown in Table 4.3. The results show that daughters provide more support than sons, though this difference only approaches statistical significance ($p < 0.06$), and married siblings provide less support than unmarried siblings. Filial responsibility does not explain sibling variation in the amount of support provided.

We speculate that filial responsibility fails to predict support because cost constraints are not directly mapped against normative preferences in this model. Further, support differentials may be detectable only when preferences and cost differences between siblings are most magnified. Thus, we focus on siblings who provide less support to their mothers than

TABLE 4.3   Fixed-Effects Regression of Instrumental Support (Log) Provided to Older Mothers in Multiple-Children Families (Observations = 241; Family Clusters = 106)

Predictors	Unstandardized estimates	SE
Female	.231[†]	.122
Age	-.018	.023
Education	.045	.051
Income	.001	.017
Married	-.356**	.115
Full-time employment	.185	.109
Has child age 16 or younger in household	.018	.115
Filial responsibility	.014	.014
Geographic distance	-.216***	.029
Constant	2.57*	1.134
R-square (within family)	.388	

*$p < .05$. **$p < .01$. ***$p < .001$. [†]$p < .06$.
Source: Longitudinal Study of Generations, 2000.

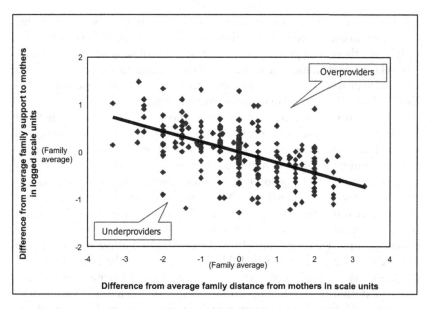

FIGURE 4.2   Scatterplot and linear trend line of logged support to mothers regressed on distance from mothers using within-family difference scores.

Source: Longitudinal Study of Generations, 2000.

their proximity would suggest *(underproviders)* and those who provide more support than their farther distance would suggest *(overproviders)*. It is important to note that because these terms denote deviations relative to expected amounts of support, it is possible that some underproviders provide more absolute support than some overproviders. We describe these two segments of the population based on residuals from the bivariate fixed-effects regression, the results of which are found in Figure 4.2. Residuals in this figure represent each sibling's departure from the amount of support one would expect based solely on the geographic distance from his or her mother (this method ensures that sibling comparisons are made within families).

We divide the sample of siblings into nine groups based on the cross-classification of relative distance from mothers and the degree of over- or undersupport to them. For distance, we created the following three categories: those who live closer than their siblings (1.5 units or less than the average family distance), those who live about the same distance as their siblings (within 1.5 units of the average family distance), and those who live farther than their siblings (1.5 units or greater than the average family distance). For deviations in support relative to distance expectations, we created the following three categories based on the exponentiated residuals in Figure 4.2: those who provided less than expected amounts of support as compared to their siblings (25% or less than the average family provision), those who provided expected amounts of support and are roughly similar to their siblings (within 25% of the average family provision), and those who provided more than expected amounts of support as compared to their siblings (25% or more than the average family provision).

We then examine the size of within-family differences in filial obligation across these nine groups with special focus on the marginal categories. These group means are shown in Figure 4.3. The results show that, as compared to their siblings, more proximate underproviders have a weaker sense of responsibility and more distant overproviders have a stronger sense of responsibility. An examination of the standard errors for these two means reveals that their 95% confidence interval does not include zero, meaning that they deviate significantly from their respective family groups. We then control for the presence of alternative roles and other characteristics shown in Table 4.3 to examine the extent to which large differences in filial obligation within these two marginal groups are due to external demands, opportunity costs, or social background characteristics. We find that the means remain statistically significant ($p < 0.05$) when adjusted by these covariates, implying that the preference profiles of

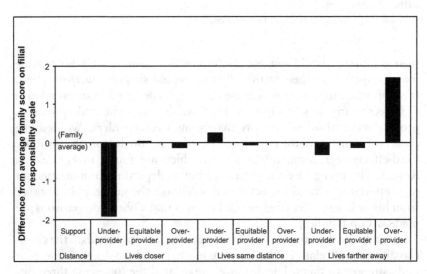

FIGURE 4.3   Filial responsibility in nine groups based on anomalousness of support to mothers (categorized residuals from Figure 4.2) and relative distance from mothers using within-family difference scores.

Source: Longitudinal Study of Generations, 2000.

siblings who under- and overprovide support to mothers are independent of role and opportunity constraints on their behaviors.

DISCUSSION

This chapter examines the allocation of intergenerational support to older mothers, bringing together lines of inquiry regarding family decision making in elder care from economics and sociology. If one can generalize that economics is concerned with preferences for action subject to cost constraints, and sociology is concerned with preferences for action subject to normative constraints, our model has synthesized elements of both traditions to demonstrate support patterns that are conceivably the result of tradeoffs between costs and norms of filial responsibility, where norms are considered revelators of underlying preferences. The central premise of this chapter is that a child's decision to support his or her aging parent is not reducible to personal cost-benefit calculations because such a decision also takes into account similar calculations made by siblings.

Filial responsibility is a cultural ideal, reinforced by religious and secular values but, as a guide to action, is tempered by the constraints of geographic distance. More strongly committed siblings will tend to contribute more care up to a threshold of cost that rises with the degree of commitment. We also found evidence for differences among siblings based on competing alternatives to providing support to older mothers. Unmarried children, ostensibly with fewer household demands on their time, provided more support to their mothers than did their married siblings. However, we found no evidence that opportunity costs related to income or having children in the household pulled adult children away from providing support. That sisters tended to provide more support than their brothers is likely the result of differential socialization to role expectations by gender since human capital and demographic characteristics on which men and women tend to vary are controlled in our models. Why would daughters remain primary caregivers even when they are equal to their brothers in resources and values? It is possible that the meaning of filial responsibility may be different for daughters and sons. Strong filial responsibility expressed by sons may mean that they feel their sisters should provide the care. In addition, if cost benefit calculations by women are more heavily weighted toward family care compared to similar calculations by men, the threshold for capitulating in care negotiations may be lower for sisters than it is for their brothers.

Unlike money exchanges, the support transfers we considered require face-to-face proximity. At closer distances, costs to children are low so that the rewards of fulfilling preferences increase "profit" quite rapidly. However, at increasingly farther distances costs rise quickly and require an extraordinary commitment on the part of children if they are to endure the sacrifices of even modest levels of support provision. Detecting these patterns required examining extremes to demonstrate the rule (what economists call *corner solutions*). Indeed, filial responsibility was only related to support in the presence of particularly high or particularly low transaction costs related to geographic distance.

We also found evidence for free-riders—adult children who live in relatively close proximity to their mothers but, as a result of their weaker filial commitment, provide less support than their more distant siblings. It may seem odd that some weakly committed children remain in close proximity to their parents. These children may rely more on their parents for support than their parents rely on them. Alternatively, the possibility remains that children who deviate from expected levels of support may adjust their values to conform to their behavior (or lack of behavior), in which case weak preferences may be considered an outcome of shirking as well as its cause.

Some scholars have suggested that intergenerational support and geographic distance from parents are jointly determined (Cox & Rank, 1992), raising concern about the possibility of another form of endogeneity in our model. Adult children may move closer to their parents in anticipation of, or in response to, impending or actual frailty (Silverstein, 1995). Some adult children remain in close proximity to their parents (rather than moving away) for the same reason. Research in Germany shows that first-born children tend to choose residence locations at a distance from their middle-aged parents and do so with the long-term strategic aim of leaving their younger siblings with a greater share of elder care duties (Konrad, Kunemund, Lommerud, & Robledo, 2002). However, because our data are from the perspective of adult children, we are able to control for their valuations of filial duty, the inclusion of which strengthens confidence in our specification.

Since our empirical specification relied on cross-sectional data, we were forced to retrospectively infer bargaining scenarios from which current support, cost, and preference structures could have reasonably emerged. We plan to extend our model using a two-stage approach along the lines suggested by Pollak (2005), in which first-stage moves set the terms for later negotiations. Since bargaining occurs both within and across generations, it would be fruitful to simultaneously include the expectations of older parents with those of multiple children, a rare feature in survey data (for an exception, see Klein Ikkink, van Tilburg, & Knipscheer, 1999). In addition, transfers among siblings, such as side payments to caregiving children, may provide greater insights into indirect strategies for fulfilling filial responsibility to parents.

As in most studies of sibling sets, there is a fair amount of nonresponse in our data; less than half of all possible adult children participated in the survey. Thus, a large number of siblings were unobserved. To the degree that nonparticipating children are systematically different with respect to key study variables, our results may be biased. Future approaches can use simulation models in which the characteristics of nonparticipants are inferred from the actions of participants under a variety of theoretical conditions, much like in physics the existence of unobserved astral bodies can be inferred by their effects on the behavior of those observed. Even with incomplete sibling samples, there are distinct advantages to examining the perspectives of adult children. Studies that rely only on parents' preferences tend to produce erratic results when predicting the amount of support received from adult children. Expectations of parents may be modified depending on the capacity of children to provide help (Peek et al., 1998) or not match with their children's intentions (Eggebeen & Davey, 1998; Lee, Netzer, & Coward, 1994). The assumption that commitment of children for the care of aging parents can be inferred from their behaviors—typically as reported by their parents—makes it difficult to detect the maneuvering (bluffing and posturing) that may precede the resolution of a care scenario as it is hashed out among siblings. Ignoring children's preferences leaves much of the bargaining story incomplete.

Our ability to ascribe bargaining behavior among siblings necessarily relies on the logic of backward induction; could the observed patterns have reasonably derived from a scenario characterized by bargaining? Certainly, a one-shot depiction of what is essentially a sequential process, and the absence of direct information on sibling negotiations, leave our interpretation as speculative. However, several features of this study, not typically found in family decision-making models, buoy confidence that our findings can be interpreted within a bargaining framework. The fact that our final two sets of analyses rely on *within-family differences* casts the allocation decision as an internal negotiation among siblings. Put another way, our findings suggest that distant children sometimes provide more support than expected because their nearer siblings feel less filial responsibility to do so. If actions were guided strictly by personal considerations, this would not hold. While it is not news that adult children act beneficently toward their older parents, our investigation suggests that such actions are contingent on trade-offs between responsibility and convenience at both individual and family levels.

REFERENCES

Arber, S., & Ginn, J. (1995). Gender differences in informal care. *Health and Social Care in the Community, 3,* 19–31.

Aronson, J. (1992). Women's sense of responsibility for the care of old-people: But who else is going to do it? *Gender and Society, 6,* 8–29.

Becker, G. S. (1991). *A treatise on the family* (enlarged ed.). Cambridge, MA: Harvard University Press.

Bengtson, V. L., Biblarz, T. J., & Roberts, R. E. L. (2002). *How families still matter: A longitudinal study of youth in two generations.* New York: Cambridge University Press.

Blieszner, R., & Mancini, J. A. (1987). Enduring ties: Older adults' parental role and responsibilities. *Family Relations, 36,* 176–180.

Bromley, M. C., & Blieszner, R. (1997). Planning for long term care: Filial behavior and relationship quality of adult children with independent parents. *Family Relations, 46,* 155–162.

Burr, J. A., & Mutchler, J. E. (1999). Race and ethnic variation in norms of filial responsibility among older persons. *Journal of Marriage and the Family, 61,* 674–687.

Cicirelli, V. G. (1988). A measure of filial anxiety regarding anticipated care of elderly parents. *The Gerontologist, 23,* 478–482.

Cicirelli, V. G. (1990). Family support in relation to health problems of the elderly. In T. H. Brubaker (Ed.), *Family relationship in later life* (pp. 212–228). Newbury Park, CA: Sage.

Cicirelli, V. G. (1993). Attachment and obligation as daughters' motives for caregiving behavior and subsequent effect on subjective burden. *Psychology and Aging, 8,* 144–155.

Cox, D., & Rank, M. R. (1992). Inter-vivos transfers and intergenerational exchange. *Review of Economics and Statistics, 74,* 305–314.

Eggebeen, D. J., & Davey, A. (1998). Do safety nets work? The role of anticipated help in times of need. *Journal of Marriage and the Family, 60,* 939–950.

Finch, J., & Mason, J. (1991). Obligations of kinship in contemporary Britain: Is there normative agreement? *British Journal of Sociology, 42*(3), 345–367.

Finley, N. J., Roberts, M. D., & Banahan, B. F., III. (1988). Motivations and inhibitors of attitudes of filial obligations towards aging parents. *The Gerontologist, 28*(1), 73–78.

Gans, D., & Silverstein, M. (2006). Norms of filial responsibility for aging parents across time and generations. *Journal of Marriage and the Family, 68,* 961–976.

Henretta, J. C., Hill, M. S., Li, W., Soldo, B. J., & Wolf, D. A. (1997). Selection of children to provide care: The effect of earlier parental transfers. *Journals of Gerontology: Series B: Psychological and Social Sciences, 52B,* 110–119.

Hequembourg, A., & Brailler, S. (2005). Gendered stories of parental caregiving among siblings. *Journal of Aging Studies, 19,* 53–71.

Himes, C. L. (1994). Parental caregiving by adult women: A demographic perspective. *Research on Aging, 16,* 191–211.

Hu, F. B., Goldberg, J., Hedeker, D., Flay, B. R., & Pentz, M. A. (1998). Comparison of population-averaged and subject-specific approaches for analyzing repeated binary outcomes. *American Journal of Epidemiology, 147*(7), 694–703.

Ingersoll-Dayton, B., Neal, M. B., Ha, J. H., & Hammer, L. B. (2003). Redressing inequity in parent care among siblings. *Journal of Marriage and the Family, 65,* 201–212.

Klein Ikkink, C. E., van Tilburg, T. G., & Knipscheer, C. P. M. (1999). Perceived instrumental support exchanges in relationships between elderly parents and their adult children: Normative and structural explanations. *Journal of Marriage and the Family, 61,* 831–844.

Konrad, K. A., Kunemund, H., Lommerud, K. E., & Robledo, J. R. (2002). Geography of the family, *American Economic Review, 92,* 981–998.

Lee, G. R., Netzer, J. K., & Coward, R. T. (1994). Filial responsibility expectations and patterns of intergenerational assistance. *Journal of Marriage and the Family, 56,* 559–565.

Little, R. J. A., & Rubin, D. B. (1987). *Statistical analysis with missing data.* New York: Wiley.

Litwak, E., & Kulis, S. (1987). Technology, proximity and measures of kin support. *Journal of Marriage and the Family, 49,* 649–661.

McMillan, J. (1979). The free-rider problem: A survey. *Economic Record,* June, 95–107.

Neuharth, T. J., & Stern, S. (2002). Shared caregiving responsibilities of adult siblings with elderly parents. *Journal of Human Resources, 37,* 441–478.

Peek, M. K., Coward, R. T., Peek, C. W., & Lee, G. R. (1998). Are expectations for care related to the receipt of care? An analysis of parent care among disabled elders. *Journals of Gerontology: Social Sciences, 53B*(3), S127–S136.

Pezzin, L. E., & Schone, B. S. (1997). The allocation of resources in intergenerational households: Adult children and their elderly parents. *American Economic Review, 87,* 460–464.

Pillemer, K., & Suitor, J. (2006). Making choices: A within-family study of caregiver selection. *The Gerontologist, 46,* 439–448.

Pollak, R. A. (1988). Tied transfers and paternalistic preferences. *American Economic Review, 78,* 240–244.

Pollak, R. A. (2000). Theorizing marriage. In L. Waite, C. Bachrach, M. Hindin, E. Thomson, & A. Thornton (Eds.) *Ties that bind: Perspectives on marriage and cohabitation.* New York: Aldine de Gruyter.

Pollak, R. A. (2005). Bargaining power in marriage: Earnings, wage rates and household production. National Bureau of Economic Research Working Paper 11239. Cambridge, MA: NBER.

Rossi, A. S., & Rossi, P. H. (1990). *Of human bonding. Parent-child relations across the life course.* New York: Aldine de Gruyter.

Silverstein, M. (1995). Stability and change in temporal distance between older parents and their children. *Demography, 32,* 29–45.

Silverstein, M., & Bengtson, V. L. (1997). Intergenerational solidarity and the structure of adult child-parent relationships in American families. *American Journal of Sociology, 103,* 429–460.

Silverstein, M., & Litwak, E. (1993). A task specific typology of intergenerational family structure in later life. *The Gerontologist, 33,* 258–264.

Silverstein, M., Parrott, T. M., & Bengtson, V. L. (1995). Factors that predispose middle-aged sons and daughters to provide social support to older parents. *Journal of Marriage and the Family, 57,* 465–476.

Sörensen, S., & Zarit, S. H. (1996). Preparation for caregiving: A study of multigeneration families. *International Journal of Aging and Human Development, 42,* 43–63.

Stark, O., & Falk, I. (1998). Transfers, empathy formation, and reverse transfers. *American Economic Review, 88,* 271–276.

Stata (2001). *Stata user's guide.* College Station, TX: Author.

Stein, C. H., Wemmerus, V. A., Ward, M., Gaines, M. E., Freeberg, A. L., & Jewell, T. C. (1998). "Because they're my parents": An intergenerational study of felt obligation and parental caregiving. *Journal of Marriage and the Family, 60,* 611–623.

Wolf, D. A., Freedman, V., & Soldo, B. J. (1997). The division of family labor: Care for the elderly parents. *Journals of Gerontology, 52B,* 102–109.

CHAPTER FIVE

Cross-National Variations in Elder Care: Antecedents and Outcomes

Ariela Lowenstein, Ruth Katz, and Nurit Gur-Yaish

INTRODUCTION

This chapter examines the national, familial, and personal factors that govern the degree to which elders expect to and actually receive needed support and care from their adult children and from formal services. Additionally, it explores cross-national differences in these two sources of support (informal and formal) on the quality of life of the elderly.

The phenomenon of an aging population is a global one (Kinsella, 2000), although its pace differs in various countries. For example, the nature of contemporary European society and its age structure are rapidly changing, which will probably affect the economy and the future financing of social welfare and health systems (Eurostat, 1996). Greater longevity also causes a secondary aging process: an increase in the number of disabled elderly who may need more care and support (World Health Organization, 2002). This adds burdens to families and states, the two major pillars of support in old age, especially in light of constrains in state spending. The global political and economic climate suggests less government responsibility to be expected in the future for elder care and increased pressure on families. Families today are entering into new intergenerational caring relationships with regard to intensity and duration, necessitating a renegotiation of relationships (Bengtson, Rosenthal, & Burton, 1996; Silverstein, Conroy, Wang, Giarrusso, & Bengtson, 2002).

In parallel with the added burden of elder care on families, marked changes have occurred in the timing of family transitions, family structures, patterns of family formation and dissolution, and the ensuing diversification of family and household forms. This diversity is related to what Stacey (1990) labeled the postmodern family, characterized by "structural fragility" and a greater dependence on the voluntary commitment of its members, which creates uncertainty in intergenerational relations. Additional structural changes include a growing number of elderly single households, increase in the proportion of childless women, and increased mobility of adult children. Other trends are changing employment patterns, especially among women, that impact family relations and caregiving. All these contribute to a shrinking pool of family support.

However similar the challenge of population aging is cross-culturally, different ways of relating to this challenge have emerged. The couple and family orientation of social life and the value attached to sociability make the family a main reference point in the aging process, as aging needs are best understood within the context of the family. Each family—and each country—may be expected to mold its solutions idiosyncratically. For example, although general family norms may be strong, there is considerable variation between families in how these norms are enacted (Daatland, 1990; Finch & Mason, 1993; Lowenstein & Katz, 2000; Rossi & Rossi, 1990). A critical step in examining elder care is adopting an approach that focuses on diverse social, familial, and cultural contexts.

Cultural diversity has emerged in recent years as a major focus of gerontology (Jackson, Brown, Antonucci, & Daatland, 2005). Cultural beliefs, values, and norms that affect an aging society determine the ways in which individuals are expected to age, their status, the role of caregiving, and the role of various family members (Burr & Mutchler, 1999). Studying older people in different countries can add to our understanding of the richness and complexity of aging, caregiving, and well-being (e.g., Chappell, 2003; Mui, Choi, & Monk, 1998).

Evidence from different cultures about the relationship between expectations by older people and the support they receive from children is equivocal. Studies carried out in Florida (Lee, G.R., Netzer, & Coward, 1994), Taiwan (Lee, Y.J., Parish, & Willis, 1994), and urban China (Chen & Adamchak, 1999), as well as analysis of data from two waves of the National Survey of Families and Households in the United States (Eggebeen & Davey, 1998) found little evidence that beliefs concerning filial responsibility influenced the amount of support received from children. Other research did find direct links between filial obligation and supportive behavior of adult children (Katz, Gur-Yaish, & Lowenstein, 2007; Parrott & Bengtson, 1999; Silverstein, Gans, & Yang, 2006; Stein et al., 1998; Whitebeck, Hoyt, & Huck, 1994). It follows that we know too little about the organizing principles and values that shape families' responses—or nonresponses—to elders' care needs and about the effect of such care transfers on the well-being of the elders.

Inconsistency across a wide set of studies suggests that important factors moderating the relationship between filial expectations and behavior have not been considered. At the micro level, such moderating factors can be personal and familial resources (e.g., family size), functioning of the elderly parent, socioeconomic status, and so on. At the meso level, they can include family relations and support and attitudes about the division of responsibility between the family and the state. At the macro level, they are social policy, availability of services for the elderly, and the existence of legal obligations for parental care.

To shed light on issues of elder care in an era of increasing demands for it and decreasing formal and informal resources, this study has three specific goals: examine the determinants associated with informal and formal service use, focusing on micro- and meso-level systems in a comparative cross-national perspective; examine the association between informal and formal service support and quality of life of frail elders (75 years and older); and identify policy-related issues.

The study addresses the following questions: (a) How much help and support is actually received by elders from different sources, informal and formal? (b) What is the impact of filial norms, attitudes toward family versus state responsibility, and family resources on elder care? (c) What role does society play, through its service systems, in family support for elders? (d) What role does family help play in the use of formal services? (e) What is the effect of use of informal and formal supports on the elders' quality of life?

To answer these research questions, we used data from the cross-national OASIS study (Old Age and Autonomy: The Role of Service Systems and Intergenerational Family Solidarity).[1] Aimed at advancing knowledge on family relations in later life, the study used a unique cross-national and cross-cultural design to discover how intergenerational family support is affected by filial expectations and conditioned by societal and cultural memberships as well as by personal and family resources. The research also examined sources of social support for the elderly within the context of societal and familial variations in the manner in which older populations are served in Israel and four European countries (Norway, Germany, England, and Spain).

The specific conceptual perspectives chosen for the current study were

- the welfare regime and family culture at the *macro* level,
- the intergenerational family solidarity at the *meso* level, and
- service use and quality of life at the *micro* level.

In the OASIS comparative study, country selection was related to various social indicators representing different social policy contexts and opportunity structures for family life, elder care, and service developments for the elderly as presented in Table 5.1 For welfare state regimes, these social indicators include the well-known typologies of Esping-Andersen (1990, 1999): legal family obligation to provide economic support to older parents versus direct responsibility of the state and access to services—in particular, home-based services—that may be alternatives to help provided by the family. The table shows that Germany and Spain are familistic welfare states that tend to favor family responsibility and give the state a subsidiary role (Germany) or a residual one (Spain). These two countries have legal obligations for elder care and relatively low levels of social care services (such as elder care). They may have, however, high levels of medical services. England and Norway have individualistic social policies, no legal obligations between adult generations within the family, and higher levels of social care services. In the mixed model of Israel, there are legal family obligations, as in Spain and Germany, but also high levels of community services, as in Norway (Daatland & Lowenstein, 2005).

Regarding family cultures, indicators of women's labor force participation, fertility rates, and percent of older persons living alone show that women's work force participation is the highest in Norway and lowest in Spain, and the fertility rate is highest in Israel and lowest in Spain and England. Living alone is lowest in Spain and highest in Norway, followed by England and Germany.

METHODOLOGY

Sample

The cross-sectional survey collected data from approximately 1,200 respondents living in the community in larger urban areas in each country. To enable a more detailed analysis of the elders' circumstances and views, the 75-years-and-older population segment was oversampled and comprised about a third of the sample (800 respondents aged 25 to

TABLE 5.1   Characteristics of the Five Countries as Welfare State Regimes and Family Cultures

	Norway	England	Germany	Spain	Israel
Welfare state model	Social-democratic	Market-liberal	Conservative-corporatist	Conservative (southern)	Mixed
Legal family obligation	No	No	Yes	Yes	Yes
Level of community services	High	Medium	Low	Low	High
Female employment rate	72%	62%	61%	45%	55%
Total fertility	1.7	1.6	1.3	1.1	2.7
Living alone[a]	38%	35%	34%	14%	24%

Note: Welfare state regime (Esping-Andersen, 1990, 1999; von Kondratowitz, 2003); female employment rate; legal obligations between adult generations (Millar & Warman, 1996); total fertility and living alone.

[a] For people 60 years and older.

74 and about 400 respondents aged 75 and older). For a detailed review of the OASIS design and model, see Lowenstein and Ogg (2003).

Research Instruments

Help from family. This variable measured the help received in the following six domains: emotional support, transportation and shopping, house repair and gardening, household chores, personal care, and financial support.

Use of formal services at home. This variable measured the use of four types of services, usually intended for frail elders: home care, home nursing, emergency aid call, and meal delivery.

Use of community services (outside the home). This variable measured the use of two types of community services for frail elders—day care centers and transportation services—and one type of community service for independent elders—pensioners' clubs.

Psychological quality of life. This variable was measured with the World Health Organization Quality of Life Assessment (WHOQOL-BREF), which measures domain-specific evaluations of the subjective living situations (WHOQOL Group, 1998). WHOQOL-BREF is a multidimensional measurement including 26 items, with four subscales: physical health, psychological well-being, satisfaction with social relationships, and satisfaction with the environment. All items are rated on a five-point Likert scale, ranging from 1 = *very dissatisfied* to 5 = *very satisfied,* relating to the preceding two weeks. Reliability and validity are good (WHOQOL Group, 1998). For the purpose of this study, we chose to focus on the subscale of psychological well-being (six items such as "How much do you enjoy life?" and "To what extent do you feel your life to be meaningful?").

Filial norms. Filial norms were measured by agreement to a four-statement familism scale based on the one developed by Lee, G.R., Peek, and Coward (1998), as follows: (a) adult children should live close to their older parents so they can help them if needed; (b) adult children should be willing to sacrifice some of the things they want for their own children in order to support their frail elderly parents; (c) older people should be able to depend on their adult children to help them do the things they need to do; and (d) parents are entitled to some return for the sacrifices they have made for their children.

The statements are expressed in universal rather than particular terms to emphasize cultural values rather than individual circumstances. Two items refer to what adult children should do, and two items articulate what elderly parents should expect. Responses for each item were on a five-point scale ranging from 1 = *strongly disagree* to 5 = *strongly agree.* A mean score was computed. Intercorrelations between the four items across all countries were moderate (ranging from 0.29 to 0.49). The alpha score for the scale was 0.79.

Family-welfare state balance. Family-welfare state balance was measured by three questions that targeted the participants' attitudes about family versus state responsibility for the elderly in the three domains of financial support, help with household chores, and personal care. The items were coded 1 = *totally family responsibility* to 5 = *totally state responsibility.* Following Daatland and Herlofson (2003), we created a family-state balance index by computing the mean score of an additive scale from –6 to 6, adding up responses (*totally state* = 2, *mainly state* = 1, *both equally* = 0, *mainly family* = –1, and *totally family responsibility* = –2.

Emotional solidarity and proximity. Three dimensions of the intergenerational family solidarity paradigm were used in the present analysis of the affective and cognitive aspects of intergenerational family solidarity (i.e., affect and consensus) and of the structural dimension of intergenerational family solidarity (i.e., proximity): (a) *affect*—feelings of emotional intimacy between parents and children, using three questions such as "How close do you feel to (this child)"? The questions were coded

1 = *not at all* to 6 = *extremely close;* (b) *consensus*—the degree of similarity of opinions and values between older parents and their children, coded 1 = *not at all similar* to 6 = *extremely similar.* The affect and consensus questions were highly correlated (r = 0.533), and therefore we computed a mean score of the affective-cognitive dimension of intergenerational family solidarity, labeled *emotional solidarity;* (c) *proximity*—the geographic distance that may constrain or facilitate interaction between older parents and their children. We computed a dichotomist variable, 1 = *at least 1 child lives less than an hour away,* 0 = *no child lives less than an hour away.*

Demographics and physical functioning. Demographics and physical functioning included the following: age—in years; gender—1 = *female,* 0 = *male;* living arrangement—1 = *living alone,* 0 = *living with a family member;* number of living children; education—measured by the highest level attained on a three-point scale in which 1 = *primary level,* 2 = *secondary level,* and 3 = *higher education;* perceived financial adequacy measured on a five-point Likert scale ranging from 1 = *very difficult* to 5 = *very comfortable;* ADL functioning—measured by the shortened version of the SF-36 health survey using 12 items (Ware & Sherbourne, 1992). The total score of the scale ranges from 0 to 100, with a higher score indicating better functioning. These attributes were selected because they were found to affect family relations and well-being in a substantial number of studies (Fernandez-Ballesteros, Zamarron, & Ruiz, 2001; Ferraro & Su, 1999; Silverstein, Burholt, Wenger, & Bengtson, 1998).

FINDINGS

Univariate Analyses

Table 5.2 presents the means and standard deviations of psychological quality of life and emotional solidarity comparing the five countries. Psychological quality of life was relatively high in all countries; it was highest in Germany and lowest in Spain. The strength of emotional solidarity (affect and consensus) was relatively high in all countries and especially high in Israel.

Table 5.3 presents the distribution of help received by elderly parents from their adult children. In all countries, emotional support was the most common type of support received from adult children. Moderate help was provided in instrumental areas, least in Israel. Relatively low rates of support in personal care and financial assistance were received. The highest levels of personal care were provided in Germany and Spain, and the lowest levels of personal care were provided in Norway. The highest rates of financial assistance were provided in Spain and Israel and the lowest in Norway and Germany.

TABLE 5.2 Means and Standard Deviations of Psychological Quality of Life and Emotional Solidarity (Emotional + Consensus) for People Who Are 75 Years and Older, by Country

	Norway		England		Germany		Spain		Israel	
	M	SD	M	SD	M	SD	M	SD	M	SD
Psychological quality of life	3.7	.03	3.6	.03	3.8	.03	3.2	.03	3.4	.04
Emotional solidarity	4.4	0.9	4.5	1.0	4.2	0.9	4.2	0.8	4.7	0.9
N	398		378		410		370		358	

Note. Mean scores on a scale of 1 (low) to 5 (high) for psychological quality of life; mean scores on a scale of 1 (low) to 6 (high) for feelings of solidarity.

Although there is no standard or norm by which to judge these levels of support, it seems reasonable to judge the support as relatively high given that total help is fairly similar across five otherwise very different countries in the areas of family traditions and welfare regimes. Some reservations are necessary, because measurements are rather crude and do not indicate volume or frequency of help. With this reservation in mind, however, another reasonable conclusion is that more generous state welfare provisions (as in Norway) do not seem to discourage family support exchanges, and the opposite is more likely.

Table 5.4 presents the distribution of use of special services for the elderly by country. Generally, a large percentage of respondents in Norway and Israel use all the different kinds of services that are available.

TABLE 5.3 Help Received From Adult Children by People Who Are Age 75 Years and Older, by Type of Help and by Country

Type of help	Norway	England	Germany	Spain	Israel
Emotional support	47	56	57	63	56
Transport/shopping	42	56	52	42	37
House repair and gardening	34	35	44	28	16
Household chores	16	31	38	39	15
Personal care	2	10	16	14	7
Financial support	3	9	3	13	12
Total help (at least one)	75	81	75	69	70
N	333	322	355	325	341

TABLE 5.4   Use of Special Services for the Elderly Age 75 Years and Older, by Country

Type of service	Norway	England	Germany	Spain	Israel
Home care	32.0	15.2	6.7	7.8	32.5
Home nursing	13.8	18.3	8.2	2.9	27.9
Emergency aid call	33.3	14.5	1.4	1.8	35.0
Meal delivery	10.4	a	7.3	.8	12.7
Day care center	5.8	5.5	3.9	1.3	24.7
Transportation	23.4	12.4	8.8	3.9	19.2
Pensioners' club	22.3	10.8	6.1	8.9	43.1
N	406	348	490	383	369

Note. Respondents were asked the following question: "In the last 12 months have you been using any services for the elderly including services at home and community services?" Response categories were yes and no.

a This question was not asked in England.

Use of day care centers and pensioners' clubs is especially high in Israel, probably because in the last decade Israel placed special emphasis on developing these types of services. Pensioners' clubs operate in almost every neighborhood in Israel's larger cities. Also notable is the higher percentage of home nursing use in Israel. In England, these services are used in moderation, while in Germany and Spain only a small number of respondents use any of the special services for the elderly.

Table 5.5 shows attitudes toward the distribution of responsibility between the family and the welfare state as well as toward mixed responsibility for elder care by country. Norway and Israel stand out as the countries where the majority of respondents perceived the welfare state as having the main responsibility in all three domains (i.e., financial, household chores, and personal care). In England, the role of the welfare state is also perceived to be more dominant but to a lesser degree. Analyzing data only from Germany and Spain (third and fourth columns) reveals that respondents from these countries perceived the state to be responsible financially to a greater degree than in the other domains. In the domains of household chores and personal care, perceptions in Germany and Spain tend toward a mix between family and the state.

Multivariate Analyses

Table 5.6 summarizes the results of three regressions of the different sources of help used by the population aged 75 years and older. The

TABLE 5.5   Family-State Balance: Attitudes Toward Family, State, and Mixed Responsibility for Elder Care for People Who Are Age 75 and Older, by Country

Areas of Responsibility		Norway	England	Germany	Spain	Israel
Financial	Family	6.7	21.5	13.3	18.2	12.7
	Both	20.9	32.6	41.1	33.4	23.2
	State	72.4	45.9	45.6	48.4	64.1
Household chores	Family	8.5	24.8	27.2	31.1	10.5
	Both	15.9	26.9	40.2	33.3	23.9
	State	75.6	48.3	32.6	35.5	65.6
Personal care	Family	7.0	31.6	27.2	38.0	8.7
	Both	11.9	20.9	39.7	32.2	23.1
	State	81.1	47.5	33.1	29.8	68.2
N		402	390	474	368	353

Note. Respondents were asked the following question: "About how much responsibility do you believe the family, the state, or both equally should have in providing three types of support (financial, household chores, and personal care) for older persons in need?"

analysis follows the model presented by Daatland and Lowenstein (2005). Norway, England, Germany, and Spain are included as dummy variables, with Israel as the reference. The model also controls for the effects of needs (physical functioning), personal resources (gender, age, education, and financial adequacy), and family resources (family solidarity, living arrangements, and number of children). The dependent variables to be explained are help from family (in the areas of instrumental help and personal care), use of services at home (home care, nursing care, and emergency buttons), and use of community services for the frail elders (day care and transportation). The three types of support were used interchangeably in the regressions—that is, for help from family as the dependent variable, the use of formal services was entered as a control. The explained variance for help from family was 26%, for use of services at home 39%, and for use of community services 25%.

The analyses show that regarding help from family, all countries had higher rates of help from family than Israel. As for services at home, the levels were significantly lower in England, Germany, and Spain. Finally, Norway, England, Germany, and Spain had lower levels of use of community services.

Family resources (family solidarity, living arrangements, and number of children) make a difference mainly in receiving help from family. The attitudinal variables (family norms and attitudes about the state-welfare

TABLE 5.6 Regressions of Help From Different Sources for People Who Are Age 75 and Older (N = 1,475)

	Help from family	Use of services at home	Use of community services
Filial norms	.156***	.042	-.054*
Family-state balance	-.078**	.027	-.011
Emotional solidarity (affect + consensus)	.106***	.022	-.003
Proximity	.171***	.002	-.008
Help from family	—	-.079***	.072**
Use of services at home	-.095***	—	.332***
Use of community services	.072**	.273***	—
Age	.066**	.103***	.012
Female	.054*	.002	-.009
Living alone	.004	.134***	.009
Number of chil-dren	.058*	.003	-.008
Education	-.009	-.028	-.064*
Financial adequacy	.031	-.002	.019
Physical functioning	-.318***	-.264***	-.120***
Norway	.180***	.025	-.120***
England	.168***	-.157***	-.208***
Germany	.261***	-.255***	-.200***
Spain	.095**	-.252***	-.231***
Total R^2	.259	.385	.254

Note. Ordinary least squares standardized regression coefficients; missing cases left out. Countries as dummy variables with Israel as reference.

 * $p < .05.$ ** $p < .01.$ *** $p < .001.$

balance) make a difference in the sense that elders in countries with higher filial norms receive more help from the family and less help from community services. Attitudes toward family-state balance show that, when family responsibility is valued more highly, more help is provided by the family.

Testing how the use of formal services at home and in the community affected help from family shows that services at home reduced family support, whereas community services elevates it.

Physical functioning is the most powerful factor among the personal resources studied here in explaining help from all sources. Other personal resources (gender, age, education, and financial adequacy) had a relatively smaller contribution and mainly toward help from family and use of services at home. Women who were older and had more children received more help from family; older respondents who lived alone used more services at home.

To study the effect of attitudes, familial resources, and the use of informal and formal supports on psychological quality of life—controlling for demographics, physical functioning, and country—a block-recursive regression with three models was applied. The findings are presented in Table 5.7. Model 3 explained 38% of the variance.

The data indicate that familial attitudes (filial norms) were a significant negative predictor of psychological quality of life in the first model only, whereas attitudes regarding the family-state balance were not

TABLE 5.7 Standardized Regression Coefficients for Psychological Quality of Life of People Who Are Age 75 and Older ($N = 1,475$)

	Model 1	Model 2	Model 3
Filial norms	-.085***	-.024	.007
Family-state balance	-.002	.012	.039
Emotional solidarity (affect + consensus)	.181***	.118***	.133***
Proximity	-.007	-.014	.013
Use of services at home	-.165***	-.074**	-.057*
Help from family	-.069**	.025	-.022
Use of community services	-.150***	-.105***	-.094***
Age		.003	-.011
Female		.018	.004
Living alone		.023	-.004
Number of children		.002	.035
Education		.123***	.053*
Financial adequacy		.279***	.237***
Physical functioning		.314***	.314***
Norway			.090**
England			.131***
Germany			.222***
Spain			-.073*
Total R^2	.112	.329	.377
R^2 Change		.217	.048

Note. For all three models, Israel is the reference.
* $p < .05$. ** $p < .01$. *** $p < .001$.

related to it. Emotional solidarity was a strong significant predictor in all three models, whereas proximity was not. Both uses of formal services (in-home and community) were negative predictors in all three models, whereas help from family was a negative predictor only in the first model. Apparently, more frail elders need and use services both at home and in the community (when available), which has a negative effect on their psychological quality of life because they are more dependent and thus forfeit some of their autonomy.

Better physical functioning, being more educated, and being in a better financial situation were positively related to psychological quality of life both in the second and third models. Gender, age, living alone, and the number of children did not make a significant contribution to psychological quality of life in any of the models. Respondents from Norway, England, and Germany reported higher psychological quality of life, while Spanish and Israeli respondents had a lower quality of life.

DISCUSSION

This chapter used data from the OASIS cross-national five-country study to investigate the idiosyncratic national, familial, and personal factors that serve as antecedents for elder care in relation to the use of informal family support and use of formal services, and the outcome of such use on the elders' quality of life.

The focus of the study was on specific types of formal services—those provided at home and those in the community (e.g., day care centers)—for frail elders needing care, rather than examining general state welfare support. To better understand the complex relationships between the use of different support types, the three sources of support were used interchangeably to test their effect on one another—that is, for help from family as the dependent variable, use of formal services was entered as a control variable, and vice-versa.

Five questions were raised at the beginning. The first question related to the help and support that older parents receive from family and from formal services, at home and in the community. The emerging pattern in this study regarding family help was that, in all countries, emotional support was the most common type of support received from adult children. It was also a strong predictor of the outcome variable of psychological quality of life. In the instrumental areas, moderate help was received, and relatively low rates of support were received in the areas of personal care and finances.

Different analyses of the OASIS data complement the above findings. For example, the emotional component in intergenerational family relations was found to be important to the life satisfaction of the older generation (Lowenstein, Katz, & Gur-Yaish, 2007). Further, a study that compared help received and provided between generations indicated that in the instrumental areas help flowed upward toward the older generation, but in the financial area it flowed downward toward the younger generation (Lowenstein & Daatland, 2006).

In the present study, use of formal services was highest in the two countries that have a large network of services for the elderly—Norway and Israel. Norway has enacted individualistic social policies and has no legal obligations between adult family generations and higher levels of social care services. Israel represents a mixed model with legal family obligations but also with high levels of home and community services. The lowest levels of formal service use were in Germany and Spain, which are familistic welfare states that tend to favor family responsibility and have relatively low levels of social care services.

The second question focused on the effect of the attitudinal variables (filial norms and attitudes toward family-state responsibility) and family resources on elder care. Generally, higher filial norms were associated with more help from the family. Empirical evidence in the literature concerning the relationship between filial norms and family support is ambiguous. Some data suggest that filial obligations play a role in the amount of care (e.g., Ikkink, Tilburg, & Knipscheer, 1999; Silverstein et al., 2006), similar to our findings. Conversely, Lee, G. R., et al. (1994), Lee, G. R., Netzer, and Coward (1995), and Eggebeen and Davey (1998) presented evidence that, in the case of older parents needing care, filial norms were not related to the actual receipt of support from adult children. The negative association found in this study between filial norms and formal services sheds light on the complex interplay between attitudes and the actual use of support from formal and informal services.

Attitudes regarding the family-state balance indicate that the welfare state has not crowded out family responsibility in elder care, although this is less true in Norway and Israel. Most elders, however, prefer the state to take a leading role, indicating that a welfare state containment policy does not seem to have support in any of the countries.

Family resources in the present study (family solidarity, living arrangements, and the number of children) make a difference mainly in receiving help from the family. Close emotional relations between generations, living in close proximity, and number of children affected the receipt of help from the family but not from the formal services.

The third question focused on the macro level, asking about the role society plays through its services in encouraging (or discouraging) family help. The data indicate that the use of services at home was negatively related to help from the family, while use of community services was positively related to it. The sharing of responsibility for elder care between formal and informal sources of support demonstrated that the two were interdependent. Use of services at home reduced help from the family, supporting the substitution hypothesis (Kunemund & Rein, 1999). At the same time, use of community services did not erode help from family, supporting the complementarity hypothesis (Lingsom, 1997). In addition to instrumental care, community services—in this case day care centers for the frail elderly and transportation—offer opportunities for social interactions, answer needs for sociability, and reduce loneliness.

The fourth question asked about the other possible direction of influence: the effect of family help on the use of formal services. The findings show that family help reduces the use of services at home, which means that the two substitute for each other; but family help does not reduce use of community services that presumably provide other benefits to the old person, such as social relations and respite to family members taking care of frail elders.

The last question related to the effect of using different types of support on the psychological quality of life of the old person, who is the recipient of assistance. The main conclusion is that the quality of life of frail older persons is low and is affected mainly by their needs—in particular, their physical functioning. This conclusion emerges also from the results showing that the two types of formal services have a negative effect on the elders' psychological quality of life and that physical functioning was a strong predictor of the use of the various support types. Additional background attributes of higher education and higher financial adequacy predicted higher levels of psychological quality of life.

Emotional solidarity was one of the strong determinants of quality of life and remained so even after controlling for the relevant macro and micro variables. These findings are congruent with those of Zhang and Yu (1998) on the importance of emotional family relations for life satisfaction among elderly Chinese. Connidis and McMullin (1993) found that parents who felt emotionally close to their children were more happy and satisfied with their lives than distant parents and those with no children.

CONCLUSION AND IMPLICATIONS

This chapter presented the antecedents and outcomes of elder care from a cross-national perspective. The increased availability and social acceptability of public services elevated the willingness by the elderly and their families to use public services when dependence begins (Daatland, 1997). Care for the aged is, therefore, a mix of informal and formal support systems, with the specific proportions of the mix varying by country and culture. Our comparative cross-national data show that the particular mix is related to two factors: (a) the family culture that guides the level of readiness and determines actual use of public services and (b) the availability and accessibility of these services.

One of the basic policy debates in this regard is whether formal services substitute for or complement informal family care. According to Hooyman (1992), a basic limitation of aging policies in most countries is that families and service systems are seen as alternatives that tend to substitute for rather than complement each other. Public opinion also tends to support the substitution idea (Daatland, 1990), whereas most research supports the complementarity hypothesis (Chappell & Blandford, 1991; Daatland & Lowenstein, 2005; Lingsom, 1997; Litwak, 1985). The findings of the current study show that substitution exists in the use of formal services at home versus family help, but that the use of community services complements help from the family.

In light of the rising costs of welfare and health services, a balance must be found between these conflicting perspectives. In a study conducted in Israel (where children are legally obligated to support their parents financially) on the impact of the Long-Term Care Insurance Law on care relations, data showed that the involvement and care of the families was not reduced; rather, the nature of the care may have changed in some cases toward providing more emotional support (Katan & Lowenstein, 1999). Similar findings from five countries were presented by Daatland and Lowenstein (2005) of "a weaker variant of the crowding-in hypothesis, namely that a generous welfare state neither reduces nor increases family efforts but allows the family to re-orient their responsibility towards less burdensome tasks" (p. 180).

It seems that more emphasis should be placed on services that strengthen and complement family care and increase the collaboration between caregiving families and the available service systems. Furthermore, we must find ways to assess good quality care from the perspectives of both the family and the formal service systems, and we must study the relationships between family networks and policy-related outcomes.

In the future, rising levels of affluence among the aged in developed countries and the introduction of state welfare provisions may provide an option of selectivity in family relationships, so that sentiment rather than obligation may increasingly govern the ties between elderly parents and younger generations. Normative obligations will continue to play a role but may become increasingly transcribed into affection and choice, giving family relationships a more personal and less structural flavor (Katz, Lowenstein, Phillips, & Daatland, 2005). At present, few caregiving role models exist, and there is a need to develop new models to guide families in an age of longevity.

There are several limitations to the present analysis. First, the data presented refer mainly to the more frail respondents who are 75 years and older; this group should be compared with the more independent elders in this group as well as with other age groups. Second, the data are cross-sectional and show a static situation of family relations; a longitudinal design would have provided a more dynamic picture about possible changes in elder care.

To enrich our understanding of family interactions, a mixed method approach combining quantitative and qualitative data collection should be used. To fully understand the complexity of family relations, a broader context of these relationships should be explored, including consideration of the points of view of the adult children, the elderly parents, and other family members. Understanding dyadic relations within the total context of family networks and roles may further help define the notion of caregiving.

Findings from the OASIS study presented here highlight the importance of comparative cross-national and cross-cultural analyses in providing new frameworks and insights for understanding idiosyncratic and intriguing differences as well as unexpected similarities between cultures and countries. Such studies should become more common.

NOTE

1. OASIS was funded under the fifth program of the European Union, contract number QLK6-TC1999–12182.

REFERENCES

Bengtson, V. L., Rosenthal, G., & Burton, L. (1996). Paradoxes of families and aging. In R. H. Binstock & L. K. George (Eds.), *Handbook of aging and the social sciences* (pp. 253–282). San Diego, CA: Academic Press.

Burr, J. A., & Mutchler, J. E. (1999). Race and ethnic variation in norms of filial responsibility among older persons. *Journal of Marriage and the Family, 61,* 674–687.

Chappell, N. L., & Blandford, A. (1991). Informal and formal care: Exploring the complementarity. *Ageing and Society, 11,* 299–317.

Chappell, N. L. (2003). Correcting cross-cultural stereotypes: Aging in Shanghai and Canada. *Journal of Cross-Cultural Gerontology, 18,* 127–147.

Chen, S., & Adamchak, D. J. (1999). The effects of filial responsibility expectations on intergenerational exchanges in urban China. *Hallym International Journal of Aging, 1,* 58–68.

Connidis, I. A., & McMullin, J. (1993). To have or have not: Parent status and the subjective well-being of older men and women. *The Gerontologist, 33*(5), 630–636.

Daatland, S. O. (1990). What are families for? On family solidarity and preferences for help. *Ageing and Society, 10,* 1–15.

Daatland, S. O. (1997). Welfare policies for older people in transition: Emerging trends and comparative perspectives. *Scandinavian Journal of Social Welfare, 6,* 153–161.

Daatland, S. O., & Herlofson, K. (2003). Norms and ideals about elder care. In A. Lowenstein & J. Ogg (Eds.), *OASIS—Old age and autonomy: The role of service systems and intergenerational family solidarity.* Haifa, Israel: University of Haifa, Center for Research and Study of Aging.

Daatland, S. O., & Lowenstein, A. (2005). Intergenerational solidarity and the family-welfare state balance. *European Journal of Ageing, 2,* 174–182.

Eggebeen, D. J., & Davey, A. (1998). Do safety nets work? The role of anticipated help in times of need. *Journal of Marriage and the Family, 60,* 939–950.

Esping-Andersen, G. (1990). *The three worlds of welfare capitalism.* Princeton, NJ: Princeton University Press.

Esping-Andersen, G. (1999). *Social foundations of postindustrial economies.* Oxford, England: Oxford University Press.

Eurostat. (1996). *Demographic statistics 1996.* Luxembourg: Office for Official Publications of the European Communities.

Fernandez-Ballesteros, R., Zamarron, M. D., & Ruiz, M. A. (2001). The contribution of socio-demographic and psychosocial factors to life satisfaction. *Ageing and Society, 21,* 25–43.

Ferraro, K. F., & Su, Y. (1999). Financial strain, social relations, and psychological distress among older people: A cross-cultural analysis. *Journals of Gerontology Series B: Psychological Sciences and Social Sciences, 54B,* S3–S15.

Finch, J., & Mason, J. (1993). *Negotiating family responsibilities.* London: Tavistock/Routledge.

Hooyman, N. R. (1992). Social policy and gender inequities in caregiving. In J. Dwyer & R. Coward (Eds.), *Gender, families, and eldercare* (pp. 181–201). Newbury Park, CA: Sage.

Ikkink, K. K., Tilburg, T. V., & Knipscheer, K. C. P. M. (1999). Perceived instrumental support exchanges in relationships between elderly parents and their adult children: Normative and structural explanations. *Journal of Marriage and the Family, 61,* 831–844.

International Labour Office (2000). *World labour report.* Geneva, Switzerland: Author.

Jackson, J. S., Brown, E., Antonucci, T., & Daatland, S. O. (2005). Ethnic diversity in aging, multi-cultural societies. In M. L. Johnson, V. L. Bengston, P. G. Coleman, & T. B. L. Kirkwood (Eds.), *The Cambridge Handbook of Age and Aging* (pp. 476–481). Cambridge, England: Cambridge University Press.

Katz, R., Gur-Yaish, N., & Lowenstein, A. (2007). *What motivates adult children to provide care to their older parents? A cross-national comparison.* Manuscript submitted for publication.

Katz, R., Lowenstein, A., Phillips, J., & Daatland, S. O. (2005). Theorizing intergenerational solidarity, conflict and ambivalence in a comparative cross-national perspective. In V. L. Bengtson, A. C. Acock, K. R. Allen, P. Dilworth-Andersen, & D. M. Klein (Eds.), *Sourcebook on family theory and research* (pp. 393–407). Thousand Oaks, CA: Sage.

Kinsella, K. (2000). Demographic dimensions of global aging. *Journal of Family Issues, 21,* 541–558.

Kondratowitz, H. J. von (2003). Comparing welfare states. In A. Lowenstein & J. Ogg (Eds.), *OASIS—old age and autonomy: The role of service systems and intergenerational family solidarity [Final report].* University of Haifa, Haifa, Israel.

Kunemund, H., & Rein, M. (1999). There is more to receiving than needing: Theoretical arguments and empirical explorations of crowding-in and crowding-out. *Ageing and Society, 19,* 93–121.

Lee, G. R., Netzer, J. K., & Coward, R. T. (1994). Filial responsibility expectations and patterns of intergenerational assistance. *Journal of Marriage and the Family, 56,* 559–565.

Lee, G. R., Netzer, J. K., & Coward, R. T. (1995). Depression among older parents: The role of intergenerational exchange. *Journal of Marriage and the Family, 57,* 823–833.

Lee, G. R., Peek, C. W., & Coward, R. T. (1998). Race differences in filial responsibility expectations among older parents. *Journal of Marriage and the Family, 60,* 404–412.

Lee, Y. J., Parish, W. L., & Willis, R. J. (1994). Sons, daughters, and intergenerational support in Taiwan. *American Journal of Sociology, 99,* 1010–1041.

Lingsom, S. (1997). *The substitution issue. Care policies and their consequences for family care.* NOVA Rapport 6/97. Oslo, Norway: NOVA.

Litwak, E. (1985). *Helping the elderly: The complementary roles of informal networks and formal systems.* New York: Guilford Press.

Lowenstein, A., & Daatland, S. O. (2006). Filial norms and family support in a comparative cross-national context: Evidence from the OASIS study. *Ageing and Society, 26,* 203–223.

Lowenstein, A., & Katan, Y. (1999). *Evaluation of the Long-Term-Care Insurance Law—A decade of operation.* Jerusalem, Israel: Center for Social Policy in Israel.

Lowenstein, A., & Katz, R. (2000). Rural Arab families coping with caregiving. *Marriage and Family Review, 30,* 179–197.

Lowenstein, A., Katz, R., & Gur-Yaish, N. (2007). Reciprocity in parent-child exchange and life satisfaction among the elderly: A cross-national perspective. Manuscript submitted for publication.

Lowenstein, A., & Ogg, J. (2003). OASIS—old age and autonomy: The role of service systems and intergenerational family solidarity [Final report]. University of Haifa, Haifa, Israel. Available online at http://www.dza.de/forschung/oasis_report.pdf

Millar, J., & Warman, A. (1996). *Family obligations in Europe.* London: Family Policy Studies Centre.

Mui, A. C., Choi, N. G., & Monk, A. (1998). *Long-term care and ethnicity.* Westport, CT: Auburn House.

Parrott, T. M., & Bengtson, V. L. (1999). The effects of earlier intergenerational affection, normative expectations and family conflict on contemporary exchanges of help and support. *Research on Aging, 21,* 73–105.

Rossi, A. S., & Rossi, P. H. (1990). *Of human bonding: Parent-child relations across the life course.* New York: Aldine de Gruyter.

Silverstein, M., Burholt, V., Wenger, G. C., & Bengtson, V. L. (1998). Parent-child relations among very old parents in Wales and the United States: A test of modernization theory. *Journal of Aging Studies, 12,* 387–409.

Silverstein, M., Conroy, S. J., Wang, H. T., Giarrusso, R., & Bengtson, V. L. (2002). Reciprocity in parent-child relations over the adult life course. *Journals of Gerontology, Series B: Psychological Sciences and Social Sciences, 57,* S3–S13.

Silverstein, M., Gans, D., & Yang, F. M. (2006). Intergenerational support to aging parents: The role of norms and needs. *Journal of Family Issues, 27,* 1068–1084.

Stacey, J. (1990). *Brave new families: Stories of domestic upheaval in late twentieth-century America.* Jackson, TN: Basic Books.

Stein, C. H., Wemmerus, V. A., Ward, M., Gaines, M. E., Freeberg, A. L., & Jewell, T. C. (1998). "Because they are my parents": An intergenerational study of felt obligation and parental caregiving. *Journal of Marriage and the Family, 60,* 611–622.

United Nations (2005). *Living arrangement of older persons around the world.* Department of Economic and Social Affairs, Population Division. New York: Author.

Ware, J. E., & Sherbourne, C. D. (1992). The MOS 36-item short-form health survey (SF-36): I. Conceptual framework and item selection. *Medical Care, 30,* 473–483.

Whitebeck, L. B., Hoyt, D. R., & Huck, S. M. (1994). Early family relationships, intergenerational solidarity and support provided to parents by their adult children. *Journal of Gerontology, 39,* S85–S95.

WHOQOL Group. (1998). The World Health Organization Quality of Life Assessment (WHOQOL): Development and general psychometric properties. *Social Science and Medicine, 46,* 1569–1585.

World Health Organization. (2002). *Active ageing—A policy framework.* Madrid, Spain: Second United National World Assembly on Ageing.

Zhang, A.Y., & Yu, L. C. (1998). Life satisfaction among Chinese elderly in Beijing. *Journal of Cross-Cultural Gerontology, 13,* 109–125.

SECTION II

Familial Contexts

CHAPTER SIX

Spouses Caring for Spouses: Untangling the Influences of Relationship and Gender

Eleanor Palo Stoller and Casey Schroeder Miklowski

For older people who are married when they encounter disease or disability, spouses are the first line of defense, providing more hours of assistance with a broader range of tasks than other family caregivers (Chappell & Kuehne, 1998). Spouses provide assistance with activities of daily living; communication, including empathy and companionship; supervision, including reminders to initiate actions; and activity and mental stimulation (Jansson, Nordberg, & Grafstrom, 2001). Over one-third of all informal caregivers of frail elderly living in community settings are spouses (Quadagno, 2005).

The higher prevalence of wife caregivers reflects gender differences in both longevity and marriage patterns: (a) Women live longer than men and generally marry men who are older than they are; and (b) when elderly men are widowed, they are much more likely than elderly women to remarry. As a result of these trends, older men are more likely than older women to be married when they encounter a need for care. Older women, on the other hand, are more likely to be widowed and, therefore, to rely on adult children, especially daughters, as caregivers.

Husbands and wives are also the most dependable caregivers, and evidence suggests that marriage provides some protection against the likelihood of institutional placement. Twenty-five percent of people who were married at the time of their death had spent some time in a nursing home, compared to 40% who were widowed, divorced or separated, or never married (Quadagno, 2005). However, married women are more frequently institutionalized than married men, so husbands may not be quite as dependable as wives in providing long-term care.

In this chapter, we explore several dimensions of spousal caregiving. We begin with a brief overview of the experiences of providing care for a frail, ill, or disabled spouse. Then we turn attention to unpacking the influence of gender—comparing the experiences of caregiving wives with the experiences of caregiving husbands as well as recognizing diversity among and between husbands and wives. The chapter concludes with a discussion of the implications of these experiences.

THE EXPERIENCES OF SPOUSE CAREGIVERS

In comparison with other caregivers, spouses tolerate greater disability for a longer time, with fewer mediating resources and at great personal cost (Seltzer & Li, 2000). The pattern of health outcomes associated with caring for a disabled spouse is most often downward, with spouses transitioning into a caregiving role exhibiting declines in self-rated health, healthy behaviors, and a range of physical and emotional health indicators (Burton, Zdaniuk, Schulz, Jackson, & Hirsch, 2003; Marks, Lambert, & Choi, 2002). When husbands and wives—rather than other family members—are primary caregivers, their efforts are less likely to be supplemented with help from other informal caregivers or from formal service providers (Chappell & Kuehne, 1998). Spouses have less discretion than other family members regarding caregiving responsibilities, since caring for an impaired partner is seen as part of the marriage contract (Miller & Montgomery, 1990), something they do out of a combination of love and duty (Davidson, Arber, & Ginn, 2000). Most spouses stop providing care only when deterioration in their own health prevents them from giving assistance. There is some evidence that wives continue providing care longer and at higher levels of disability than do husbands (Stoller, 1992). This difference can reflect a somewhat lower tolerance threshold among husbands in comparison to wives, but it can also indicate that husbands are better able to recognize a care situation that exceeds both their own resources and resources available to them in the community (Hooker, Manoogian-O'Dell, Monahan, Frazier, & Shifren, 2000).

Empirical research on the difficulties—or burden—experienced by caregiving spouses has yielded some conflicting results. Several researchers contend that spouse caregivers experience less role conflict and lower levels of burden than other caregivers (Young & Kahana, 1989). Others, however, report that caregiving has a greater negative impact on spouses in comparison with other caregivers (George & Gwyther, 1986). In part, this divergence reflects the multidimensionality of caregiver burden, which includes emotional, social, financial, and physical dimensions (Mui, 1995; Stoller, 1992).

GENDER DIFFERENCES IN CAREGIVING

Divergent findings may also reflect a failure to consider differences between husbands and wives. Gender is a key dimension of social organization in society, and men and women face different expectations and obligations and encounter different internalized and structural barriers in fulfilling their roles. While the task structure facing caregiving husbands and caregiving wives may be similar, the gender of a spouse has a significant impact on the meaning and consequences of the caregiving role.

Researchers have documented a range of gender differences in the experience of providing care. Women provide more hours of informal care than do men, including more assistance with activities of daily living—which encompasses housework, meal preparation, and personal care (including incontinence care) (Allen, 1994; Navaie-Walier, Spriggs, & Feldman 2002). Women also report more difficulty with care; greater feelings of burden, anxiety, stress, and depression; and more physical symptoms associated with caregiving, including sleep disruption, chronic fatigue, weight change, and gastrointestinal problems (Amberg, Jansson, Grafstrom et al., 1998; Kramer & Kipnis, 1995; Navaie-Walier et al., 2002; Yee & Schulz, 2000).

COMPARING THE CAREGIVING EXPERIENCES OF HUSBANDS AND WIVES

To what extent are gender differences reflected in the experiences of husbands and wives caring for an ill or disabled spouse? We will focus on comparisons in six areas: (a) caregiver burden, (b) the meaning of care, (c) the household division of labor, (d) financial impact, (e) social support, and (f) coping strategies.

Caregiver Burden

Most studies indicate that caregiving husbands report lower levels of burden and higher levels of well-being than caregiving wives (Marks et al.,

2002; Rose-Rego, Strauss, & Smyth, 1998; Yee & Schulz, 2000). Even as they transition into the caregiving role, wives report lower levels of autonomy and purpose in life than husbands (Marks et al., 2002). This gender difference in reported burden is smallest during the initial stages of caring but appears to increase over time, with more experienced husband caregivers reporting lower levels of strain than husbands who recently assumed their caregiving responsibilities. Mui (1995) suggests that husbands' limited experience with many caregiving tasks make the early stages of care more challenging, but that task-related strain diminishes with experience.

With respect to specific dimensions of caregiver burden, research indicates that wives experience higher levels of emotional and physical strain associated with caregiving responsibilities than do husbands. Wives are also more likely than husbands to report that caregiving impinges on their social and personal lives. Perhaps because caregiving is often seen as "natural" for women, wives are less likely than husbands to receive supplementary assistance, both from family members and from formal service providers. Although wives report more strain directly related to the experience of caregiving, there is some evidence that caregiving husbands tend to report higher rates of unhappiness and more strain in the marital relationship (Kramer & Lambert, 1999).

There are also some differences between husbands and wives in the predictors of caregiver burden. Even though wives are more likely than husbands to experience a conflict between caregiving and other roles, when husbands experience this conflict, it has a stronger negative impact on their perceptions of the burden. Wives are also more negatively affected by their husband's behavioral problems, including making excessive demands, falling down, and asking repetitive questions (Ingersoll-Dayton & Raschick, 2004; Mui 1995).

The Meaning of Care

Caring for an impaired spouse has different meanings for husbands and wives. Although both husbands and wives consider spousal caregiving part of the marriage contract—inspired by a combination of love and duty—some researches argue that women emphasize the obligation to care, whereas men perceive more latitude in assuming the caregiving role (Chappell & Kuehne, 1998). In citing the marriage contract, wives were more likely to mention "in sickness and in health" as the "foundation for caring, whereas men were more likely to cite the 'for worse' part of the marriage vow to describe what they had to 'endure' in caring for their wives" (Davidson, Arber, & Ginn, 2000, p. 545).

In describing the consequences of caregiving in their own lives, wives tend to focus on changes in the relationship brought about by the husband's illness, whereas husbands focus more on specific tasks (Chappell & Kuehne, 1998; Miller, 1987). Wives are also more likely to feel personal responsibility for maintaining their husband's safety and for reducing his suffering. Perhaps as a result, wives also have more trouble setting limits to their caregiving and are more likely to feel guilty about not doing enough (Stoller, 1992).

Wife caregivers were more likely than husband caregivers to describe strategies for bolstering their husbands' sense of independence and self-esteem (Jansson et al., 2001). For example, the wives in Miller's (1987) qualitative study devised strategies for supporting their husbands' sense of control, even as they assumed more and more responsibility for task management and decision-making. They tried to keep life as "normal" as possible, arranging activities that preserved as much as possible of their husband's past self (Jansson et al., 2001).

Despite the greater burden experienced by wives, there is some evidence that elderly husbands are more highly invested in the caregiving role than are elderly wives, perhaps reflecting their view of caring as a choice rather than an obligation (Navon & Weinblatt, 1996; Yee & Schulz, 2000). Pruchno and Resch (1989) interpret this difference within the context of reciprocity, explaining that husbands express a "greater sense than did the wives that the care they currently provide to their spouses was due them in return for years of prior support and nurturing" (p. 163). Lobo-Prabhu, Molinari, Arlinghaus, Barr, and Lomax (2005) refer to this process as delayed quid pro quo reciprocity. Husbands are also more likely than wives to report that caring for their spouses bolsters their self-esteem—a positive outcome reflecting pride in their own accomplishments, gratitude of their spouse, and praise from both family members and professional care providers. In contrast, caring by wives is more likely "an extension of the invisible daily routine of noticing, interpreting and responding to the needs of the partner" (Davidson et al., 2000, p. 546).

Research on the meaning of care has also included the care recipient. An important finding of these studies addresses the fit between the amount of support received and the recipient's need for independence (Martire, Stephens, Druley, & Wojno, 2002). These studies suggest that too much support can be detrimental to care recipients, especially to dependent wives. Receiving more assistance than is needed or wanted undermines perceptions of competence and control, particularly in domains with high salience for care recipients. Wives who felt less competent as a result of their husbands' assistance with domestic responsibilities exhibited lower well-being over time, particularly among those women for whom it was important to complete these instrumental tasks on their own (Martire et al., 2002).

The Impact of Caregiving on the Division of Labor

The consequences of caregiving on the couple's division of household labor depends on both the extent and range of incapacity experienced by each spouse and by the couple's division of labor prior to the onset of disability. Unfortunately, longitudinal data showing changes in the division of household labor over time do not exist, so we know very little about how current cohorts of elderly couples handled household work when they were younger. This makes it difficult to disentangle the impact of stage of life (or age-related) changes from cohort effects. Some insights can be gained, however, by reviewing current research on the gender division of domestic work.

This literature, consisting primarily of cross-sectional studies, demonstrates that the cultural assignment of domestic production has remained fairly consistent in response to women's increased labor force production over the past 40 years. Although there has been some increase in men's household production, particularly when wives are employed outside the home, women still perform the majority of household work. Women with higher incomes can reduce their workload by delegating tasks to hired help or by purchasing market equivalents ("outsourcing"), a pattern that appears to be increasing among younger cohorts today (Blair-Loy, 2003). Nevertheless, they still retain responsibility for most domestic tasks, with husbands' contributions defined as "helping."

Tasks performed by husbands share certain features that distinguish them from women's household work. Tasks most often performed by husbands are characterized by clearly defined boundaries (e.g., mowing the lawn), flexible scheduling and an element of discretion as to when tasks would be done (e.g., doing household repairs and handling finances), and greater leisure components (e.g., playing with children) (Miller & Cafasso, 1992). As a result, husbands have more control over their time, whereas women's work is more likely to lock them into a rigid (or at least externally controlled) schedule.

What happens after retirement? Although there is some evidence that retired husbands increase somewhat their participation in some household tasks, elderly wives continue to bear a greater share (Solomon, Acock, & Walker, 2004) and to feel responsible for managing household work (Altschuler, 2004). These findings suggest that the impact of a spouse's disability is gender specific. Incapacity of a husband means that wife caregivers assume greater responsibility for male-stereotypic tasks, such as yard work, household repairs, and financial management. When a wife becomes ill or disabled, husband caregivers are faced with a need to assume responsibility for more routine household chores. This involves mastering specific instrumental tasks, developing skills such as cooking and provisioning without instructions provided by their wives. But taking on a wife's household responsibilities also means less autonomy and less flexibility of scheduling. Because the wife is almost always responsible for the home, even if she delegates some tasks, the disability of a wife means the couple has lost its manager of household production.

Although husbands do increase the hours devoted to household tasks when their wives become impaired, their household work prior to their wives' illness remains a significant predictor of their contribution after their wives become ill or impaired. As Allen and Webster (2001) explain, "husbands who are most helpful prior to their wives' impairment are also most helpful afterward" (p. 913). Marital happiness is also a predictor of a husband's involvement in household work, but only among men with egalitarian attitudes toward gender and marital roles (Allen & Webster, 2001).

Perhaps because of the assumption that domestic work is the woman's responsibility, wife caregivers receive less help with household chores from their husbands than husband caregivers receive from their wives, and this assistance from the care recipient resulted in more stress reduction for husband caregivers than for wife caregivers (Ingersoll-Dayton & Raschik, 2004). Husband caregivers also receive more supplemental assistance than wife caregivers from other family members. This is an important difference, because evidence indicates that receiving help with household tasks is associated with reduced levels of stress for both caregiving husbands and caregiving wives (Ingersoll-Dayton & Raschik, 2004).

Learning to perform tasks previously handled by the impaired spouse is a challenge, but it is also an opportunity to demonstrate competence and experience a sense of achievement. Spouse caregivers have the potential for more emotional support from their spousal care recipient than other caregivers, which can reduce stress related to providing care (Mak, 2005). Some couples report becoming closer as they work together on devising new strategies for handling responsibilities. Studies of caregiving wives suggest that ongoing support from their impaired husband enhances wives' well-being and marital satisfaction (Franks & Stephens, 1996; Wright & Aquilino, 1998).

However, this potential benefit can be eroded if the dependent spouse is reluctant to give up responsibility or criticizes the caregiver's task performance (Townsend & Franks, 1997). Disagreements can emerge around standards of cleanliness, the degree of detail required to manage finances, or the way the family car should be maintained. Although these are seemingly minor disputes when viewed from the outside, these disagreements can be infuriating to the care recipient who has lost control over areas of life previously managed without interference and frustrating to the care provider who is trying to juggle the work of both spouses. Conflicts also can arise when the disabled spouse tries to assist with tasks he or she is no longer able to perform. For example, a study by Ingersoll-Dayton and Raschik (2004) reported that, when care-receiving wives exhibit behavior problems, their efforts to assist their husbands with domestic tasks actually interfered with the husband's caregiving activities and increased stress levels.

Impact on Social Support Networks

Disability of a spouse produces gender-specific outcomes on both socio-emotional and instrumental support provided. First, older men are more likely than older women to rely exclusively on their wives for empathy, affection, and companionship (Kramer, 1997), so their wives' impairment can undermine their primary source of socioemotional support. In contrast, women are more likely to have developed a wider range of close friendships with other women that supplement their relationship with their husband. Second, the illness of a wife means that the couple has lost the person who traditionally maintained contact with kin networks, including arranging visits, organizing holiday gatherings, and maintaining relationships (DiLeonardo, 1992). The work of maintaining kinship ties takes both time and skill and is difficult to delegate to other people. Caregiving husbands, therefore, more frequently experience declines in contact with family and friends. Maintaining social involvement appears to be especially important for husbands who have been in a caregiver role for longer periods of time, with evidence suggesting that husband caregivers who are less satisfied with their social participation report the highest levels of strain (Kramer, 1997). But even for women, the initial advantages of larger support networks disappear if the husband's escalating care needs isolate the wife caregivers and impede their ability to fulfill expectations for reciprocity that characterize informal networks (Wright & Aquilino, 1998).

Impact on Financial Resources

Since out-of-pocket expenses are drawn from a common pool, husbands and wives share the economic costs of care. However, the financial impact of a spouse's care needs is a cost more often borne by wives, at least in the long run, since wives usually outlive their husbands. Husbands who are receiving care are more often distressed over the future financial impact of their illness on their wives, since husbands are more likely than wives to have internalized responsibility for providing economically for their families. Particularly in current cohorts of elderly men, providing for their families was an important way in which men fulfilled their perceived gender role.

Caregiving responsibilities can discourage labor force participation, particularly for older wives (Szinovacz & Davey, 2004). For many older women, leaving the work force to care for a husband during his final illness amounts to early retirement, especially given the low probability of reemployment among older workers (Szinovacz & Davey, 2005). Early exit from the labor force results not only in lost wages but also in the opportunity to develop higher earnings profiles and subsequent retirement benefits (Johnson & Lo Sasso, 2000).

Differences in Coping Resources

Coping resources and strategies can moderate the negative impact of caregiving stress. Wives tend to have larger informal networks at the onset of caregiving than do husbands, but this initial advantage in network support can also be diminished by their greater tendency to limit social involvement as caregiving demands escalate (Navaie-Walier et al., 2002). Women are also more likely than men to increase involvement in religious activities as a strategy for dealing with caregiving challenges (Neal, Ingersoll-Dayton, & Starrels, 1997; Picot, Debanne, Namazi, & Wykle, 1997), and several studies have identified both physical and mental health benefits of religious coping among diverse groups of caregivers (Haley et al., 2004).

Some evidence suggests that women use less effective coping strategies than men, particularly for stresses involving family problems and negative events in their social networks (Yee & Schulz, 2000). They are more likely to rely on emotion-based strategies such as escape avoidance coping—that is, relying on wishful thinking, selective ignoring, and behavioral efforts to avoid the problem (Rose, Strauss, Neundorfer, Smyth, & Stuckey, 1997). Wives tend to internalize responsibility for their husband's safety and well-being, and therefore have more difficulty setting limits, are less likely to leave their husbands alone, and are more likely to feel engulfed in caregiving. Caregiving stress is also negatively related to self-care behaviors (Haley et al., 2004), and there is some evidence that wife caregivers are less likely than husband caregivers to maintain appropriate self-care and preventive health behaviors, including finding time to exercise, rest when sick, and take medications (Burton, Newsom, Schulz, Hirsch, & German, 1997).

Husbands exhibit greater reliance on instrumental or problem-solving coping strategies (Kramer, 1997). These strategies are more effective in coping with interpersonal problems, financial problems, and health-related problems (Barusch & Spaid, 1989) and contribute to greater personal efficacy and positive affect (Kramer, 1997). Husband caregivers are more likely than wives to conceptualize caregiving as "work" and to adopt a task-oriented, care management orientation. They are more likely than women "to 'do caregiving' by compartmentalizing and by avoiding the experience of being swallowed by the caregiving situation" (Thompson, 2002, p. 34). Although their management approach to spousal care is sometimes dismissed as uncaring, this strategy provides greater perceived control, feelings of self-efficacy, and protection from the intense stress and burnout that often characterize wife caregivers (Szabo & Strang, 1999). However, too much emphasis on the work of care can be a symptom of strain. Men are more likely than women to hide negative emotions and to mask grief and anger by immersing themselves in activity (Kramer, 2002). Men are also more likely to exhibit excess anger (e.g., starting fights, driving aggressively) or to use alcohol or other drugs as a coping strategy (Gwyther, 1990; Kramer, 1997). Furthermore, there is some evidence that instrumental problem-focused strategies favored by men are associated with more positive outcomes than the emotion-focused coping that is more prevalent among women (Kramer, 1997). Emotional responses provide at best temporary relief, whereas more proactive problem-focused strategies reinforce feelings of mastery and control (Seltzer, Greenberg, & Kravss, 1995).

OTHER SOURCES OF VARIATION IN THE EXPERIENCE OF SPOUSE CAREGIVERS

In addition to recognizing differences between husbands and wives, it is essential to emphasize variation among husbands and variation among wives. Research describing families has deconstructed the image of "The American Family," pointing instead to the diversity of family experiences across social class, ethnicity, nature of disability, duration of marriage, and age/cohort differences.

Social Class

The well-established link between socioeconomic resources and health means that economically advantaged older couples enter old age with fewer health problems and more resources than their more privileged counterparts (O'Rand, 1996; Ross & Wu, 1996). Middle- and upper-class couples are able to supplement spousal caregiving through purchasing additional services—outsourcing some of the domestic production or care responsibilities—when they need more assistance than a spouse can provide. More affluent younger couples already demonstrate higher levels of this type of outsourcing to assist in child care (Blair-Loy, 2003), so it is likely that at least some will continue this pattern when they encounter frailty in late life.

Ethnicity

Gerontologists are beginning to understand the impact of ethnicity on the experience of family care. European American elders are more likely to rely on spouses for long-term care. Spouses account for 28% of the caregivers of White elders, 20% of Hispanic elders, and 15% of African American elders (Quadagno, 2005).

A number of studies have found that African American caregivers tend to exhibit lower levels of stress, burden, and depression than other groups of caregivers—a difference that has been attributed to cultural meanings attached to caregiving, cultural differences in support resources, and faith and religion as a way of coping with burden (Haley et al., 2004; Janevic & McConnell, 2001). African Americans are more likely to turn to informal supports and prayer and to use more effective coping strategies, including positive appraisals, reframing the situation in positive terms, and deriving higher levels of day-to-day meaning from caregiving (Dilworth-Anderson, Williams, & Cooper, 1999; Farran, Miller, Kaufman, Donner, & Fogg, 1999; Janevic & McConnell, 2001).

Gerontologists and policymakers have long assumed that African American families were advantaged in informal network resources, but more recent evidence indicates that these networks can demand more support than they provide and often diminish when members can no longer fulfill reciprocity obligations. Rochelle (1997) warns that continuing structural, economic, and social discrimination has begun to erode traditional networks of African Americans. Few studies, however, have explored differences between African American husbands and wives, despite evidence that the gendered division of household labor is more flexible in African American than in White households (McAdoo, 1986).

Nature of Illness or Disability

The experience of spousal caregiving varies with the nature of the care recipient's disability (Townsend & Franks, 1997; Wright & Aquilino, 1998). In general, cognitive impairment generates greater stress than physical impairment, especially for wives (Hooker et al., 2000). Cognitive impairment can result in personality changes that strain relationships, and indeed destroy the foundation of long-lasting relationships. Although physical impairment requires spouses to learn new roles and redefine aspects of their relationship, both partners can participate in this renegotiation if social skills remain intact. Balanced exchanges in emotional support reduce burden and increase marital satisfaction among caregiving wives when their husbands experience low to moderate levels of disability but are less effective at higher levels of impairment, when the demands of caregiving dominate everyday life (Wright & Aquilino, 1998).

For conditions with a gradual onset, spouses have an opportunity to learn new skills gradually (Davidson et al., 2000). Furthermore, the impaired spouse can continue to handle some of his or her responsibilities. Such arrangements not only reduce the workload of the caregiving spouse but also enhance the self-esteem of the care recipient.

Duration of Marriage

Duration of marriage can moderate the experience of spousal caregiving. Evidence suggests that wives in second or third marriages express greater burden in caregiving than wives facing a husband's illness or disability after many years of marriage. The age gap between husbands and wives increases with subsequent marriages, and middle-aged wives caring for very old husbands encounter the added stress associated with negative events that occur "off time"—that is, at unexpected stages of the life cycle (Gwyther, 1990).

Interpreting Age Differences

There is some evidence that younger caregivers report greater disruptions in schedules and role strain than older caregivers. Nijboer and colleagues (2000) suggest that younger caregivers may experience more secondary role strains involving work and social activities or that older spouses may more easily accept responsibilities that are anticipated at their stage of life. We need to exercise caution when considering age differences in the experience of spouse caregivers and in generalizing the experiences of today's older couples to future cohorts. For example, marriage rates are lower among baby boomers than among previous generations, and, among baby boomers who marry, divorce rates are high in comparison to previous cohorts (Easterlin, 1996). These trends will affect the availability of spouses as potential caregivers as baby boomers move into late life.

The distinction between age and cohort is a central dimension of the life course perspective, which directs our attention to the powerful connection between individual lives and the historical context in which these lives unfold (O'Rand & Henretta, 1998). Most research on elderly caregivers examines the experiences of people born during the first third of the twentieth century. Future cohorts of spouse caregivers will have experienced a different historical period. Two-earner families are increasingly prevalent at all stages of the family life cycle and at all social locations, although changes in the division of domestic labor are occurring more slowly. More parents are relying on formal help or commercial substitutes for housework and child care. While women retain responsibility for domestic production, the growing gap between the rich and poor has enabled affluent women to relieve themselves of some aspects of domestic work by becoming managers of domestic work done by other women (Cole, 1986). Care must be taken that the experiences of current cohorts of spouse caregivers not constrain the research questions posed by investigators in the coming decades.

PRACTICE IMPLICATIONS

Research on spousal caregiving suggests some specific practice guidelines for supporting spouse caregivers. Some guidelines address the spouse's role in the caregiving situation, and others address differences between husbands and wives.

First, the quality of the marital relationship is an important predictor of caregiving outcomes. Problems in the relationship between husbands and wives spill over into the caregiving experience, a finding that highlights the ongoing need to help couples to alleviate care-related stresses as well as addressing longstanding conflicts. Old conflicts often resurface around caregiving demands and can aggravate negative consequences for both the care provider and care recipient. In contrast, women in high-quality relationships report more positive outcomes in providing care to a disabled spouse (Yee & Schulz, 2000). Assessing communication patterns and exchanges of support between husbands and wives will enhance providers' ability to counsel caregiving couples (Dorfman, Holmes, & Berlin, 1996).

Second, family caregiving is a normative stage of the family life cycle, not an indicator of family pathology. Family caregivers view themselves as competent adults seeking personally relevant solutions to problems in living. Wives caring for an impaired husband could benefit from accessible and affordable respite services designed to alleviate the demands of routine household tasks (Rose-Rego et al., 1998). They are more likely to seek and adhere to professional advice if caregivers are treated as consumers who need more information to make informed decisions rather than as patients or clients who need "treatment" (Gwyther, 1990). This appears to be especially true of husband caregivers.

From a programmatic perspective, men have long been underrepresented in interventions designed to assist caregivers, even considering their lower prevalence in the caregiving population (DeVries, Hamilton, Lovett, & Gallagher-Thompson, 1997), a pattern that Kramer (2002) attributes to the gendered nature of most caregiving interventions. Many programs focus on sharing and expressing feelings, an approach that tends to be more attractive to women than to men. Women are more likely than men to make use of support help lines or support groups. Programs for men caregivers are likely to be more successful when they emphasize educational interventions and information relevant to specific caregiving problems (Thompson, 2002). Men are more likely to respond to labels such as "seminar" or "forum" and focus on training for instrumental tasks and strategies for maintaining social involvement (Kramer, 1997).

Research on spousal caregiving can guide the content of interventions aimed at husbands and wives caring for an ill or disabled partner. In designing programs for spouse caregivers, Quadagno (2005) emphasizes the importance of teaching clients how to accept help and set limits, maintain healthy life-styles, and take time for relaxing and pursuing pleasurable activities. Such programs need to address strategies for managing multiple responsibilities (often with additional assistance), for giving oneself permission to take time away from caregiving, and for developing more effective coping styles (Rose et al., 1997). Recognizing differences between husbands and wives can assist service providers in emphasizing gender-specific concerns. Whereas some programs—such as support groups—focus on the caregiver, others can involve both caregivers and care recipients. For example, in addition to teaching wives about financial management, husbands can be encouraged to explain the techniques they have employed in handling family resources. This example also sensitizes us to the impact of social class differences. While portfolio management is a concern for affluent families, other couples struggle to meet everyday expenses.

As Burton and colleagues (2003) emphasize, designing appropriate educational programs and other interventions benefits caregivers by alleviating or moderating the impact of burden and it helps their impaired spouses, who may otherwise be left without their primary source of assistance. Evidence-based practice that recognizes characteristics of the spousal relationship, as well as the ways in which gender and other dimensions of diversity shape this relationship, will be most likely to enhance the ability of the couple to manage disease and disability while maintaining for as long as possible the quality of the relationship.

REFERENCES

Allen, S. M. (1994). Gender differences in spousal caregiving and unmet need for care. *Journals of Gerontology: Social Sciences, 49,* 187–195.

Allen, S. M., & Webster, P. S. (2001). When wives get sick: Gender role attitudes, marital happiness and husbands' contribution to household labor. *Gender & Society, 15,* 898–916.

Altschuler, J. (2004). Meaning of housework and other unpaid responsibilities among older women. *Journal of Women and Aging, 16,* 143–159.

Amberg, B., Jansson, W., Grafstrom, M., et al. (1998). Differences between and within genders in caregiving strain: A comparison between caregivers of demented and non-caregivers of non-demented elderly people. *Journal of Advanced Nursing, 28,* 849–858.

Barusch, A. S., & Spaid, W. M. (1989). Gender differences in caregiving: Why do wives report greater burden? *The Gerontologist, 29,* 667–676.

Blair-Loy, M. (2003). *Competing devotions: Career and family among women executives.* Cambridge, MA: Harvard University Press.

Burton, L. C., Newsom, J. T., Schulz, R., Hirsch, C. H., & German, P. (1997). Preventive health behaviors among spousal caregivers. *Preventive Medicine, 26,* 162–169.

Burton, L. C., Zdaniuk, B., Schulz, R., Jackson, S., & Hirsch, C. (2003). Transitions in spousal caregiving. *The Gerontologist, 43,* 230–241.

Chappell, N. L., & Kuehne, V. K. (1998). Congruence among husband and wife caregivers. *Journal of Aging Studies, 12,* 239–254.

Cole, J. (1986). *All American women: Lines that divide, ties that bind.* New York: Free Press.

Davidson, K., Arber, S., & Ginn, J. (2000). Gendered meanings of care work within late life marital relationships. *Canadian Journal on Aging, 29,* 536–553.

DeVries, H. M., Hamilton, D. W., Lovett, S., & Gallagher-Thompson, D. (1997). Patterns of coping preferences for male and female caregivers of frail older adults. *Psychology and Aging, 12,* 263–267.

DiLeonardo, M. (1992). The female world of cards and holidays: Women and families and work of kinship. In B. Thorne & M. Yalom (Eds.), *Rethinking the family.* Boston: Northeastern University Press.

Dilworth-Anderson, P., Williams, S. W., & Cooper, T. (1999). Family caregiving to elderly African Americans: Caregiver types and structures. *Journals of Gerontology: Social Sciences, 54B,* 237–241.

Dorfman, L. T., Holmes, C. A., & Berlin, K. L. (1996). Wife caregivers of frail elderly veterans: Correlates of caregiving satisfaction and caregiver strain. *Family Relations, 45,* 46–55.

Easterlin, R. (1996). Economic and social implications of demographic patterns. In R. Binstock & L. K. George (Eds.), *Handbook of aging and the social sciences* (pp. 73–93). San Diego, CA: Academic Press.

Farran, C. J., Miller, B. H., Kaufman, J. E., Donner, E., & Fogg, L. (1999). Finding meaning through caregiving: Development of an instrument for family caregivers of persons with Alzheimer's disease. *Journal of Clinical Psychology, 55,* 1107–1125.

Franks, M., & Stephens, M. A. P. (1996). Social support in the context of caregiving: Husbands' provision of support to wives involved in parent care. *Journal of Gerontology, 51,* 43–52.

George, L. K., & Gwyther, L. P. (1986). Caregivers for dementia patients: Complex determinants of well-being and burden. *The Gerontologist, 26,* 253–259.

Gwyther, L. P. (1990). Letting-go: Separation-individuation in a wife of an Alzheimer's patient. *The Gerontologist, 30,* 698–702.

Haley, W. E., Gitlin, L. N., Wisniewski, S. R., Mahoney, D. F., Coon, D. W., Winter, L., Corcoran, M., Schinfeld, S., & Ory, M. (2004). Well-being, appraisal, and coping in African-American and Caucasian dementia caregivers: Findings from the REACH study. *Aging & Mental Health, 8,* 316–329.

Hooker, K., Manoogian-O'Dell, M., Monahan, D. J., Frazier, L. D., & Shifren, K. (2000). Does type of disease matter? Gender differences among Alzheimer's and Parkinson's disease spouse caregivers. *The Gerontologist, 40,* 568–573.

Ingersoll-Dayton, B., & Raschick, M. (2004). Relationship between care-recipient behaviors and spousal caregiving stress. *The Gerontologist, 44,* 318–327.

Janevic, M. R., & McConnell, C. M. (2001). Racial, ethnic and cultural differences in the dementia caregiving experience: Recent findings. *The Gerontologist, 41,* 334–347.

Jansson, W., Norberg, G., & Grafstrom, M. (2001). Patterns of elderly spousal caregiving in dementia care: An observational study. *Journal of Advanced Nursing, 34,* 804–812.

Johnson, R. W., & Lo Sasso, A. T. (2000). *The trade-off between hours of paid employment and time assistance to elderly parents at midlife.* Washington, DC: Urban Institute.

Kramer, B. J. (1997). Differential predictors of strain and gain among husbands caring for wives with dementia. *The Gerontologist, 37,* 239–249.

Kramer, B. J. (2002). Husbands caring for wives with dementia: A longitudinal study of continuity and change. *Health and Social Work, 25,* 97–107.

Kramer, B. J., & Kipnis, S. (1995). Eldercare and work-role conflict: Toward an understanding of gender differences in caregiver burden. *The Gerontologist, 35,* 340–348.

Kramer, B. J., & Lambert, J. D. (1999). Caregiving as life course transition among older husbands: A prospective study. *The Gerontologist, 39,* 658–667.

Lobo-Prahbu, S., Molinari, V., Arlinghaus, K., Barr, E., & Lomax, J. (2005). Spouses of patients with dementia: How do they stay together "till death do us part"? *Journal of Gerontological Social Work, 44,* 161–174.

Mak, W. W. (2005). Integrative model of caregiving: How macro and micro factors affect caregivers of adults with severe and persistent mental illness. *American Journal of Orthopsychiatry, 75,* 40–53.

Marks, N. F., Lambert, J. D., & Choi, H. (2002). Transitions to caregiving, gender and psychological well-being: A prospective U.S. national study. *Journal of Marriage and the Family, 64,* 657–667.

Martire, L. M., Stephens, M. A. P., Druley, J. A., & Wojno, W. C. (2002). Negative reactions to received spousal care: Predictors and consequences of miscarried support. *Health Psychology, 21,* 167–176.

McAdoo, H. (1986). Societal stress: The Black family. In J. Cole (Ed.), *All American women: Lines that divide, ties that bind* (pp. 187–197). New York: Free Press.

Miller, B. (1987). Gender and control among spouses of the cognitively impaired: A research note. *The Gerontologist, 27,* 447–453.

Miller, B., & Cafasso, L. (1992). Gender differences in caregiving: Fact or artifact? *The Gerontologist, 332,* 498–507.

Miller, B., & Montgomery, A. (1990). Family caregivers and limitations in social activities. *Research on Aging, 12,* 72–93.

Mui, A. C. (1995). Caring for frail elderly parents: A comparison of adult sons and daughters. *The Gerontologist, 35,* 86–93.

Navaie-Walier, M., Spriggs, A., & Feldman, P. H. (2002). Informal caregiving: Differential experiences by gender. *Medical Care, 40,* 1249–1259.

Navon, L., & Weinblatt, N. (1996). "The show must go on": Behind the scenes of elderly spousal caregiving. *Journal of Aging Studies, 10,* 329–342.

Neal, M. B., Ingersoll-Dayton, B., & Starrels, M. E. (1997). Gender and relationship differences in caregiving patterns and consequences among employed caregivers. *The Gerontologist, 37,* 804–816.

Nijboer, C., Triemstra, M., Tempelaar, R., Mulder, M., Sanderman, R., & van den Bos, G. (2000). Patterns of caregiver experiences among partners of cancer patients. *The Gerontologist, 40,* 738–746.

O'Rand, A. M. (1996). The precious and the precocious: Understanding cumulative dis/advantage over the life course. *The Gerontologist, 36,* 230–238.

O'Rand, A. M., & Henretta, J. C. (1998). Age and inequality: Diverse pathways through later life. Boulder, CO: Westview Press.

Picot, S. J., Debanne, S. M., Namazi, K. J., & Wykle, M. L. (1997). Rewards, costs and coping of African American caregivers. *Nursing Research, 44,* 147–152.

Pruchno, R. A., & Resch, N. L. (1989). Husbands and wives as caregivers: Antecedents of depression and burden. *The Gerontologist, 29,* 159–165.

Quadagno, J. (2005). *Aging and the life course* (3rd ed.). Boston: McGraw-Hill.

Rochelle, A. (1997). *No more kin: Exploring race, class, and gender in family networks.* Thousand Oaks, CA: Sage.

Rose, S. K., Strauss, M. E., Neundorfer, M. M., Smyth, K. A., & Stuckey, J. C. (1997). The relationship of self-restraint and distress to coping among spouses caring for persons with Alzheimer's disease. *Journal of Applied Gerontology, 16,* 91–103.

Rose-Rego, S. K., Strauss, M. E., & Smyth, K. A. (1998). Differences in the perceived well-being of wives and husbands caring for persons with Alzheimer's disease. *The Gerontologist, 38,* 224–230.

Ross, C., & Wu, C. (1996). Education, age, and the cumulative advantage in health. *Journal of Health and Social Behavior, 37,* 104–120.

Seltzer, M. M., Greenberg, J. S., & Krauss, M. W. (1995). A comparison of coping strategies of aging mothers of adults with mental-illness or mental-retardation. *Psychology and Aging, 10,* 64–75.

Seltzer, M. M., & Li, L. W. (2000). The dynamics of caregiving: Transitions during a three-year prospective study. *The Gerontologist, 40,* 165–178.

Solomon, C., Acock, A., & Walker, A. (2004). Gender ideology and investment in housework: Postretirement change. *Journal of Family Issues, 25,* 1050–1071.

Stoller, E. (1992). Gender differences in the experiences of caregiving spouses. In J. W. Dwyer & R. T. Coward (Eds.), *Gender, families and elder care* (pp. 49–64). Newbury Park, CA: Sage.

Szabo, V., & Strang, V. (1999). Experiencing control in caregiving. *Image: Journal of Nursing Scholarship, 31,* 71–75.

Szinovacz, M. E., & Davey, A. (2004). Retirement transitions and spouse's disability: Effects on depressive symptoms. *Journal of Gerontology: Social Sciences, 59B,* S333–S342.

Szinovacz, M. E., & Davey, A. (2005). Predictors of perceptions of involuntary retirement. *The Gerontologist, 45,* 36–47.

Thompson, E. (2002). What's unique about men's caregiving? In B. Kramer & E. Thompson (Eds.), *Men as caregivers: Theory, research and service implications* (pp. 20–47). New York: Springer.

Townsend, A., & Franks, M. (1997). Quality of the relationship between elderly spouses: Influence on spouse caregivers' subjective effectiveness. *Family Relations, 46,* 33–39.

Wright, D. L., & Aquilino, W. M. (1998). Influence of emotional support exchange in marriage on caregiving wives' burden and marital satisfaction. *Family Relations, 47,* 195–204.

Yee, J. L., & Schulz, R. (2000). Gender differences in psychiatric morbidity among family caregivers: A review and analysis. *The Gerontologist, 40,* 147–164.

Young, R. F., & Kahana, E. (1989). Specifying caregiver outcomes: Gender and relationship aspects of caregiving strain. *The Gerontologist, 29,* 660–666.

CHAPTER SEVEN

Division of Care Among Adult Children[1]

Adam Davey and Maximiliane E. Szinovacz

Adult children play a central role within the family context of care for frail elders. As the preceding chapter by Stoller and Miklowski indicated, older married adults turn first to a spouse for assistance. However, rising divorce rates during the past decades may decrease the availability of spouses as caregivers in the future, and, as the gender gap in longevity closes and more couples age together, both spouses may experience frailty or cognitive decline and thus require support from other family members. After spouses, the next preferred group of potential family caregivers is adult children (Cantor, 1975). Today's cohort of older adults is unique with regard to their high fertility, which produced the baby boom cohorts. As a result, these parents have, on average, more children than generations that precede or follow them. While children of today's older adults tend to have more siblings than older and younger cohorts, they also have more parents who survived into old age than earlier cohorts, and thus more potential occasions to provide care. Both the availability of multiple adult children as potential caregivers and the potential care needs of multiple parents or parents-in-law likely heighten the complexity of care networks and the need to negotiate and navigate multiple relationships, requiring greater coordination of care activities and enhancing opportunities for conflict over the allocation of care responsibilities.

Two recent national studies have examined the involvement of adult children in care for parents. Wolff and Kasper (2006) used data from the 1989 and 1999 National Long-Term Care Surveys to update earlier estimates by Stone, Cafferata, and Sangl (1987) and to provide a national profile of caregivers for frail older adults. These authors used linked data from disabled (defined as having at least one limitation in activities of daily living [ADLs] or instrumental activities of daily living [IADLs] or institutional residence) older adults (ages 65 and older) and their primary informal caregivers. The latter construct was defined as the individual providing the most assistance with personal activities of daily living (or instrumental activities of daily living in the absence of ADLs). According to these data, the estimated number of chronically disabled, community-dwelling older adults increased from 5.3 million in 1989 to 5.6 million in 1999. Interestingly, they found that 29.5% (22.3% in 1989) of disabled older adults reported receiving no human help. Between 1989 and 1999, adult children replaced spouses as the most common primary caregivers (an increase from 35.9% to 41.3% of primary caregivers). Nearly three-quarters (76.5% in 1989 and 73.3% in 1999) of adult child caregivers were women, but the proportion of sons as primary caregivers increased over this time. Adult children also had the highest rates of employment among all caregivers. Finally, just under half of adult children (less than one-third in 1989) were sole caregivers.

As large as these numbers are, they are much lower than those reported in another nationally representative survey that relied on a somewhat different methodology. A study by the National Alliance for Caregiving and AARP (2004) collected data from 1,247 caregivers among a larger sample of 6,139 individuals contacted. Extrapolating to the U.S. population suggests that fully 16% of the population, or more than 33 million individuals, provide care to someone 50 years of age or older. This study found that 44% of caregivers to an older adult reported providing assistance to a parent. As well, 37% indicated that they were the sole caregiver during the past 12 months. Of those who were not the sole caregiver, 68% said that another helper was an adult child of the care recipient. There was also considerable evidence of a preference for same-sex care, with 35% of men providing care to a man versus 28% of women. It should be noted that there are many more women than men who receive care. Finally, 30% of caregivers reported providing assistance to more than one individual.

Part of the wide discrepancy between the estimates in these two studies is due to the time frame considered. Eligibility to be considered a caregiver in Wolff and Kasper's study (2006) required provision of assistance within the previous week, whereas the time frame for the National Alliance study encompassed the past 12 months. Although participation in caregiving is dynamic, this alone cannot entirely account for the difference. Definitional issues are also important. The definition of caregiving was limited to assistance to individuals 65 and older with personal and instrumental activities of daily living in the former study but was defined more broadly—including help with household chores, finances, outside services, and visits—in the latter study, in which older adults were considered to be 50 years and older. Both studies, however, suggest considerable involvement of adult children in care for older parents and present largely similar estimates of the characteristics of adult child caregivers.

In their review of the predictors of instrumental assistance between generations, Davey, Janke, and Savla (2005) called for greater recognition that the family is often the most central context in which to consider intergenerational support networks. Yet much of the previous literature on family caregiving has focused on identification of a primary caregiver—the person who provides the most support to an older adult or who bears primary responsibility for coordination of care efforts (Stone et al., 1987; Wolff & Kasper, 2006). The issue of who becomes a primary caregiver is interesting in itself, but as a result the caregiving literature largely overlooks the role of family history and family context. More importantly, a focus on the primary caregiver directs attention away from the secondary and supportive roles that families as systems provide in sustaining older adults in the community. Emphasis on the family context implies a set of research questions that are only rarely considered when the focus is exclusively on the primary caregiver. What factors determine whether specific children provide assistance to parents in times of need? How commonly are multiple children or their spouses involved in care? How much stability and change is there in care networks over time, and what predicts change in caregivers over time? What are the implications of changes in these care networks for caregiver well-being?

This chapter on the division of care among adult children is organized into three main sections. The first section considers research on multiple children as caregivers within the same family. The second section focuses on the division of care for parents and parents-in-law between spouses. The final section presents some new data regarding the implications of changes in care networks for caregiver well-being.

ADULT CHILDREN AS CAREGIVERS

A variety of conceptual approaches have been used to understand children's involvement in parent care. Parental need for assistance is central in both economic and behavioral health care utilization models (Stark, 1995). Other common constraints include the opportunity costs associated with providing care, the potential to substitute one form of assistance for another (see the chapter by Johnson in this volume), reciprocity for previous help and relationship quality (Henretta, Hill, Li, Soldo, & Wolf, 1997; Silverstein, Conroy, Wang, Giarusso, & Bengtson, 2002;

Whitbeck, Hoyt, & Huck, 1994), as well as constraints on time (Johnson & Lo Sasso, 2000; Sarkisian & Gerstel, 2004), and what Campbell and Martin-Matthews (2003) refer to as "legitimate excuses" and "caring by default." A complex set of factors, then, determine the likelihood of care, and they include paid employment and other care obligations such as for dependent children and other living parents and parents-in-law. In addition to parents' care needs and constraints, other characteristics of the care situation, such as coresidence, are also important, as are the care recipients' and caregivers' resources to obtain alternative supports (Coward & Dwyer, 1991; Engers & Stern, 2002; Wolf, Freedman, & Soldo, 1997).

Involvement of Multiple Children as Caregivers

As the national profiles cited above indicate, care for most older adults involves assistance from more than one individual. This potential for involvement of multiple caregivers has not been well represented in the literature to date, although there are notable exceptions (e.g., Johnson & Lo Sasso, 2000; Wolf et al., 1997; Wong, Kitayama, & Soldo, 1999).

Matthews (1987) was one of the first researchers to conceptualize the family as the primary caregiver and to examine the distribution of assistance within the family as a result. She considered families in which at least one parent was 75 years of age or older and living in the community and that had at least two daughters, both of whom were interviewed. A further requirement was that at least one daughter had to be employed. Several important insights emerged from the findings. First, siblings often disagreed regarding the relative efforts of themselves and their siblings, a finding that is echoed by more recent quantitative studies (e.g., Pillemer & Suitor, 2006; Suitor & Pillemer, 2007). Systematic exploration of the nature and implications of these perceptual biases have important implications, especially in recent nationally representative studies such as the Health and Retirement Study (HRS), in which a single informant provides information for many family members. A second theme that emerged from Matthews's work was that family structure (i.e., number of siblings, gender composition) has implications for how care is divided among siblings. While suggesting that important differences are likely to be present, this study cannot provide general guidance, because the research design (limited to families with at least two daughters) precludes more general inferences. Another important implication of this study is that it suggests that the way in which care is divided does not directly predict its perceived adequacy. Of course, it is just as likely that a specific arrangement is selected to achieve adequate support for an older parent.

In related analyses from the same data set, Matthews and Rosner (1988) identified five primary parent care styles among adult siblings, considered as individual patterns of involvement rather than family constellations of support. Routine assistance reflected regular ongoing assistance provided as part of the sibling's routine. Backup assistance was support provided on an intermittent basis, reliably elicited as needed. Circumscribed assistance was limited in scope but provided predictably and reliably, subject to clear expectations. Sporadic assistance is provided at a sibling's convenience and is not typically coordinated with support provided by the other siblings. This lack of integration was not necessarily problematic, however. Finally, dissociation reflected siblings who were reliably uninvolved in assistance to parents.

Matthews and Rosner (1988) also identified several factors associated with a particular child's style of involvement. Circumscribed, sporadic, and dissociative styles were less prevalent among families with only two daughters. Larger sibships promoted greater diversity in the patterns of assistance, often with some siblings taking primary roles and others serving more supportive or auxiliary functions. Gender differences also emerged, with sons more likely to exhibit the less involved patterns of assistance. Even when sons are involved, their efforts may be secondary to a lone daughter who assumes primary responsibility or be seen to be less important than those of daughters by both siblings (Matthews, 1995). Efforts of sons also may be directed toward fostering parents' independence to a greater extent than support from daughters and daughters-in-law (Matthews & Heidorn, 1998). Factors related to family ties and birth order were also implicated, but the patterns were not simple ones. In some families, more responsibility fell on oldest siblings, and in others a favorite child emerged.

These qualitative observations agree well with recent quantitative investigations that show that unobserved heterogeneity may be present in within-family models and that caregiving decisions of adult children are interdependent, suggesting the importance of unmeasured variables in differentiating patterns of support across different families (Checkovich & Stern, 2002; Suitor & Pillemer, 2007; Wong et al., 1999). This should not be surprising given the extent to which roles within support networks appear to be negotiated (Finch & Mason, 1993).

A number of extrafamilial influences also appeared to affect a particular sibling's style of assistance, also suggestive of considerable heterogeneity. Several factors were important. Geographic proximity can limit the ability of a sibling to be involved in hands-on assistance, but there are also endogeneity considerations. Employment status poses time constraints but also contributes additional financial resources. The presence of a spouse can pose a competing tie or obligation, but spouses also can serve as a support for care responsibilities. Overall, then, while pointing to factors of potential influence on individual and sibling patterns of assistance, the direction of influence of particular factors is not always clear-cut. Nevertheless, both qualitative and quantitative studies suggest that a focus on primary caregivers misrepresents the structure and important features of care networks.

Assistance by Multiple Children in the Same Family

Previous research has adopted a variety of approaches to the study of care networks for older adults. Some studies have focused, for example, on the diverse composition of care networks, often including multiple individuals and spanning several generations of caregivers (Dilworth-Anderson, Williams, & Gibson, 2002; Ingersoll-Dayton, Neal, Ha, & Hammer, 2003; Orel & Dupuy, 2002; Szinovacz, 2003; Wolf et al., 1997). Focusing on a single (usually primary) caregiver is insufficient to capture informal care as it most often occurs.

Other studies have focused on the decision by family members to participate in care and predictors of the extent of their involvement in care (Caron, Griffith, & Arcand, 2005; Henretta et al., 1997; Marks, 1996; McGarry & Schoeni, 1997; Wolf et al., 1997). Because they consider caregivers at a specific point in time, they capture diverse caregivers at different stages of the caregiving career (Aneshensel, Pearlin, Mullan, Zarit, & Whitlatch, 1995). As a result, these studies confound factors predicting the care entries and exits of specific adult children with factors that predict whether any adult child participates in parent care. These studies also tend to over-represent individuals involved in care for a longer time period who are likely to differ from caregivers who are involved for shorter periods of time.

Qualitative and quantitative inquiries focusing on how care decisions are negotiated among adult children (Finch & Mason, 1993; Hequembourg & Brallier, 2005; Matthews, 1992) have shown that adult children's participation in care derives from a combination of factors, including normatively founded negotiations among adult-child siblings based on perceived filial responsibility, each child's ability and willingness to provide care, structural characteristics of the entire sibling network, and parent's characteristics (Finch & Mason, 1993; Henretta et al., 1997; Laditka & Laditka, 2001; Marks, 1996; McGarry & Schoeni, 1997; Wolf et al., 1997). On balance, these studies demonstrate clear gender differences, with daughters more involved in care than sons (Henretta et al., 1997; Wolf et al., 1997). Similarly, children with more competing obligations or greater care costs—such as those who are married, employed, or live farther away from parents—tend to be less involved in care (see chapters by Johnson and by Silverstein, Conroy, & Gans in this volume). These studies show that characteristics of one's siblings affect one's own likelihood of involvement in care. Individuals with sisters tend to provide less assistance, although parents experience a net benefit in overall support from having more children available (Wolf et al., 1997).

Another group of studies focused not on actual care provided but rather on expectations of care. Pillemer and Suitor (2006) used a within-family design to investigate characteristics of adult children that are associated with mothers' expectations of assistance. They considered four sets of predictor variables, including similarity between mothers and children, emotional closeness, past patterns of intergenerational exchanges, and the children's availability in terms of residential proximity and other responsibilities or commitments. Among their Boston-area sample of 566 individuals between 65 and 75 years of age, daughters and children to whom the mother felt closer were the most likely expected source of support. Children who lived farther away and who were employed were somewhat less likely to be selected; there was some evidence for expectations of continuity of support. However, neither marital nor parental status was a significant predictor of expected support.

An interesting pair of studies by Lawrence, Goodnow, Woods, and Karantzas (2002) examined the importance of gender, work, marital, and parental roles on how older adults would ideally allocate a variety of care tasks. Their approach involved perceptions of hypothetical care situations and was experimental in nature. Daughters were generally assigned more tasks than sons; however, gender differences were diminished when additional information was provided regarding other commitments. As well, they found that the match between parent and child gender was particularly important for some tasks, such as bathing. In general, employment status was a more important consideration than either marital or parental status.

There is also evidence of distinctions among biological and stepchildren as potential care providers. Using a vignette approach, Ganong and Coleman (2006) found that stepparents acquired later in life were not deemed true family members so that norms of filial obligation did not apply. Consequently, responses to the question of whether adult children should help parents with ADLs were considerably more favorable for biological parents than for stepparents. Furthermore, those who expressed some obligation toward helping stepparents did so either as a support to the biological parent (helping the biological parent care for the stepparent) or contingent on past relationship history.

Whereas studies on adult-child caregivers have focused on adult-child and parent characteristics that predict assumption of care, most longitudinal studies emphasized transitions between informal and formal care (Kelman, Thomas, & Tanaka, 1994; Lyons, Zarit, & Townsend, 2000; Miller & McFall, 1991; Stoller, 1990). Although the general type of care provided (formal versus informal) tends to be relatively stable, some changes in network composition over time did occur. For example, networks have been shown to shift toward greater involvement of women in care over time (Stoller, 1990). Other longitudinal research has focused on "caregiving careers" or "trajectories," usually with an emphasis on duration and intensity (Andrieu et al., 2005; Seltzer & Li, 2000) or caregiver well-being (Aneshensel et al., 1995; Gaugler, Davey, Pearlin, & Zarit, 2000; Lawton, Moss, Hoffman, & Perkinson, 2000; Seltzer & Li, 2000). These studies have tended to focus on changes within individuals rather than adopting an emphasis on the entire care network. As a result, they capture only part of the change in care over time.

Limited research is available with a focus on changes in specific caregivers. A study by Jette, Tennstedt, and Branch (1992) found that approximately one-quarter of their sample experienced a change in the primary caregiver over a 4-year period. When changes occurred, they most often reflected shifts from a spouse to an adult child, or from one adult child to another, and were most common when the caregiver and care recipient lived separately. Another study focused on beginning or ending care by adult children (Dwyer, Henretta, Coward, & Barton, 1992). Adult children who assumed the caregiving role were more likely to be younger, daughters, unmarried, live proximally, and not involved in full-time employment. Adult children who stopped providing care, on the other hand, were more likely to be sons, to have become married, and not live proximally. This study also considered characteristics of the entire sibling network, and found that one child's transitions affected the transitions of the other siblings, making it difficult to differentiate between changes in care and changes in responsibilities. These findings do suggest, however, the importance of considering the entire care network for understanding care provided by specific individuals.

Changes in Adult-Child Caregiver Networks

Although older adults typically have more than one child, we still know little about what predicts children's involvement in care to parents, and little research has characterized the structure, emergence, and stability of these care networks. Szinovacz and Davey (2007) used longitudinal data from the HRS to examine the extent of change in adult-child care networks, as well as factors associated with these changes.

Nearly half (43.2%) of all parents received care from an adult child at some point during the 8-year period covered by this study, and this proportion differed by parent's gender and whether the parent was alive for the entire period. Over half of mothers who died received care from adult children, compared with nearly one-quarter of fathers, with between 14% and 22% receiving care in any wave. Thus, the risk of becoming a caregiver is cumulative and cross-sectional snapshots considerably underestimate lifetime risk. The size of the adult-child care network differs somewhat for mothers and fathers. In 47% of cases for fathers and 54% of cases for mothers, a single adult child provided assistance. Care from two or three children was more likely for fathers (43%) than mothers (36%), and both mothers and fathers were equally likely (10%) to receive help from four or more children.

We examined changes in adult-child care networks based on the question of whether the respondent or his/her siblings provided care with basic needs such as bathing or dressing a parent since the previous interview.[2] Comparing the participation of each adult child over two waves (2 years), we found that change in any adult-child caregiver occurred in slightly more than half of the care occasions for families including at least two adult children and reporting continuing care over two HRS waves. Change in the primary adult-child caregiver was reported for more than a quarter of care occasions. In 19.9% of all these networks, a child was added to the network; in 21.1%, a child was dropped from the network; and in 13.4% of networks, both adding and dropping of at least one adult child occurred simultaneously over the 2-year period. These data clearly demonstrate the fluidity of adult-child support networks over time.

Although selected parent (e.g., whether the parent can be left alone or died between waves) and child characteristics (e.g., whether they also provided financial aid to a parent) were significant predictors of change, characteristics of the sibling network played an important part as well. Foremost among these characteristics was the number of living siblings, the number of siblings involved in care at time 1, and the gender distribution of the sibling care network. Based on our earlier analyses that controlled for race, socioeconomic context, and selected parent and adult-child characteristics, we estimated the probability of network change for specific care scenarios. The results are shown in Figures 7.1 and 7.2. Both number of living brothers and number of living sisters increase the probability of change in caregivers (Figure 7.1), although the number of sisters is more important. Specifically, in networks with no female adult child, the predicted probability of network change is 41.8% compared to 47.1%, 52.6%, and 57.9% for those with one, two, or three female adult children, respectively. In contrast, change occurs in 51.2% of networks with no male adult children compared to 58.1% for those with three adult male children.

Even more pronounced differences occur when considering both the number of initial caregivers and the gender composition of caregivers

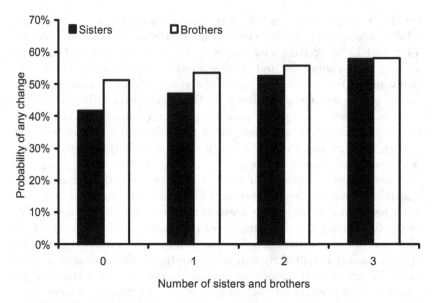

FIGURE 7.1   Predicted probability of change in any caregiver, by number of sisters and brothers. Original calculations based on analyses presented in Szinovacz and Davey (2007).

(Figure 7.2). Network change is more likely as the number of initial care-givers rises (mostly due to dropping of caregivers from the network) and in networks that include men. Considering both characteristics together, we find, for example, that change in caregivers occurred in 45.1% of net-works with a single female caregiver at time 1, but in 55.4% of networks with a single male. If there are three caregivers initially, then the probabil-ity of change rises to 57.6% if there were initially only female caregivers, to 67.3% if there were only male caregivers, and to 72.8% for networks that included both male and female caregivers.

There were systematic differences in how networks changed. The likelihood of adding an adult child to the care network seemed to be en-tirely determined by their availability, because only the number of living sisters and brothers predicted the likelihood of adding adult children to the network. The probability of dropping a sibling from the network was greater in mixed-gender and larger care networks as well as in networks that included married adult children. Exchange of one caregiver for an-other prevailed among networks including sons, among minorities, and among families with multiple living children.

In summary, change in the composition of adult-child care networks appeared to be the norm rather than the exception over the 2-year windows

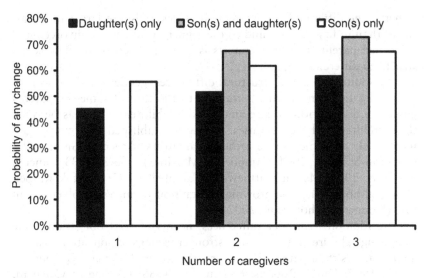

FIGURE 7.2   Predicted probability of change in any caregiver, by initial number of caregivers and gender composition of caregiver network. Original calculations based on analyses presented in Szinovacz and Davey (2007).

studied. To some extent, the possibilities for change are constrained by family structure, with the greater availability of siblings predicting a greater likelihood of change, and networks involving both daughters and sons appear to be more volatile than those involving daughters or sons alone. It is somewhat less common for changes to occur in the adult child providing the most care. When it does occur, it is more common for sons than daughters and in larger sibling networks.

THE GENDER MANDATE OF CARE: SOCIAL STRUCTURE AND NORMS OF FILIAL OBLIGATION

As described in the previous section, the division of care among family members reflects a complex set of factors. One of these factors is the greater involvement of women than men in caregiving. This gender difference evolves from social structural and normative factors. Because women tend to outlive men, and because men tend to marry women who are younger than themselves, women are less likely to have a living spouse to provide care assistance later in life. This suggests that adult children will be more involved in providing assistance to mothers than fathers. Age differences between spouses generally are larger in remarriages than in first unions, and so the higher prevalence of divorced and remarried parents in future cohorts is likely to accentuate these social structural differences.

In addition to social structural differences, gender norms, norms of filial obligation, and norms pertaining to the care of same-sex parents guide the distribution of care among adult children as well as between these children and their spouses. It is well established that women are more likely than men to be primary caregivers (Arber & Ginn, 1991; Calasanti & Slevin, 2001; Campbell & Martin-Matthews, 2003; Cancian & Oliker, 2000; Martin Matthews & Campbell, 1995; Wolff & Kasper, 2006), although there is growing recognition of men's involvement in care (Kramer & Thompson, 2002).

In addition to gender differences, norms of filial obligation guide caregiving. Children typically have stronger feelings of obligation to assist ailing parents than parents-in-law or stepparents (Coleman, Ganong, & Cable, 1997; Finley, Roberts, & Banahan, 1988; Ganong & Coleman, 2006; Lawton, Silverstein, & Bengtson, 1994; Lee, G.R., Peek, & Coward, 1998; Rossi & Rossi, 1990), and the strength of these feelings is an important predictor of how involved they are likely to become in care for a parent (Campbell & Martin-Matthews, 2003; Lee, G.R., et al., 1998; Walker, Pratt, Shin, & Jones, 1990; see also Silverstein et al. in this volume).

A third norm pertains to gender fit of care recipients and caregivers. Same-gender care is favored over cross-gender care. Because more care recipients are women, this norm also drives women into caregiving roles (Campbell & Martin-Matthews, 2003; Cicirelli, 1995).

The interplay of these norms is illustrated in Figure 7.3. Solid arrows indicate assistance to each spouse's own parents in line with norms of filial obligation, whereas dashed lines indicate assistance to the same gender in line with norms of same-gender care. As indicated in the figure, the interplay of both norms favors care for husbands' fathers on the part of husbands and care for wives' mothers on the part of wives. Because fathers tend to be married and receive primary care from their spouses and because gender role norms assign care responsibilities more to women than men, the balance of responsibility for parent care rests more heavily on women than men (Lee, E., Spitze, & Logan, 2003; Shuey & Hardy, 2003; Soldo, Wolf, & Henretta, 1999). However, husbands may be drawn into caregiving to support their caregiving wives. Husbands and wives can also influence one another's behavior. Gerstel and Gallagher (2001) found, for example, that when wives provided more assistance, so did their husbands. In contrast, couples acted most independently when support was most obligatory (i.e., to own parents) or most voluntary (i.e., to friends). This suggests a complementary model rather than one of substitution.

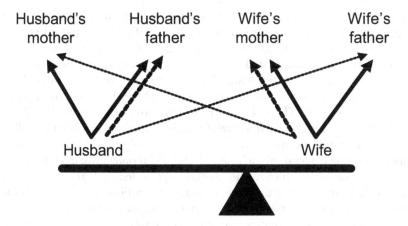

FIGURE 7.3 Gender differences in opportunities for care and care norms. Solid arrows indicate assistance to each spouse's own parents in line with norms of filial obligation, whereas dashed lines indicate assistance to the same gender in line with norms of same-gender care.

Overall, this literature suggests that the social structural and normative contexts of care favor women's and wives' involvement in care activities, and that husbands are sometimes drawn into care activities as helpers to their wives. However, not all husbands are supportive. Matthews and Rosner (1988), for instance, distinguished among three groups of husbands: those who were directly involved in caregiving, those who were indifferent but did not hinder their wives' caregiving, and those who were antagonistic. That husbands' support is important can be seen from studies indicating that the extent of support husbands provide and the extent of stress spillover from caregiving to marital roles are linked to caregivers' well-being and their marital quality (Franks & Stephens, 1996; Suitor & Pillemer, 1996).

Division of Parent Care Between Spouses

As previously noted, little research has assessed spouses' division of parent care. We recently pursued this issue with pooled data from the 1992 through 2000 waves of the HRS (Szinovacz & Davey, 2006). Our analyses of 1,449 care occasions showed that, for nearly two-thirds of couples, care to parents and parents-in-law was shared to some extent between spouses. Our results confirmed the interplay among normative factors, as shown in Figure 7.4. Exclusive care was provided by 48.2% of wives for care to their mothers, compared to 1.8% for care to husbands' fathers. On the other hand, 26.1% of husbands provided exclusive care to their own fathers, but fewer than 1% cared exclusively for the wife's mother. Among couples in which both spouses participated in care, the relative participation of husbands also reflected the combined influences of gender norms, filial obligation, and preference for same-gender care (see Figure 7.5). More involvement on the part of wives predominated for wives' mothers (71.9%), followed by care for wives' fathers (60.4%). Husbands carried the heavier care load for their own fathers in 40.8% of couples and for their own mothers in 35.6% of couples. These data confirm that normative contexts exhibit a strong influence on husband's relative involvement in parent care. In line with gender role norms, wives provided relatively more assistance (and more assistance overall) than husbands did. Filial obligation leads to greater involvement of each spouse in assistance provided to their own parents, and same-gender norms promote greater participation of wives in care for mothers and more involvement of husbands in care for fathers.

In addition to normative contexts, our analyses (Szinovacz & Davey, 2006) also revealed the influence of selected spouse and marital relationship variables on spouses' relative participation in parent care. Wives' perceptions of the couple's involvement in joint activities had a positive effect on husbands' contributions to care, but primarily for care to wives' own parents. Husbands were relatively more involved in care as the total hours of help provided by the couple increased, and this was particularly true for help to the husband's own parents. Relative commitments and

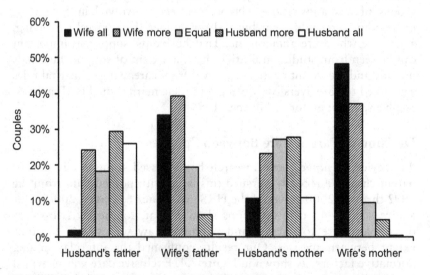

FIGURE 7.4 Division of parent care between spouses by parent's gender and kinship. Original computations based on the Health and Retirement Study and data prepared for Szinovacz and Davey (2006).

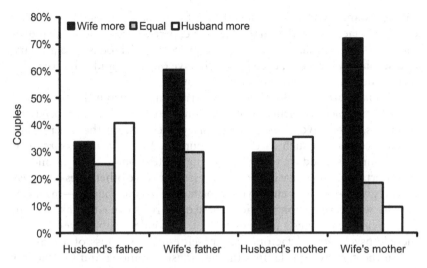

FIGURE 7.5   Division of parent care between spouses in couples where both spouses contribute to care, by parent's gender and kinship. Original computations based on the Health and Retirement Study and data prepared for Szinovacz and Davey (2006).

abilities of the spouses—such as employment or health—had more influence on husbands' participation in care.

In sum, then, we find that care responsibilities are shared by a majority of couples and that this is particularly true for husbands' parents and especially husbands' fathers. Our results also point to the important role of normative contexts in moderating the effects of spouses' marital relationship and of other commitments and ability on couples' division of parent care. Specifically, they suggest that a couple's commitment to joint activities can override the gender mandate and filial obligation pertaining to care for wives' parents, whereas care for husbands' parents is more flexible in regard to spouses' relative commitments and abilities.

EFFECTS OF CHANGES IN CARE NETWORKS ON DEPRESSIVE SYMPTOMS

Despite nearly 25 years of family caregiving research, there is still no unifying theoretical perspective guiding the literature. Several perspectives have been presented, each differing in the constructs emphasized. The stress process model (e.g., Aneshensel et al., 1995), for example, seeks to understand variability in the effects of care experiences. Why do two caregivers faced with the same objective experience respond in such dramatically different fashions? The stress process model focuses on primary and secondary stressors, each of which have objective and subjective elements and contribute to caregiving outcomes.

Primary stressors are those that derive directly from the context of care. Their objective elements include limitations of ADLs and behavior problems. Subjective elements of primary stressors, on the other hand, capture constructs such as caregiver burden. *Secondary stressors* arise from sources secondary to the caregiving context but are not secondary in importance. Objective secondary stressors involve other roles occupied by caregivers—such as employment or family responsibilities—that may conflict with care responsibilities. These other roles can either exacerbate or support the caregiver in his or her role. Secondary subjective stressors include psychological factors such as self-esteem and loss of a sense of self in the caregiving role. It is the relationships among and satisfaction with these roles that can moderate or mediate the influence of primary stressors on well-being.

In addition to primary and secondary stressors, a variety of background characteristics and resources are also important in predicting caregiving outcomes. Factors such as social support, coping style, and personality can moderate the effects of stress proliferation and containment on caregiver adaptation. The stress process model is important for understanding many of the key contextual factors in caregiving over time, as well as illustrating differences between caregivers at different stages of the caregiving career.

Although the stress process model has served a central role in predicting caregivers' adjustment to the assistance they provide, research guided by this perspective has tended to focus on a primary caregiver. As a result, it has not generally been applied within a network context. Other roles such as marriage or competing obligations are typically considered in terms of secondary stressors. Relationships with other individuals, particularly with regard to "support" broadly conceived, fall under the category of moderators such as social support. In fact, it can be difficult to consider how the stress process model should be extended to a network framework.

A second difficulty with research applying the stress process model to caregiving is that it is often based on samples of individuals who are already selected for their involvement in care and who continue their involvement over time. As such, it is difficult to evaluate the effects of beginning or ending involvement in care. Even when models and data are longitudinal, continuous involvement in care removes one key aspect of potential variability from the care situation.

It is beyond the scope of this chapter to review the large literature using the stress model or similar frameworks to predict caregiver well-being (for reviews, see Schulz & Beach, 1999; Schulz, O'Brien, Bookwala, & Fleissner, 1995; Schulz, Visintainer, & Williamson, 1990). However, some recent studies based on the HRS, including our own analyses, deserve mention. Chumbler, Pienta, and Dwyer (2004) used data from the 1992 wave of the HRS to compare depressive symptom scores between adult-child caregivers and noncaregivers. These authors worked from a role theoretical perspective, focusing on role strain and role enhancement. Chumbler et al. identified 252 individuals providing care (defined as help with basic personal needs for at least 100 hours over the past 12 months) to a mother and 57 individuals providing care to a father. They found that depressive symptoms were higher in caregivers than noncaregivers, but that these effects were limited to care for fathers and were also moderated by the effects of having a spouse and being employed. However, their models did not control for hours of care provided, which were quite diverse in their sample. Reid and Hardy (1999) also found that caregiving women reported higher depressive symptoms than noncaregivers, but that this effect was no longer significant once other roles such as work and parenting were controlled.

Dunlop, Song, Lyons, Manheim, and Chang (2003) used data from individuals aged 54 to 65 in the 1996 wave of the HRS, restricting analyses to the 7,690 individuals who completed the Composite International Diagnostic Interview Short Form (see Kessler, Andrews, Mroczek, Ustun, & Wittchen, 1998), a diagnostic interview to assess clinical depression. In their multivariate model predicting the probability of a major depressive episode, these authors found that providing care to a frail parent was associated with a 37% higher risk of experiencing depression relative to those who did not provide this assistance. Because their analyses were not limited exclusively to caregivers (or even those with living parents), their models did not control for the extent of involvement in assistance to parents.

Another HRS-based study by Amirkhanyan and Wolf (2003) found evidence that having a disabled parent was associated with depressive symptoms among noncaregivers. Building on these early cross-sectional analyses, Amirkhanyan and Wolf (2006) applied a stress process framework to the study of parental disability on adult children longitudinally. In particular, this approach allowed them to separate the older adult's need for assistance from the adult children's response to those needs. Data for their study were drawn from three waves of the HRS (1996, 1998, and 2000). For both men and women, parents' need for care predicted higher depressive symptoms. However, for women only, providing care had a separate association with higher depressive symptoms. These results suggest that nonprovision of assistance to a needy parent may undermine both men's and women's well-being, whereas provision of assistance was mainly detrimental to women's well-being.

Effects of Network Changes on Caregiver Depression

Based on our recent research suggesting that care is most often a shared experience and that there is considerable change in the composition of care networks over time, we used data from the HRS to investigate how changes in the composition of sibling support networks over time affect the well-being of adult children. The HRS includes some information on background characteristics and primary and secondary stressors. In addition, the HRS contains data about respondents' and each of their siblings' provision of help with basic needs to a parent. This allows the assessment of changes in individual siblings' participation in care to parents over time. We considered data from all respondents in cases that assistance was provided to parents by at least one adult child over two waves. Our primary research question was: Are care transitions by the respondents and their siblings related to changes in respondents' depressive symptoms?

Data. Our data were drawn from the first five waves of the HRS (1992 to 2000). To obtain sufficient cases for analyses, data were pooled across consecutive waves. Longitudinal data were also necessary to capture changes in care networks between waves. From the larger HRS sample, we selected all individuals with at least one living parent across two waves, who had at least one living sibling, and who provided assistance to a parent in at least one of those two waves. As a result, care could be provided to multiple parents, and care could be provided to the same parents in multiple waves. Consequently, all analyses adjust for nonindependence of observations from the same family and for the complex survey sampling design (for a description of the HRS, see Juster & Suzman, 1995). Overall, our models included data on 580 care occasions. To address issues of missing data, we created five multiple imputation data sets using routines described in Schafer (1997). Data from each imputation set were analyzed separately and results combined to provide a single set of estimates.

Measures. Our primary *outcome* variable was the eight-item dichotomously scored version of the Center for Epidemiologic Studies Depression (CES-D) Scale (Radloff, 1977; Steffick, 2000), measured at time 2. All other variables were drawn from the preceding wave of data collection or refer to transitions that occurred between waves.

Our analyses included several *background characteristics.* Depressive symptoms from the previous wave served as a covariate. Scaling of this construct was modified from the 1992 to subsequent waves. Consistent with our previous research using this variable (Szinovacz & Davey, 2004), we used a rescaled version of the CES-D for the 1992 wave. Other background characteristics included gender (*female* = 1, *male* = 0), race (dummy coded as Black, Hispanic, and other race with White as the reference category), whether the parent was female (*mother* = 1, *father* = 0), years of education, logged household income, and the number of brothers and number of sisters.

The HRS data contained a limited number of indicators that could be considered as *primary stressors*. These included the respondent's hours of help, whether the respondent provided the most help among his or her siblings (1 = *yes*, 0 = *no*), whether the parent lived with the respondent (1 = *yes*, 0 = *no*), whether the parent moved out from the respondent's house (1 = *yes*, 0 = *no*) or moved in with the respondent (1 = *yes*, 0 = *no*) between waves, whether the parent was married (1 = *yes*, 0 = *no*), and whether the parent could be left alone (1 = *yes*, 0 = *no*).

Limited information was available regarding *secondary stressors*. Included in our models based on preliminary analyses were whether the respondent also provides assistance to another parent (1 = *yes*, 0 = *no*) and whether the respondent's spouse was also in poor health (1 = *yes*, 0 = *no*).

To capture the *family context of care*, we constructed a set of dummy-coded indicators representing all possible combinations of respondents and siblings beginning, continuing, or stopping care, with continuous care on the part of both siblings and respondents as the reference category. We were particularly interested in the situation in which one sibling started care while another sibling stopped.

Analyses and results. Because of the highly positively skewed nature of depressive symptoms, we estimated interval regression (i.e., censored) models, adjusting for survey design effects and nonindependence that could result from multiple care occasions for the same parent or simultaneous care to multiple parents. Complete results from the model are presented in Table 7.1. As can be seen in the model, there was considerable evidence for stability in levels of depressive symptoms over time. As well, levels of depressive symptoms were lower among respondents with more education and higher incomes. Interestingly, there were no effects on depressive symptoms of any of the primary or secondary stressors. The only other significant effect pertained to the family context of care. Specifically, the situation in which the respondent initiated care between waves while a sibling stopped providing assistance was associated with significantly and substantially higher levels of depressive symptoms on the part of the respondent. This suggests that assumption of care to substitute for a sibling is particularly difficult. It may be that such care occurs under more difficult circumstances, such as more conflicting role obligations that initially precluded the respondent's participation in care, and takes on a more nonvoluntary character that has been linked to lowered well-being for spouse caregivers (Szinovacz & Davey, 2004).

TABLE 7.1 Interval Regression Model Predicting Time 2 Depressive Symptoms ($N = 580$)

Predictor	Estimate	Estimated SE	M	SD
Background characteristics				
Time 1 depressive symptoms	0.73**	0.06	1.84	2.01
Female	0.28	0.29	0.72	0.45
Black	-0.20	0.34	0.20	0.40
Hispanic	-0.73	0.47	0.10	0.30
Other race	-0.99	1.42	0.01	0.08
Parent female	-0.12	0.32	0.83	0.38
Years of education	-0.11*	0.04	12.15	3.34
Income (logged)	-0.16*	0.08	10.17	1.70
Number of brothers	0.02	0.09	1.67	1.55
Number of sisters	0.04	0.09	1.72	1.56
Primary stressors				
Respondent's hours of help	0.00	0.00	605.00	1002.84
Respondent provides most help	0.26	0.34	0.57	0.50
Parent lives with respondent	-0.15	0.37	0.15	0.36
Parent moved out	0.05	0.74	0.03	0.17
Parent moved in	0.00	0.72	0.03	0.17
Parent married	0.31	0.36	0.19	0.40
Parent can be left alone	0.21	0.26	0.66	0.47
Secondary stressors				
Respondent provides help to other parent	-0.13	0.48	0.09	0.29
Respondent's spouse in poor health	0.12	0.32	0.17	0.38
Sibling context of care				
Respondent begins care, sibling begins	0.44	0.57	0.06	0.24
Respondent begins care, sibling continues	-0.08	0.60	0.06	0.24
Respondent begins care, sibling stops	1.29*	0.55	0.06	0.24
Respondent stops care, sibling begins	0.65	0.64	0.04	0.20
Respondent stops care, sibling continues	0.31	0.61	0.05	0.23
Respondent stops care, sibling stops	-0.59	0.66	0.04	0.20

Continued

TABLE 7.1   Interval Regression Model Predicting Time 2
Depressive Symptoms (N = 580) (Continued)

Predictor	Estimate	Estimated SE	M	SD
Respondent continues care, sibling begins	0.30	0.33	0.17	0.38
Respondent continues care, sibling stops	0.47	0.35	0.17	0.38
Intercept	2.06	1.10		
$\chi^2(27)$	237.24**			

* $p < .05$. ** $p < .0001$.

The HRS has several limitations relevant to examining the effects of
network changes on caregiver well-being. First, care questions are retrospective, referring to the time since the previous wave. As a result, it is possible for caregivers to have provided extensive supports between waves but
not to be a current caregiver. Related to this, there is very little information
about the timing of transitions. It is not possible, for example, to know
when within the period between interviews care commenced or ceased. It
is highly likely that both of these factors have important implications for
caregiver well-being, but they are not possible to tease out from these data.
Finally, although previous research has pointed to the important moderating influences on the association between stressors and psychological
outcomes of factors such as coping and social support, they are not well
represented in the HRS. Given these limitations, then, it is surprising that
we were able to identify even a single network transition that was robustly
associated with changes in depressive symptoms over a 2-year period.

IMPLICATIONS OF CARE NETWORKS FOR
RESEARCH AND PRACTICE

As the chapter by Uhlenberg and Cheuk at the beginning of this volume makes clear, there are rising concerns about the future availability
of informal caregivers for the baby boom cohort (see also Jette et al.,
1992). Uhlenberg and Cheuk attribute this decline to both the increased
prevalence of divorce among baby boomers and lower fertility among
children of the baby boom cohorts. This scenario raises the significance
of studying family care networks and the extent to which family members share care or substitute for each other over time. Because so much
of the caregiving literature has relied on analyses of cross-sectional data

and had an overwhelming focus on the primary caregiver (Soldo, Wolf, & Agree, 1990), it will become increasingly important to address both shortcomings, examining factors associated with longitudinal transitions in care networks, broadly conceived.

The analyses presented in this chapter show that care is often shared between spouses or among adult children, and that specific types of network changes can undermine caregiver well-being. They also document considerable fluctuation in care networks over time. Thus, the prevailing emphasis on identifying and following a primary caregiver might misrepresent the structure and functioning of care networks over time. As well, an emphasis on a primary caregiver fails to capitalize on available but untapped resources available to older adults (Zarit, Davey, Edwards, Femia, & Jarrott, 1998).

The preceding review of the literature on adult children as caregivers, as well as our own analyses, point to several future research needs. Because most of what we know about care is focused on the assistance provided directly to older adults, for example, we know very little about the supports that caregivers might provide to one another. These forms of indirect caregiving have not been examined in much detail to date, but better understanding of them is likely to be one key to helping families provide the best care possible for older adults. Similarly, our existing theories provide only a starting point for thinking about the implications of care networks for well-being, in contrast to the standard assumptions regarding a primary caregiver. Until our measures and data are improved in this regard, we are unlikely to gain significant insights into the diversity of family care arrangements and their impact on caregivers' and care recipients' well-being.

Finally, a shift in focus toward network considerations of caregiving opens up a host of new research possibilities to identify the constellations of support that best support older adults in the community and that are most likely to lead to (or delay) outcomes such as institutionalization. It will be particularly important to pinpoint those characteristics of care networks that provide the greatest benefit for older adults as they experience greater disability and frailty.

Moving to a network conceptualization of caregiving also requires a shift in thinking for practitioners. In dealing with caregivers, for example, it is important to establish the composition of the caregiver network and who has responsibility for which tasks (the caregiver accompanying the patient to the office may not be the primary caregiver or the one who purchases and administers medications). Instructions to caregivers should be addressed to the primary caregiver and any other caregiver who may be involved in relevant care tasks. Because change in care networks appears to be the norm, practitioners need to be aware that caregivers may change from one visit to another. For this reason, it may be important to establish and then reestablish the composition of the caregiver network at each visit. This can help to assess the adequacy of care as well as to identify the individual (or individuals) to whom specific instructions should be addressed. In addition, it is essential to assess the network of potential caregivers. Patients with small networks may be particularly vulnerable to inadequate care or potential negative effects of caregiver stress on patient outcomes. On the other hand, large networks can entail considerable negotiation and renegotiation of care responsibilities among network members. If such negotiations create conflict, this can contribute to caregiver stress and negatively impact patient outcomes.

Demographic projections for the aging baby boom cohorts' care needs and resources suggest a shift toward more complex support networks than those typical for current cohorts of elderly. Although families are likely to remain central in supporting frail older adults, they may increasingly use formal helpers or assistance from a wider range of relatives and friends. As informal care networks become more complex, so will the magnitude of the task of coordinating and sustaining these networks. Providing practitioners and policymakers with a sound scientific base to accomplish this task constitutes a formidable challenge to research on family caregiving.

NOTES

1. Preparation of this chapter was funded in part by a grant from the National Institute on Aging, R01 AG024045, Maximiliane E. Szinovacz, P.I.
2. Our presentation of changes in adult-child care networks is based on Szinovacz and Davey (2007). The analyses rely on data from the Health and Retirement Study (HRS), which were collected and managed by the University of Michigan's Institute of Social Research and funded by the National Institutes of Health (NIH). Our research was funded by NIH grant R01 AG024045, Maximiliane E. Szinovacz, P.I.

REFERENCES

Amirkhanyan, A. A., & Wolf, D. A. (2003). Caregiver stress and noncaregiver stress: Exploring the pathways of psychiatric morbidity. *The Gerontologist, 43*, 817–827.

Amirkhanyan, A. A., & Wolf, D. A. (2006). Parent care and the stress process: Findings from panel data. *Journals of Gerontology: Social Sciences, 61B*, 248–255.

Andrieu, S. H., Bocquet, A. J., Gillette-Guyonnet, S., Nourhashem, F., Salva, A., Grand, A., et al. (2005). Changes in informal care over one year for elderly persons with Alzheimer's disease. *Journal of Nutrition, Health, and Aging, 9*, 121–126.

Aneshensel, C. S., Pearlin, L. I., Mullan, J. T., Zarit, S. H., & Whitlatch, C. J. (1995). *Profiles in caregiving: The unexpected career.* San Diego, CA: Academic Press.

Arber, S., & Ginn, J. (1991). *Gender and later life.* London: Sage.

Calasanti, T. M., & Slevin, K. F. (2001). *Gender, social inequalities, and aging*. Walnut Creek, CA: Alta Mira Press.

Campbell, L. D., & Martin-Matthews, A. (2003). The gendered nature of men's filial care. *Journals of Gerontology: Social Sciences, 58B*, S350–S358.

Cancian, F. M., & Oliker, S. J. (2000). *Caring and gender*. Walnut Creek, CA: Alta Mira Press.

Cantor, M. H. (1975). Life space and the social support system of the inner city elderly of New York. *The Gerontologist, 15*, 23–27.

Caron, C., Griffith, J., & Arcand, M. (2005). How family caregivers perceive their interactions with health care providers in long-term-care settings. *Journal of Applied Gerontology, 24*, 231–247.

Checkovich, T. J., & Stern, S. (2002). Shared caregiving responsibilities of adult children with elderly parents. *Journal of Human Resources, 37*, 441–478.

Chumbler, N. R., Pienta, A. M., & Dwyer, J. W. (2004). The depressive symptomatology of parent care among the near elderly. *Research on Aging, 26*, 330–351.

Cicirelli, V. G. (1995). *Sibling relationships across the life-span*. Newbury Park, CA: Sage.

Coleman, M., Ganong, L., & Cable, S. M. (1997). Beliefs about women's intergenerational family obligations to provide support before and after divorce and remarriage. *Journal of Marriage and the Family, 59*, 165–176.

Coward, R. T., & Dwyer, J. W. (1991). A longitudinal study of residential differences in the composition of the helping networks of impaired elders. *Journal of Aging Studies, 5*, 391–407.

Davey, A., Janke, M. C., & Savla, J. S. (2005). Antecedents of intergenerational support: Families in context and families as context. In M. Silverstein, R. Giarrusso, & V. L. Bengtson (Eds.), *Annual review of gerontology and geriatrics: Intergenerational relations across time and place* (pp. 29–54). New York: Springer.

Dilworth-Anderson, P., Williams, I. C., & Gibson, B. E. (2002). Issues of race, ethnicity, and culture in caregiving research: A 20-year review (1980–2000). *The Gerontologist, 42*, 237–272.

Dunlop, D. D., Song, J., Lyons, J. S., Manheim, L. M., & Chang, R. W. (2003). Racial/ethnic differences in rates of depression among preretirement adults. *American Journal of Public Health, 93*, 1945–1952.

Dwyer, J. W., Henretta, J. C., Coward, R. T., & Barton, A. J. (1992). Changes in the helping behaviors of adult children as caregivers. *Research on Aging, 14*, 351–375.

Engers, M., & Stern, S. (2002). Long-term care and family bargaining. *International Economic Review, 43*, 73–114.

Finch, J., & Mason, J. (1993). *Negotiating family responsibilities*. New York: Tavistock/Routledge.

Finley, N. J., Roberts, M. D., & Banahan, B. F. (1988). Motivators and inhibitors of attitudes of filial obligation towards aging parents. *The Gerontologist, 28*, 73–78.

Franks, M., & Stephens, A. (1996). Social support in the context of caregiving: Husbands' provision of support to wives involved in parent care. *Journal of Gerontology: Social Sciences, 51*, P43–P52.

Ganong, L. H., & Coleman, M. (2006). Obligations to stepparents acquired in later life: Relationship quality and acuity of needs. *Journals of Gerontology: Social Sciences, 61B*, 80–88.

Gaugler, J. E., Davey, A., Pearlin, L. I., & Zarit, S. H. (2000). Modeling caregiver adaptation over time: The longitudinal impact of behavior problems. *Psychology and Aging, 15*, 417–436.

Gerstel, N., & Gallagher, S. K. (2001). Men's caregiving: Gender and the contingent character of care. *Gender and Society, 15*, 197–217.

Henretta, J. C., Hill, M. S., Li, W., Soldo, B. J., & Wolf, D. A. (1997). Selection of children to provide care: The effect of earlier parental transfers. *Journals of Gerontology: Social Sciences, 52B,* S110–S119.

Hequembourg, A., & Brallier, S. (2005). Gendered stories of parental caregiving among siblings. *Journal of Aging Studies, 19,* 53–71.

Ingersoll-Dayton, B., Neal, M. B., Ha, J., & Hammer, L. (2003). Redressing inequity in parent care among siblings. *Journal of Marriage and the Family, 65,* 201.

Jette, A. M., Tennstedt, S. L., & Branch, L. G. (1992). Stability of informal long-term care. *Journal of Aging and Health, 4,* 193–211.

Johnson, R. W., & Lo Sasso, A. T. (2000). *The trade-off between hours of paid employment and time assistance to elderly parents at midlife.* Washington, DC: Urban Institute.

Juster, F. T., & Suzman, R. (1995). An overview of the Health and Retirement Study. *Journal of Human Resources, 30,* 7–56.

Kelman, H. R., Thomas, C., & Tanaka, J. S. (1994). Longitudinal patterns of formal and informal social support in an urban elderly population. *Social Science and Medicine, 38,* 905–914.

Kessler, R. C., Andrews, G., Mroczek, D., Ustun, B., & Wittchen, H.-U. (1998). The World Health Organization Composite International Diagnostic Interview Short-Form (CIDI-SF). *International Journal of Methods in Psychiatric Research, 7,* 171–185.

Kramer, B. J., & Thompson, E. H. (2002). *Men as caregivers: Theory, research, and service implications.* New York: Springer.

Laditka, J. N., & Laditka, S. B. (2001). Adult children helping older parents: Variations in likelihood and hours by gender, race, and family role. *Research on Aging, 23,* 429–456.

Lawrence, J. A., Goodnow, J. J., Woods, K., & Karantzas, G. (2002). Distributions of caregiving tasks among family members: The place of gender and availability. *Journal of Family Psychology, 16,* 493–509.

Lawton, L., Silverstein, M., & Bengtson, V. L. (1994). Solidarity between generations in families. In V. L. Bengtson & R. A. Harootyan (Eds.), *Intergenerational linkages: Hidden connections in American society* (pp. 19–42). New York: Springer.

Lawton, M. P., Moss, M., Hoffman, C., & Perkinson, M. (2000). Two transitions in daughters' caregiving careers. *The Gerontologist, 40,* 437–448.

Lee, E., Spitze, G., & Logan, J. (2003). Social support to parents-in-law: The interplay of gender and kin hierarchies. *Journal of Marriage and Family, 65,* 396–403.

Lee, G. R., Peek, C. W., & Coward, R. T. (1998). Race differences in filial responsibility expectations among older parents. *Journal of Marriage and the Family, 60,* 404–412.

Lyons, K. S., Zarit, S. H., & Townsend, A. L. (2000). Families and formal service usage: Stability and change in patterns of interface. *Aging and Mental Health, 4,* 234–243.

Marks, N. F. (1996). Caregiving across the lifespan: National prevalence and predictors. *Family Relations, 45,* 27–36.

Martin Matthews, A., & Campbell, L. D. (1995). Gender roles, employment, and informal care. In S. Arber & J. Ginn (Eds.), *Connecting gender and ageing: A sociological approach* (pp. 129–143). Buckingham, England: Open University Press.

Matthews, S. (1992). Placing filial behavior in the context of the family. In B. Bauer (Ed.), *Conceptual and methodological issues in family caregiving research* (pp. 55–62). Toronto, Canada: University of Toronto Press.

Matthews, S. H. (1987). Provision of care to older parents: Division of responsibility among adult children. *Research on Aging, 9,* 45–60.

Matthews, S. H. (1995). Gender and the division of filial responsibility between lone sisters and their brothers. *Journals of Gerontology: Social Sciences, 50B,* 312–320.

Matthews, S. H., & Heidorn, J. (1998). Meeting filial responsibilities in brothers-only sibling groups. *Journals of Gerontology: Social Sciences, 50B*, 278–286.

Matthews, S. H., & Rosner, T. T. (1988). Shared filial responsibility: The family as the primary caregiver. *Journal of Marriage and the Family, 50*, 185–195.

McGarry, K., & Schoeni, R. F. (1997). Transfer behavior within the family: Results from the Asset and Health Dynamics study. *Journals of Gerontology: Psychological and Social Sciences, 52B*, 82–92.

Miller, B., & McFall, S. (1991). Stability and change in the informal task support network of frail older persons. *The Gerontologist, 31*, 735–745.

National Alliance for Caregiving and AARP. (2004). *Caregiving in the U.S.* Washington, DC: Author.

Orel, N. A., & Dupuy, P. (2002). Grandchildren as auxiliary caregivers for grandparents with cognitive and/or physical limitations: Coping strategies and ramifications. *Child Study Journal, 32*, 192–213.

Pillemer, K., & Suitor, J. J. (2006). Making choices: A within-family study of caregiver selection. *The Gerontologist, 46*, 439–448.

Radloff, L. (1977). A self-report depression scale for research in the general population. *Applied Psychological Measurement, 1*, 385–401.

Reid, J., & Hardy, M. (1999). Multiple roles and well-being among midlife women: Testing role strain and role enhancement theories. *Journals of Gerontology: Social Sciences, 54B*, 329–338.

Rossi, A. S., & Rossi, P. H. (1990). *Of human bonding: Parent-child relations across the life course.* New York: Aldine de Gruyter.

Sarkisian, N., & Gerstel, N. (2004). Explaining the gender gap in help to parents: The importance of employment. *Journal of Marriage and the Family, 66*, 431–451.

Schafer, J. L. (1997). *Analysis of incomplete multivariate data.* London: Chapman & Hall.

Schulz, R., & Beach, S. (1999). Caregiving as a risk factor for mortality: The caregiver health effects study. *Journal of the American Medical Association, 282*, 2215–2219.

Schulz, R., O'Brien, A., Bookwala, J., & Fleissner, K. (1995). Psychiatric and physical morbidity effects of dementia caregiving: Prevalence, correlates, and causes. *The Gerontologist, 35*, 771–791.

Schulz, R., Visintainer, P., & Williamson, G. M. (1990). Psychiatric and physical morbidity effects of caregiving. *Journal of Gerontology: Psychological Sciences, 45*, 181–191.

Seltzer, M. M., & Li, L. W. (2000). The dynamics of caregiving: Transitions during a three-year prospective study. *The Gerontologist, 40*, 165–178.

Shuey, K., & Hardy, M. A. (2003). Assistance to aging parents and parents-in-law: Does lineage affect family allocation decisions? *Journal of Marriage and the Family, 65*, 418–431.

Silverstein, M., Conroy, S. J., Wang, H., Giarrusso, R., & Bengtson, V. L. (2002). Reciprocity in parent-child relations over the adult life course. *Journals of Gerontology: Social Sciences, 57B*, 3–13.

Soldo, B. J., Wolf, D. A., & Agree, E. M. (1990). Family, households, and care arrangements of frail older women: A structural analysis. *Journal of Gerontology: Social Sciences, 45*, S238–S249.

Soldo, B., Wolf, D., & Henretta, J. (1999). Intergenerational transfers: Blood, marriage, and gender effects on household decisions. In J. P. Smith & R. J. Willis (Eds.), *Wealth, work and health: Innovations in measurement in the social sciences.* Ann Arbor: University of Michigan Press.

Stark, O. (1995). *Altruism and beyond: An economic analysis of transfers and exchanges within families and groups.* Cambridge, England: Cambridge University Press.

Steffick, D. E. (2000). *Documentation of affective functioning measures in the Health and Retirement Study* [HRS/AHEAD Documentation Report]. Ann Arbor, MI: Institute for Survey Research, University of Michigan.

Stoller, E. P. (1990). Males as helpers: The role of sons, relatives, and friends. *The Gerontologist, 30,* 228–235.

Stone, R., Cafferata, G. L., & Sangl, J. (1987). Caregivers of the frail elderly: A national profile. *The Gerontologist, 27,* 616–626.

Suitor, J. J., & Pillemer, K. (1996). Sources of support and interpersonal stress in the networks of married caregiving daughters: Findings from a 2-year longitudinal study. *Journal of Gerontology: Social Sciences, 51,* S297–S306.

Suitor, J. J., & Pillemer, K. (2007). Mothers' favoritism in later life. *Research on Aging, 29,* 32–55.

Szinovacz, M. E. (2003). Dealing with dementia: Perspectives of caregivers' children. *Journal of Aging Studies, 17,* 445–472.

Szinovacz, M., & Davey, A. (2004). Retirement transitions and spouse's disability: Effects on depressive symptoms. *Journals of Gerontology: Social Sciences, 59B,* S333–S342.

Szinovacz, M. E., & Davey, A. (2006). Division of care between spouses: Variations by kin relationship. Manuscript submitted for publication.

Szinovacz, M. E., & Davey, A. (in press). Changes in adult-child caregiver networks. *The Gerontologist.*

Walker, A. J., Pratt, C. C., Shin, H. Y., & Jones, L. L. (1990). Motive for parental caregiving and relationship quality. *Family Relations, 39,* 51–56.

Whitbeck, L., Hoyt, D. R., & Huck, S. M. (1994). Early family relationships, intergenerational solidarity, and support provided to parents by their adult children. *Journal of Gerontology: Social Sciences, 49,* 585–594.

Wolf, D. A., Freedman, V., & Soldo, B. J. (1997). The division of family labor: Care for elderly parents. *Journals of Gerontology: Social Sciences, 52B,* S102–S109.

Wolff, J. L., & Kasper, J. D. (2006). Caregivers of frail elders: Updating a national profile. *The Gerontologist, 46,* 344–356.

Wong, R., Kitayama, K., & Soldo, B. J. (1999). Ethnic differences in time transfers from adult child to elderly parents: Unobserved heterogeneity across families. *Research on Aging, 21,* 144–175.

Zarit, S. H., Davey, A., Edwards, A. B., Femia, E. E., & Jarrott, S. E. (1998). Family caregiving: Research findings and clinical implications. In A. S. Bellack & M. Hersen (Series Eds.) & B. A. Edelstein (Vol. Ed.), *Comprehensive clinical psychology: Vol. 7. Clinical geropsychology* (pp. 499–523). Oxford, England: Elsevier Science.

CHAPTER EIGHT

Children in Caregiving Families

Maximiliane E. Szinovacz

Involvement of children and adolescents in work in general and in care activities in particular was established practice historically and is still relatively common in some non-Western societies. In postindustrial societies, on the other hand, childhood is viewed as a separate life stage devoted foremost to educational and play activities (Ariès, 1962; Jurkovic, 1997), and children's involvement in adult-type work activities is deemed inappropriate and is, for the most part, prohibited (e.g., through child labor laws). However, caregiving by children is usually unpaid and occurs within the family, rendering it invisible and sometimes outside the realm of legislation, service agencies, and formal care providers (Becker, 1995; Dearden & Becker, 1997; Newman, 2002; Thomas et al., 2003).

This invisibility also pertains to the caregiving literature. Until the late 1980s, care by children tended to be treated either from a psychological and therapy perspective or from a medical and clinical perspective. This research typically relied on case studies and focused on the physical disability and psychiatric conditions exhibited by caregiving children or their families (Aldridge & Becker, 1999; Chase, 1999; Jurkovic, 1997; Olsen, 1996). Impetus for research on children as carers came from the United Kingdom, resulting in special programs for young carers, legislation to protect them, and several large-scale surveys based on youths enrolled in young carers projects (Dearden & Becker, 1995, 1998, 2000, 2004). Since the 1990s, young caregivers became a special focus of study in other countries, including Australia and the United States (Beach, 1994, 1997; Carers Australia, 2001; Orel & Dupuy, 2002; Orel, Dupuy, & Wright, 2004; Szinovacz, 2003). A recent U.S. survey commissioned by the National

Alliance for Caregiving (2005) is, to my knowledge, the only representative study specifically devoted to young caregivers.

Despite these efforts, research on children in caregiving families remains scarce. With the exception of the National Alliance survey, studies have relied on either small convenience samples or larger surveys of specific population groups such as children involved in the British young carers projects. These studies not only differ in what they considered "young carers," but many of them also tended to emphasize negative care outcomes partially to secure funding for programs and to promote legislative changes (Newman, 2002; Olsen, 1996). Particularly lacking is theoretically informed research that explores the conditions leading to children's involvement in care and especially the outcomes, both positive and negative, of such involvement. In addition, few investigations have explored the family dynamics resulting from the presence of children in caregiving families. Caregiving research has, for the most part, assessed caregiving by spouses and adult children with an emphasis on the primary caregiver. This perspective ignores that caregiving is often a family enterprise. Not only is caregiving usually shared among multiple family caregivers such as the care recipient's adult children, but family members of each caregiver are directly or indirectly involved as well.

To the extent possible with current research, this chapter adopts a contextual approach to children's involvement in caregiving that integrates past research findings with previously unpublished data from my research.[1] It also adds a brief section on the impact of children on adults' caregiving decisions and outcomes.

BACKGROUND: DEFINITIONS AND PREVALENCE

Considerable debate has surrounded the question of what constitutes caregiving by children and adolescents. This debate results from reliance on divergent criteria for definitions of children's caregiving. While some research emphasized the care tasks performed by children, other studies focused on the age appropriateness of the children's care activities, the extent of their care activities, or the impact of caregiving on the children (Dearden & Becker, 2000). For the purposes of this chapter, I adopt a broad definition of children's involvement in caregiving (see Table 8.1), differentiating children's involvement along two dimensions—direct or indirect and active or passive. Direct involvement occurs when the child is directly affected by work for or exposure to the care recipient, whereas indirect involvement is restricted to situations in which the child's life is influenced only by the caregiver's demands or reactions to the care situation. The distinction between active and passive involvement rests on whether the child performs work for the care recipient or for the caregiver. Direct active involvement implies caregiving activities on the part of the child. These can range from primary care responsibilities to minor chores. In the case of indirect active involvement, the child is assigned tasks other than caregiving that are normally performed by the caregiver and do not constitute regular household responsibilities of the child. Direct passive involvement refers to influences of the care recipient's illness or presence on the child—for example, if a child's friends are prohibited from visiting as a result of the care recipient's presence in the home. The fourth category, indirect passive involvement, recognizes the system character of families and the impact of life changes for one family member on the lives of all other family members. Even if children do not perform care tasks or tasks that support the caregiver and have no direct exposure to the care recipient, they may still be affected by a parent's or other relative's caregiving. For instance, stressed caregivers may become less patient when children misbehave, or conflicts between spouses over caregiving may take their toll on the children as well. Many studies do not differentiate clearly among these divergent types of children's involvement or focus exclusively on one type. The British studies have emphasized children as primary caregivers (Becker, 1995), but other research has adopted broader definitions that include indirect and passive involvement (National Alliance for Caregiving, 2005). Because the focus of this volume is on care for the elderly, I further emphasize children's involvement in care for the elderly or at least for adults rather than their contributions to care for other family members, especially siblings.

Partly due to divergent definitions and partly due to lack of data, it is difficult to estimate the prevalence of children's involvement in care-

TABLE 8.1 Types of Children's Involvement in Caregiving

	Active	Passive
Direct	Children perform care tasks for the care recipient.	Children's lives are influenced by the care recipient's illness and/or his or her presence in the home.
Indirect	Children perform tasks that support the caregiver but do not involve care for the care recipient.	Children's lives are influenced only by the parent's (or other relative's) caregiving.

giving. According to 2001 U.S. census data, 4.78 million children lived in multigenerational households that included at least one parent and a grandparent. These children represent 6.9% of all children under age 18 (Kreider & Fields, 2001). However, these data ignore care outside children's households and they include coresidence situations formed to support the adult children rather than care for older parents. Several nationally representative data on caregivers also offer some information on children's involvement in care. The survey conducted in 2003 on behalf of the National Alliance for Caregiving indicates that 37% of all caregivers had a child under age 18 in the household. This proportion was considerably higher among African Americans (53%) than among other racial and ethnic groups (National Alliance for Caregiving, 2004, p. 26). According to the National Long-Term Care Survey (NLTCS) conducted in 1999, 11.3% of caregivers had coresiding children under age 15. This proportion was higher among adult-child caregivers (18.0%) than among spouse caregivers (3.8%) (Wolff & Kasper, 2006, p. 352). The survey of young caregivers in the United States suggests that 3.2% of households with children 8 to 18 years of age include a child caregiver. This yields an estimate of 906,000 households with young caregivers in the United States (National Alliance for Caregiving, 2005, p. 11). These figures demonstrate that prevalence estimates may vary considerably due to differences in definitions, survey methods, or estimation procedures. They also provide a cross-sectional view that may underestimate the risk of children's involvement in care throughout their childhood years. For example, Szinovacz (in press), using data from the Health and Retirement Study (HRS). showed that, while only a relatively small proportion of women (under 15% for any racial and ethnic group) age 51 to 61 in 1992 with living parents provided care to parents at any one point in time, this proportion rose to about one-third for White and Black women and to over one-quarter for Hispanic women if care over a 10-year period was considered. Thus, the proportion of children ever involved in caregiving is probably considerably higher than the proportion indicated in cross-sectional surveys.

RESEARCH ON CAREGIVING CHILDREN

Because the literature on child caregivers is largely atheoretical, I present results of previous studies and of my own research within a conceptual framework that is informed by life course and family system theories and builds upon the so-called stress process model used in research on adult caregivers (Pearlin, Aneshensel, Mullan, & Whitlatch, 1996). Some of the crucial concepts in life course theory are contextual embeddedness of life transitions, linked lives, and life course development (Bengtson & Allen, 1993; Elder, 1995). Family systems theorists also have emphasized the interconnectedness among family members and the impact of individual family members' experiences on the system as a whole. According to the stress process model, outcomes of caregiving reflect the influence of primary stressors (the care situation) and secondary stressors (strains associated with other roles that may be affected by and influence caregiving). These stressors and their outcomes are contingent on selected social and economic characteristics (contextual embeddedness) and affected by moderators such as social support (Pearlin et al., 1996) or coping strategies. In line with life course theory, it is also essential to integrate ontological factors or individual development into models assessing the effect of care involvement on children (Jurkovic, 1997). Several studies suggest that care activities can impede individual development or guide it in specific directions. Furthermore, parents' development may promote or hinder reliance on their children's supports for themselves or for the care of other relatives (Jurkovic, 1997).

As shown in Figure 8.1, this suggests a conceptual framework consisting of the following main dimensions: contexts (cultural, socioeconomic, familial, personal), primary and secondary stressors, moderators consisting of coping strategies and social supports, and outcomes. It should be noted that this conceptual model remains essentially untested for child caregiving. Existing qualitative studies provide some insights into possible associations among major concepts but lack generalizability, whereas quantitative research lacks multivariate models that account for interrelationships among major model concepts. Furthermore, practically all studies were cross-sectional, rendering causal interpretation problematic. I use this framework to integrate findings from past research. This account will be augmented by mainly unpublished insights and quotes from a small qualitative study of adolescents assisting in the care of relatives with dementia ($N = 17$) I conducted in the late 1990s (see endnote 1).

Contexts

The life course concept of contextual embeddedness points to the importance of contextual factors that shape caregiving experiences. These contexts impinge on how care is distributed among family members, how care responsibilities are perceived, whether and which secondary stressors hinder adaptation to care, or which specific difficulties caregivers face and which supports they can enlist. Past research identified four major care contexts: cultural, socioeconomic, familial, and personal.

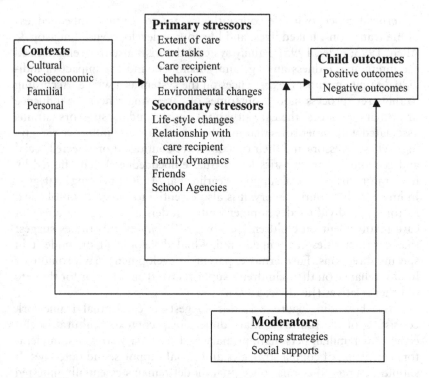

FIGURE 8.1   Conceptual framework for the analysis of child caregiving.

Cultural Contexts

Cultural contexts may influence the extent of children's involvement in caregiving as well as the outcomes of their involvement. Children's assumption of caregiving roles occurs by default when adults are not available or willing to participate in care or in response to parental authority (Lackey & Gates, 2001). Whether parents require children's contributions to care will depend on societal norms concerning the age appropriateness of such involvement as well as on the availability of alternative care sources. A European report on child carers suggests, for instance, that children's involvement especially in physical care activities may be less common in Sweden than in Germany, France, or the United Kingdom due to differences in these countries' welfare systems (Becker, 1995).

Another cultural norm impinging on child caring is gender ideology. Several studies suggest that girls are more often assigned caregiving tasks than their brothers (Dearden & Becker, 1995; Jacobson & Wood, 2004), and the extent of this gender bias may vary across countries (Dietz & Clasen, 1995).

As far as the influence of cultural contexts on outcomes is concerned, there can be little doubt that the non-normative character of children's caregiving in Western postindustrial societies contributes to adaptation problems. Child caregiving is not only off-time, but when children take on major responsibility—especially for parent care—it can also violate child protection laws or school attendance regulations. Consequently, those parents who may be most in need of formal supports may be reluctant to seek such help due to worries about punitive interventions (Becker & Aldridge, 1995; Dearden & Becker, 2000; Thomas et al., 2003). Even if such interventions are not a concern, secrecy about child caregiving reflects embarrassment on the part of the young carers and fears on the part of the parents that they may be deemed inadequate (Becker, 1995; Newman, 2002; Thomas et al., 2003). Such secrecy and embarrassment, as well as the relatively low incidence rate at any one point in time, further prevent caregiving children from turning to friends or securing other informal supports. Studies indicate that caregiving children are usually reluctant to tell others about their situation (Lackey & Gates, 2001) or find them to be nonsupportive (Beach, 1994; Dellmann-Jenkins, Blankmeyer, & Pinkard, 2001). For example, one of the girls (age 15) in my study commented:

> They just say, oh, you know, I really feel sorry for you, but there is this thing that's wrong in my life and . . . a lot of them aren't able to (be) sympathetic.

It is telling that this adolescent describes her caregiving experience as something "wrong in [her] life," a clear indication of her awareness that this situation contradicts standards of young adolescents' "normal" life-styles. As studies on adult caregivers suggest (Pearlin et al., 1996), lack of supports is likely to render adaptation to caregiving more difficult.

Socioeconomic Contexts

Both British studies and the U.S. survey of young caregivers indicate that child caregiving prevails among lower socioeconomic status families (National Alliance for Caregiving, 2005). It is not clear, however, to what extent socioeconomic status is confounded with other family character-istics such as minority status or having a single parent. Furthermore, the over-representation of lower-income families among young caregivers may reflect greater reluctance of upper-status families to participate in surveys on child caregiving. Certainly, lower-income families have fewer resources to secure paid help with care and other household services. No data are available that link families' socioeconomic status to the out-comes of child caregiving.

Family Contexts

Little is also known about how preexisting family structures and relationships impinge on children's involvement in care. Especially children's assumption of the main caregiver role sometimes evolves from family disruption or dysfunctional family dynamics (Chase, 1999; Dearden & Becker, 2004; National Alliance for Caregiving, 2005). Because these circumstances are in themselves stressful for children, they may intensify the effects of caregiving. When the care recipients are relatives outside the nuclear family unit (e.g., grandparents), past relationships with these relatives, both on the part of the caregiving children and their parents, can influence children's willingness to help (Piercy & Chapman, 2001) as well as their response to the care situation. However, as discussed later, caregiving also can alter relationships with such relatives as well as family dynamics within the nuclear family unit.

Personal Contexts

Children's responses and adaptation to their caregiving responsibilities will further depend on their personality and especially the developmental stage at which caregiving starts. Younger children may have difficulty understanding the care situation and care recipients' behaviors, especially if care is for a relative with mental illness or dementia. They also may be physically challenged by some care tasks such as lifting the care recipient (Becker & Aldridge, 1995) or lack the skills to perform selected care tasks (Gates & Lackey, 1998). In addition, care involvement may hinder ego development particularly among adolescents (Beach, 1997) and interfere with selected developmental tasks such as the establishment of close emotional relationships or education (Beach, 1997; Dellmann-Jenkins et al., 2001). Clinical and retrospective accounts suggest that such impingement on developmental tasks may have long-ranging effects, including lack of individuation, problems with adult relationships, difficulty with jobs due to educational problems, choice of careers in helping professions, or unresolved anger and fear (Chase, 1999; Dearden & Becker, 2000; Lackey & Gates, 2001; Orel & Dupuy, 2002). Because some of the conditions prompting children to assume caregiving roles also may affect their development, prospective studies will be necessary to ascertain the relative importance of specific contexts on the long-term outcomes of child caregiving.

Primary Stressors

As shown in Figure 8.1, primary stressors reflect features of the care situation and their direct impact on children's life-style. Particularly important seem to be the extent of required care, the types of tasks performed by children, the care recipients' condition and behaviors, as well as changes in the home environment necessitated by coresidence with the caregiver.

Extent of Care

The extent of care reported in studies on child caregivers varies widely, mainly due to differences in the definition of child carers used for sampling purposes. For instance, over a third of British young carers with primary care responsibility spend over 15 hours per week with caregiving tasks (Dearden & Becker, 2004, p. 9). Of the children surveyed in the United States, over 40% said that they had "a lot" of responsibility, but this percentage did not differ significantly between caregiving and noncaregiving children (National Alliance for Caregiving, 2005, p. 31). It remains unknown how long children are involved in caregiving roles. Those assuming primary or secondary care for disabled or mentally ill parents may spend considerable time periods in the caregiving role, whereas care for other relatives may be of much shorter duration. Retrospective accounts suggest increased depressive symptoms later in life among children with longer care duration (Shifren & Kachorek, 2003).

Caregiving Tasks

Children's caregiving activities include a wide range of tasks. Some may just increase their contributions to regular domestic chores, while others take on general as well as personal care, watch over and spend time with their ailing relative, provide emotional support, or participate in the care of their siblings to relieve the caregiving parent (Dearden & Becker, 1998, 2004; Jacobson & Wood, 2004; Lackey & Gates, 2001; National Alliance for Caregiving, 2005; Orel et al., 2004). According to the British young carer survey, emotional support and domestic chores are the most commonly performed activities, whereas involvement in personal care and care for siblings is rare (Dearden & Becker, 2004). Other researchers note that children's participation in personal care activities tends to be avoided and is the most stressful (Dearden & Becker, 1998; Gates & Lackey, 1998; Lackey & Gates, 2001; Orel et al., 2004). My research confirmed that adolescents take on multiple care tasks. Many had to watch relatives who may otherwise wander off, a task they called "grandma sitting," while others engaged in more personal care tasks. For example, a 13-year-old girl complained about the many chores she had to do:

> There's a whole lot of stuff that has to be done. I have to feed her and get her into bed at night and get her up in the morning and get her clothes on so she can go to the place [day care] and stuff like that.

As was the case in other investigations, adolescents in my study felt particularly uncomfortable with personal care tasks, and some care recipients resisted the adolescents' help, perhaps in an effort to preserve their dignity and to reduce role reversal.

> She used to fight me because I was a guy taking her to the bathroom. Like when I try to give her a bath, she doesn't really like that. The nurses have no problem giving her a bath, but when I try to give her a bath it's a different story.

Care Recipient Behaviors

It is not only caregiving chores that can contribute to children's stress but also the behaviors of the care recipient. As others have observed, children are often frustrated and angered by behaviors of relatives who are mentally ill or who have dementia (Aldridge & Becker, 1993a; Orel et al., 2004). Specifically noted by the children in my study were care recipients' invasion into their life space, incontinence, exhibition of anger, redundancy, telling on the adolescent, wandering, unusual ("weird") behaviors, creating disorder in the home, being overly demanding, and resisting help. Several adolescents complained about care recipients' invasion into their life space. This behavior was particularly common when adolescents shared their room with the care recipient but occurred in other cases as well. Care recipients "got into" or "messed with" the adolescents' personal possessions, hid items around the house, or occupied common space such as bathrooms for long time periods. Such invasions disrupted normal household routines.

> When she's in the room she'll change things around, we'll never find them and stuff like that. When we ask her where they are she won't tell us. And like when we have to go to the bathroom, she'll take the toilet paper and hide it in the room somewhere so we can't find it. And like she'll hide my school clothes, and when I get up in the morning I can't find them.

Although incontinence was quite common among care recipients, only a few adolescents viewed this condition as an issue. Care recipients' incontinence could become a problem when adolescents had to clean up after their relatives' accidents or the accident happened in the presence of friends. It is not uncommon for care recipients with dementia to exhibit anger and engage in aggressive behaviors. Adolescents reported that their relatives "screamed" or even became physically abusive. Such anger can trouble adolescents who may not understand why their relative is mad. For example, a 15-year-old girl whose father had Alzheimer's disease noted: "It's just weird, 'cause he has no idea why he's mad, and he's just mad as anything."

Many adolescents were considerably bothered when their relatives told parents about the adolescents' misdeeds. While some of these complaints were based on behaviors exhibited by the adolescents, many others were fantasies created in the care recipients' diseased minds. These "untrue stories" confused the adolescents and got them "in trouble" with their parents. "She'll tell lies about things and it will cause one big argument between everybody."

Several adolescents further mentioned unusual (what they usually refer to as "weird" or "crazy") behaviors on the part of their ailing relatives. Adolescents reacted to these exhibitions in various ways: some were confused, others annoyed, and one girl (age 13) noted that she had to learn not to laugh when her grandmother started to sing and believed she was Shirley Temple. Some care recipients were perceived as overly demanding. Whether this is a personality trait or a consequence of their illness is not always clear. Whatever the cause for these demanding behaviors, adolescents got upset when the care recipients' demands restricted the adolescents' own activities, when the care recipients complained to parents about adolescents' inadequate help, or when, as a 13-year-old girl put it, the care recipient "constantly picks on me."

Environmental Change

Changes in the home environment are common when the care recipient coresides with the caregiving family. Dens and family rooms were altered to become the relative's bedroom, additions to the home were built, or, in cases where the family moved in with the relative, the house was redecorated. When other adequate space was not available, adolescents had to share their room with the relative. Although this was relatively rare (noted by two adolescents), it seemed to be particularly troublesome. The care recipients woke the adolescents at night, disturbed their possessions, or had "accidents" in the shared room. Even the mere presence of another household member and the sharing of living space could be perceived as intrusion into the family's life-style or the adolescent's life space. Adolescents had to adapt to their relatives' habits and standards, and they had to take consideration of the relative's mental condition. For example, some of the Alzheimer's patients would get confused or disoriented if the house was "cluttered," or parents would insist on an orderly house because of frequent visitors:

> My mom is more hard about it [cleanliness] because more people come
> over here to see my grandmother we don't know. They don't like call,
> it's like out of the blue people come, like her old friends, or my aunts
> or something like that. So she wants the house to look kind of nice for
> that.

However, adolescents also can benefit from their relative's presence. One
girl (age 12) felt safer with her grandmother in the house.

These illustrations demonstrate that children's adaptation to caregiving is influenced by features of the care situation. Available evidence
suggests that care situations are particularly difficult if they involve intensive and long-lasting care and if they include personal care tasks. As
is the case for care by adults (Ory, Hoffman, Yee, Tennstedt, & Schulz,
1999), care for relatives with mental health problems is more problematic than care for relatives with physical health problems. In the case
of children, such care is particularly difficult because children may have
difficulty understanding the meaning and implications of dementia or
other psychiatric conditions, and their parents may accept information
from relatives who have dementia and discipline children based on these
relatives' invalid complaints. When care recipients coreside with young
caregivers, changes to the home environment can become an additional
source of stress.

Secondary Stressors

Secondary stressors "arise in areas of life lying beyond the boundaries of
caregiving" (Pearlin et al., 1996, p. 292). Research suggests that young
carers' main secondary stressors consist of changes in their life-style, family dynamics, and relationships with friends. They also include competing
obligations (especially school demands) and reactions of teachers.

Lifestyle Changes

The responsibilities and chores associated with caregiving require several
adaptations in young carers' life-style. Most often noted are decreases
in leisure time and restrictions on activities (Aldridge & Becker, 1993a;
Becker & Aldridge, 1995; Dearden & Becker, 2000; Gates & Lackey,
1998). Children often have to forgo extracurricular activities and other
leisure pursuits because they have to watch over the care recipient at
home. For example, one of the adolescents in my study noted:

> I know I can't stay after school 'cause then no one's here to get my
> grandmother. And there's a lot of things I want to do after school and
> I can't do it, like cheerleading tryouts.

Others noted that they had to adjust their behaviors to demands posed by the relative's presence in their home or to the care recipients' attitudes:

> You can't listen to music even softly, we have to just totally shut up. It's really hard.

> We have to like be more calm.

> She's really old fashioned, [and] like I'm a very affectionate person and I have my fiancé around all the time and I have to stay distant around him with her. And it gets hard for us because he doesn't understand quite how it is and the whole affection thing, that's hard.

Even when time for leisure is available, these activities are often interrupted to attend to care recipients' needs. In addition, care recipients' behaviors may interrupt the children's activities or even disturb their sleep, leading to fatigue:

> Like when she wakes me up in the middle of the night and talks to me, and then I don't have time to sleep and stuff like that, and I be real tired in school.

These examples illustrate the invasive effect caretaking can have on children's life-style. Many children took these limitations in stride, but others resented the curtailing of cherished activities.

Relationship With the Care Recipient

Relatives' illness or coresidence can bring about profound changes in their relationships with the caregiving children. Such changes pertain both to the structure of relationships as well as to their quality. The most frequently noted structural changes in relationships are role reversal (including parentification) and a decline in the care recipient's authority. These structural changes have been of concern to family therapists and are reflected in the growing literature on parentification. Role reversal—that is, children who are main caregivers especially for a parent—is noted consistently in the literature on young carers (Aldridge & Becker, 1999). Such instances of role reversal were also evident in my study. Some adolescents felt ambivalent about their assumption of parent-like roles vis-à-vis their relatives, but some of this ambivalence also reflected empathy for the care recipient:

> Sometimes I have to, you know: "Hey grandma you're not supposed to be doing that." It's kind of hard, it's just kind of like dealing with a child. It is really, and that's hard.

> It's really hard to tell her and to watch her without having to explain why I'm watching her, because she's older and that gets hard 'cause I don't know what to say.

Other children, on the other hand, took advantage of the situation and enjoyed exerting authority over the care recipient:

> Now it's easy because I can tell her what to do, I can tell her to shut up, and she'll shut up.

Other structural changes in the relationships between child caregivers and care recipients pertain to the frequency of interactions and joint activities. In some cases, interactions became more frequent as relatives who had been seen only rarely moved into the household, but, in many other cases, care recipients' dementia precluded interactions and joint activities.

In addition to structural changes, there is ample evidence of qualitative changes in relationships. Some children felt closer to their ailing relatives, while others reported that relationships became more distant (Orel & Dupuy, 2002). My data showed that most adolescents (70%) perceived a deterioration in the relationship, based on retrospective comparisons of their relationship with the care recipient before and after he or she became ill or moved into the household. However, close to a quarter of the adolescents (23%) saw an improvement in the relationship, mostly as a consequence of having more contact with the care recipient. One adolescent reported no change in the relationship. Similar to the quantitative results, the qualitative analyses revealed both positive and negative features of adolescents' relationship with the care recipient. In addition to role reversal, negative relationship features included "mean" or other negative acts toward the care recipient.

Positive relationship features refer to the relationship as a whole (closeness), to the adolescents' attitudes and behaviors toward the care recipient (reciprocity, helpfulness, empathy), or to the care recipient's attitudes and behaviors toward the adolescents (helpfulness, gifts, consideration). Some adolescents became closer to a grandparent they had hardly known before because the grandparent either lived far away or had little interaction with the family. These adolescents also seemed to gain some added sense of family and family history. Others reported positive exchanges between the relative and themselves. Some adolescents specifically mentioned gifts from the grandparents; others noted that care recipients helped with chores and took over duties previously assigned to the adolescents by their parents. In other cases, the adolescents just appreciated a cooperative or considerate attitude on the part of their relatives:

> Like if we're in the room playing Nintendo or something and she wants to watch TV, she always asks: "Is the TV going to bother you?" you know.

These gestures helped to preserve a positive relationship between care recipients and adolescents despite the many negative behavioral and cognitive manifestations of the relatives' disease. Adolescents also engaged in positive behaviors toward the relative. They helped their relatives, talked with them, and expressed sympathy for their condition:

> I'm closer to my grandmother. I get to help her with different things. Even though she has Alzheimer's or whatever, when she has trouble remembering I can help her.

Especially (although not exclusively) adolescents who had a close relationship with the care recipient in the past viewed helping their relative as acts of reciprocation. However, notions of reciprocity were further reinforced by feelings of obligation to help a grandparent. One male adolescent (age 19) said

> She used to help me all the time, why shouldn't I? But that wouldn't be the only thing, that's my grandmother, I would help her anyway.

The overall picture evolving from these case descriptions and from findings reported in other studies is perhaps one of ambivalence. On the one hand, adolescents are sometimes shocked and appalled by their relatives' erratic behaviors and demands. On the other hand, they demonstrate considerable empathy and sympathy for the care recipients and often engage in positive exchanges that can benefit both the care recipient and the adolescent. It is only in rare cases that relationships are nearly exclusively negative. This occurred when the care recipients had reached advanced stages of dementia or other diseases that prohibited real communication or when a negative relationship history precluded feelings of closeness or understanding on the part of the adolescent.

Family Dynamics

Both family systems theory and the life course perspective point to the interconnectedness among family members' experiences. Yet studies on young carers rarely address their relationships with other family members or the impact of caregiving on the family unit. Those that do address such relationships indicate that care tasks are sometimes shared among family members and that caregiving can alter family relationships.

Positive influences on family relationships include empathy especially for the main caregiving parent, bonding, increased closeness, and restraint (Beach, 1994, 1997; Dellmann-Jenkins et al., 2001; Lackey & Gates, 2001; Szinovacz, 2003; Thomas et al., 2003). Children appreciate their parents' efforts as carers and show understanding for the stresses of caregiving. Such empathy is often tied to children's own involvement in caregiving—that is, because they know how caregiving affects them, they also realize how caregiving can affect their parents. Joint participation in caregiving chores and parents' willingness to include children in care decision-making also contribute to closer relationships and bonding between the main caregiver (typically the mother) and the children. More rarely, the care recipient's presence in the home and concerns that loud arguments would upset the care recipient can lead to more restraint in parent-child interactions (Szinovacz, 2003).

There are numerous negative effects of caregiving on parent-child relationships as well. These include lack of attention by the parent, fewer family activities, increased strictness, and more family tensions (Beach, 1994; Szinovacz, 2003). Most of these negative effects reflect the parents' caregiver stress and preoccupation with care. Some parents who are main caregivers become so involved in their caregiving responsibilities that they "forget" about their children. Caregiving families also have less time for family activities and are more restrained in what activities they can pursue (Dearden & Becker, 2000; Gates & Lackey, 1998; Szinovacz, 2003). For example, a 13-year-old girl in my study complained

> 'Cause like, Harborfest and all that stuff . . . we'd always go to it, but now we can't. We want to go to a movie before, we just leave . . . and now we have to wait for my aunt to stay with my grandma.

In addition, caregiving can increase family tensions and reduce the quality of family relationships (Beach, 1994; Hamill, 1994; Lackey & Gates, 2001; MaloneBeach, Degenova, & Otani, 1998; MaloneBeach, Otani, & Degenova, 1999). Such tensions might be reflections of the stresses experienced by caregiving family members, but they can also revolve around whether the care recipient should be moved to a nursing home, how much time the main caregiver devotes to care activities, or the distribution of care among the children in the family (Gates & Lackey, 1998; Szinovacz, 2003). For example, stresses experienced by the caregiving parent are sometimes taken out on other family members, including the children. Indeed, some of the children I studied reported that they were afraid about how mad their parent could get (Szinovacz, 2003). Others expressed astonishment when parents expressed anger toward the care recipient. This situation troubled the children because they observed a role reversal in the grandparent-parent relationship that violated their expectations of parent-child authority. In addition, conflicts may arise when family members perceive the care situation differently (Hamill, 1994; Pruchno, Burant, & Peters, 1997; Pruchno, Peters, & Burant, 1995).

The Effect of Parental Status on Caregiving

Although the main focus of this chapter is on the effects of family caregiving on children, it is important to keep in mind that parental status and especially the presence of dependent children in the household can influence parents' decision to assume care as well as parents' caregiver stress.

Evidence regarding the effect of responsibilities to one's own children on assumption of the caregiver role is not clear. On the one hand, older children may serve as backup encouraging care; on the other hand, parents with dependent children have less time for caregiving and may also feel reluctant to expose their children to elder care or to rely on them for support (Gallagher & Gerstel, 2001). Reflecting these opposing forces, some studies showed that childless caregivers or those without dependent children were more likely to assume care (Pezzin & Schone, 1999; Wolf, Freedman, & Soldo, 1997), whereas others found the opposite trend (Johnson & Lo Sasso, 2000). There is some evidence linking the presence of children to the time parents spend caregiving. Some research suggests that the number of children is linked to reduced care hours (Wolf et al., 1997), but others reported variations by gender of the caregiver (Sarkisian & Gerstel, 2004) or the child. For example, Gallagher and Gerstel (2001) showed that the presence of young boys constrained the time mothers spent on care for their parents-in-law, whereas the presence of an older daughter increased time devoted to care for mothers' own parents. Fathers with young daughters spent more time caring for other relatives, while fathers with young boys devoted less time to parent-in-law care, and fathers with older boys spent more time with parent care. In contrast, Henz (2006), using British national data, found that women's involvement in care was negatively related to the number of their children, whereas fathers' participation in care was more influenced by children's age. Furthermore, relationships with children have been associated with caregiver stress. Stephens and Townsend (1997) showed, for example, that parent care led to decreased life satisfaction among mothers who also experienced high stress in the relationships with their children.

Overall, these studies confirm that family caregiving can have profound effects on the family unit. On the one hand, caregiving decisions and performance are influenced by parental status; on the other hand, family dynamics are influenced by caregiving. While caregiving may be particularly important for children's relationships with the primary caregiver (who is usually the mother), relationships with other family members are affected as well. That caregiving can also impinge on children's activities and roles outside the family unit is shown in the following sections.

Friends and Peers

Friends constitute an important part of adolescents' social networks. Consequently, friends' reactions to the caregiving situation or to adolescents' problems with this situation can facilitate or hinder adolescents' adaptation. Past research reveals three general themes related to caregiving children's interactions with peers. The first theme pertains to knowledge about caregiving, the second to effects on the quality of peer relationships and friends' supports, and the third to the extent of time devoted to activities with friends.

My research indicated that most adolescents lacked peers who had caregiving experiences, a fact that often leads adolescents to expect that their friends will not understand or will react negatively to the adolescent's caregiving experiences. One 17-year-old girl reported how she felt when the mother of one of her friends apparently had mental health problems:

> I understand how my friends feel because . . . before my grandmother [got sick] I knew there was a lady—I don't even remember who she is, it was one of my friends' mother or something—[who] freaked me out. It was like I don't want to come around her, she was kind of weird asking me all these questions and stuff. So I can understand how they feel and I don't expect them to understand.

This reluctance to share caregiving experiences with their friends is sometimes well justified. Some children receive little comfort and understanding from friends (Beach, 1994; Dellmann-Jenkins et al., 2001). Adolescents in my study reported that their friends were unable to empathize with their situation or even made fun of the care recipient's condition. When friends are unsupportive, adolescents not only lack the comfort that empathy from their friends could provide but sometimes become apprehensive about their own role and about the family's image:

> No, they don't really understand and sometimes, you know, when they come over it's kind of embarrassing sometimes because [of] his condition. If he ever, you know, went off on a tangent and saw something— 'cause sometimes he does that and it's not really there—then they kind of, I don't know, they don't understand.

They say "tell her it's Christmas, tell her it's Christmas," and I'll go tell her it's Christmas, and she's like "Oh, I better go and get you something." It's really dumb.

Such reactions may create some distance between the adolescent and his or her friends or at least a feeling of being different or set apart from one's peers. It is thus not surprising that some children keep their friends away from the care situation (Beach, 1994) and do not share their experiences with them.

However, some adolescents are fortunate enough to have friends who demonstrate sympathy and support (Beach, 1997). Such friends can have a calming influence on children who are upset about their relatives' condition or behaviors, and they help adolescents gain some perspective on their predicaments or, as one adolescent put it, "vent their frustrations":

When things happen and I just need someone to talk to and get advice from, it's like comfort, you know.

Oh yeah, they (friends) ask about my grandmother, ask how's she's doing, they know she's sick. They make little jokes about her, but, you know, it's all in jest, no hard feeling or anything. But just the fact that they ask about her is heartwarming enough for me.

In some cases, friends even became directly involved in care activities to help the adolescent. Especially adolescents' boy- or girlfriends established relationships with the care recipients and helped looking after them.

Studies that addressed the influence of caregiving on the amount of time children spend with friends document consistently that caregiving interferes with peer activities. Caregiving children have less time for activities with friends (Beach, 1994; Lackey & Gates, 2001; Orel & Dupuy, 2002; Thomas et al., 2003) and sometimes are also restrained in terms of the types of activities they can pursue:

Because like grandma's here and when she's sleeping and stuff, and when I have friends stay the night I can't have like [more than] one or two now because we wake her up.

I can't have friends over as much as I could because he has to be in the right state of mind, and if he's not in the right state of mind they can't come over.

Friends, then, can lighten children's burden when they empathize and show support, but they can also render the care situation more difficult. Having unsupportive friends contributes to caregiving children's feelings of being different from their peers, and such reactions may keep them from reaching out to others who may be more understanding.

School

Caregiving not only influences children's family and leisure experiences but also their school performance and attendance. Especially children assuming a primary caregiver role reported various ways in which caregiving impinged on school attendance and performance. Caregiving responsibilities led them to miss school or leave early, and some even dropped out of school altogether (Aldridge & Becker, 1993b; Dearden & Becker, 1995, 2000, 2004). In addition, school performance may suffer. Children with extensive care responsibilities may be too tired to do their school work, experience too many interruptions when care recipients require immediate assistance, or experience depressed moods that keep them from completing home assignments (Aldridge & Becker, 1993a; Lackey & Gates, 2001; Thomas et al., 2003). For example, one of the adolescents in my study commented

> Sometimes I'm just like, you know, too tired, I don't want to do it. It's because I'm too tired of the situation, and I'll just want to be lazy and not do my homework and not really want to do anything with the school.

It is not clear, however, to what extent school problems reported by caregiving children are really attributable to caregiving. The U.S. survey suggests that most school problems are mentioned equally often by caregiving and noncaregiving children. Young caregivers (ages 8 to 15 years) and caregiving children who coreside with relatives were more likely to not submit homework than noncaregiving children and caregiving children living separately. Furthermore, children involved in assistance with an elder's activities of daily living tended to miss school more than children involved in helping an elder with instrumental activities of daily living or other tasks (National Alliance for Caregiving, 2005). Even though caregiving responsibilities can result in decreased school attendance, going to school also serves as a reprieve from the caregiving situation at home (Gates & Lackey, 1998; Lackey & Gates, 2001). Some authors have suggested that care-related school problems eventually reduce young carers' job opportunities (Dearden & Becker, 2000). However, the long-range effects of care on employment will require careful longitudinal research that adjusts for other potential influence factors such as socioeconomic background.

Moderating Factors

How well children adapt to caregiving depends not only on the stressors themselves but also on moderating forces—namely, coping strategies and social supports. Because informal supports were already addressed previously, this section deals with coping and formal supports.

Coping

Despite the interest in how caregiving affects children, there has been little exploration of what strategies children use to cope with their caregiving responsibilities. A notable exception is Orel and Dupuy's (2002) small study of children involved in the care of their grandparents. Their interviews with six children from three families revealed three types of coping: behavioral, cognitive, and emotional. Behavioral coping strategies consisted of behaviors through which children either distanced themselves physically from the care situation (e.g., leaving the room, involvement in other activities) or used the care recipient's disability to their own advantage (e.g., by pretending they could not understand the grandparent's request). Cognitive coping involved denial of the care recipient's illness or ignoring of the care recipient's demands as well as the development of a positive definition of the situation. Emotional coping responses included empathy and religious involvement.

The two major themes on coping emerging from my research were active and passive coping. Although labeled differently, several of these strategies correspond to those described by Orel and Dupuy (2002). Coping responses classified under active coping included handling the situation, control, patience, and behavioral adaptations. Several adolescents emphasized that they had learned to deal with or handle either the care situation itself or specific features of the care situation. As the following quotes illustrate, some adolescents did not explicitly specify how they accomplished this, but implicit in their answers was that they had made an effort to adjust and gained some feeling of self-worth from this effort. Other adolescents were more specific about how they coped with the situation: they spoke of having learned self-control and patience or of having altered their behaviors.

> When I'm around my grandmother . . . I have more patience, have more patience with her, have more patience with my mom, my sister, just that way. I have more patience.

> I'm not trying to praise myself for being able to handle the situation, [but] then there are a lot of people who I know in church who wouldn't be able to handle it as best as I did.

> I think I know how to deal with the illness a little bit better, the Alzheimer's. I know how to deal with the side effects of it . . . I've also talked to her doctor, and he says, you know, just let her live, let her do what she wants to do.

An additional behavioral coping strategy involved adaptations to care recipients' problematic behaviors:

> See that tape recorder, just bought it, right, she'll say it's hers. Then she'll say, "well I got it from Egypt . . . like about 50 years ago . . . and it's like valuable and I need it." Then you'll have to give it to her to make her shut up, and you'll have to steal it back.
> I try to be happy around her, so I don't worry her, 'cause if she sees any hint of getting upset or sad or anything, she'll pick up on it and she'll constantly tell you about it.

The second type of coping that emerged from the interviews was passive coping. Some adolescents seemed to adapt to the care situation either by avoiding it or by getting used to it over time. What distinguishes these scenarios from active coping strategies is that the adolescents are not taking any direct steps to deal with the situation. Three forms of passive coping were evident from the interviews: distancing, ignoring, and habituation. A few adolescents coped essentially by fleeing the premises—they distanced themselves from the care recipient by going to another place in the house, or they engaged in activities that took them outside the home. Typical for these situations is that the adolescent leaves the care recipient's presence until feelings of stress are alleviated: "I'll just go in my room and chill out." Others mentally distanced themselves by ignoring the care recipients or their behaviors. They block out what the care recipient does or have learned not to become upset with their relatives' behaviors:

> At first it was really hard, but now I can kind of like single it out. It doesn't bother me as much as it used to.

In some cases, adaptation simply occurred over time—the adolescents got used to the care situation. Such habituation sometimes followed periods of pronounced stress and indicated that adolescents' responses changed over time.

These examples leave little doubt that many adolescents attempt to deal with their relative's presence and behaviors in numerous and sometimes quite creative ways. In many cases, these adaptations require considerable effort on the adolescents' part and occur over a long period of time. Because their relatives' presence, as well as parents' demands and stress reactions, put continuous strain on the adolescents, their coping efforts did not always succeed.

Formal Supports

Schools' and teachers' responses to young carers seem, at best, ambivalent. Although some teachers try to be supportive, others either ignore the children's situation or become overintrusive (Beach, 1994; Dearden & Becker, 1995; Thomas et al., 2003). One of the main issues seems to be that school personnel's primary concern is the children's school attendance and performance, and violations of attendance rules are seen as misbehaviors on the part of the children or as a problem requiring formal intervention (Dearden & Becker, 1995; Thomas et al., 2003). Both scenarios imply a sort of punishment of caregiving children. In the first case, children are held responsible for a situation over which they have little control; in the latter case, families and children fear that schools may initiate legal proceedings due to violation of attendance rules or disabled parents may be deemed unfit and the caregiving children removed from the family (Becker & Aldridge, 1995).

Similar difficulties exist in obtaining valuable supports for children from health care professionals. Because health care professionals focus on patients and are used to dealing with adults, caregiving children are sometimes ignored because they are children and thus not given medical information necessary for their caregiving activities (Becker & Aldridge, 1995; Dearden & Becker, 1995). This is particularly problematic when children are the main caregivers. Health care workers visiting homes have also been reported to ignore children, even though they must be aware of their involvement in care activities. In the worst case scenario, community care assistance may be withdrawn because children are available as carers (Becker & Aldridge, 1995).

In addition, most support services targeting caregivers are geared toward adults. Such services rarely fulfill the needs of young carers (Becker & Aldridge, 1995; Dearden & Becker, 1995) and may, in some cases, even undermine children's family supports. For example, one adolescent in my study complained that her mother was always going to support group meetings and had no time for her. Fear of punitive interventions further prevents many families from seeking supports from social agencies.

Outcomes

Much of the literature on caregivers in general and on child caregivers in particular stresses negative outcomes. However, for child caregivers, the evidence to support overwhelmingly negative outcomes is problematic. Available studies typically lack comparison groups and fail to compare children's well-being prior to and after they assumed caregiving roles. One exception is the U.S. survey on child caregivers, which includes a comparison group of noncaregivers. This survey showed no significant differences in mood between caregiving and noncaregiving children. However, these analyses do not adjust for the extent of children's involvement in care or other factors that may influence mood. The adolescents in my study were asked how their life was now and how it had been prior to their assumption of the caregiving role (scored on a 10-point scale). Almost two-thirds of the adolescents (65%) indicated that their life had changed for the worse after the care recipient became ill or moved into the household, but some adolescents perceived either no change (18%) or an improvement in their lives (18%). Qualitative studies attest to ambivalent outcomes: they demonstrate both positive and negative effects of caregiving on children's well-being.

Positive Outcomes

Positive consequences of caregiving reported in previous studies and evident from my research consist of developmental change, learning experiences, enhanced self-concept, financial profit, and positive attitudes toward older people. One of the consequences of assuming adult roles is increased maturity (Dearden & Becker, 2000; Gates & Lackey, 1998; Lackey & Gates, 2001; Orel & Dupuy, 2002). Such maturity manifests itself in more independence and responsibility and is often based on positive learning experiences from exposure to the illness and the need to deal with the situation (Dearden & Becker, 2000; Lackey & Gates, 2001; Orel & Dupuy, 2002; Thomas et al., 2003). Some adolescents in my study also noted that they had learned more about dementia. The following quotes illustrate these positive outcomes, although some ambivalence is notable as well:

> Well, I'm more aware of getting old. And I don't want to get to where he's going. That scares me, 'cause I don't want to live that long, if that's how it ends up.

> I'm coming out of it with more education and more wisdom into what's going on with the situation. I'm aware of what happens with Alzheimer's.

> It helped me a lot. Just in the world it will help me get through stuff.

Children further noted that they derive a sense of gratification, satisfaction, and enhanced self-esteem from their care experiences. Such improvements in children's self-concept evolve from successful coping, feelings of usefulness, and fulfillment of obligations (Dellmann-Jenkins et al., 2001; Gates & Lackey, 1998; Lackey & Gates, 2001; Orel & Dupuy, 2002).

Although relatively rare, some children reported material gains. Care recipients' income may help the children's parents pay for family expenses. Other adolescents received money or gifts from the care recipients.

The development of more positive attitudes toward older people is another positive outcome of children's caregiving (Beach, 1997). It should be noted, however, that some children become more prejudiced toward the aged (Orel & Dupuy, 2002). The following quote from a 17-year-old girl in my study illustrates this ambivalence:

> I look at them (older people) almost as babies, I mean that sounds bad, but just seeing how you enter the world as this thing that needs help and basically you exit the world and you need help. And so it's just looking at elderly people, I have more sympathy for them. I'm able to look at them in a different way. Before I used to be "Oh gosh, that person is so slow." Now I'm just, "No, I really do understand why they are [slow]." That it's not their fault. It's, you know, what has happened to them.

Negative Outcomes

Although many children derive some benefit from their caregiving experiences, many report negative outcomes as well. As is the case with adult caregivers, caregiving children experience considerable stress. This stress manifests itself in different ways, ranging from feelings of frustration and anger, to worry, anxiety, and sadness or grief (Dearden & Becker, 2000; Gates & Lackey, 1998; Orel et al., 2004; Thomas et al., 2003). Children in my study indicated that they felt "stressed out," had mood swings, became angry, frustrated, upset, resentful, or sad and depressed. While some adolescents kept their feelings to themselves, others directed their frustrations and anger against the care recipient or other family members and friends:

> It makes me go off on her [care recipient] and I like start cussing all the time.

> I've been less patient with my friends 'cause I'm using up all my patience on him [care recipient].

While some adolescents reacted with anger or mood swings, others exhibited negative self-feelings. These negative self-feelings arose when adolescents felt guilty about doing too little for the care recipient or had difficulty coping with the situation. Some adolescents reacted to the care situation with negative self-feelings, but others became sad or displayed depressive symptoms. Depressive symptoms tended to occur when adolescents were overwhelmed by the care situation, whereas sadness was often a response to the care recipients' deteriorating condition and in anticipation of their death. For example, a 13-year-old girl who was very close to her grandmother said

> It's kind of sad because, you know, when people like don't want to do anything for themselves, it makes you think that they just want to sit there and just die.

To summarize, caregiving involves both costs and benefits for children. Benefits include maturation and positive self-feelings, whereas negative outcomes manifest themselves in negative affect, negative self-feelings, depressive symptoms, perceived coping difficulties, and behavioral stress reactions.

CONCLUSION

Children's involvement in caregiving differs in significant ways from caregiving by adults. These differences influence children's caregiving experiences as well as the availability of and access to formal supports. They also may have contributed to the relative neglect of children in the caregiving literature up to the 1990s.

In contrast to care by adults, caregiving by children is non-normative and often involuntary. Most Western nations frown on children's involvement in stressful labor. In addition, children take on caregiving roles either because their family situation forces them to do so (e.g., when a single parent requires care) or because their parents assign caregiving tasks to them. Only very rarely are children the initiators of their caregiving activities (Orel et al., 2004). These features of children's caregiving mean, first, that most caregiving children are trapped in a situation (they would have to leave the parental home to escape), whereas overwhelmed adult caregivers have the option to shift the care of ailing relatives to other helpers or to an institution. While some parents may attend to their children's stress in care decisions, they do not necessarily do so. Indeed, as described above, at least some parents become so involved in their caregiving that they pay little attention to their children's needs. As life course theorists have pointed out, the off-time and usually involuntary character of children's caregiving may render it particularly stressful.

The second implication of these special features of child caregiving is that access to formal services is both problematic and contingent on adults' interventions. Children do not have the means or the authority to obtain formal help but rather depend on their parents to access such supports. Parents, however, may be reluctant to turn to formal helpers precisely because their children's involvement in care is non-normative and may lead to punitive actions (either on the basis of laws pertaining to "unfit" parents or on the basis of regulations pertaining to abused and neglected children) on the part of welfare or health care agencies (Newman, 2002). Both parents and children thus often hide child caregiving from the outside world. It is consequently not surprising that support programs for caregivers have rarely attended to children.

Support services for child caregivers have become widespread in Britain but are in their early stages in most other countries. Apart from clinicians' therapeutic interventions, British researchers first engaged in concerted efforts to investigate and develop support programs for child caregivers. These efforts eventually resulted in legislation and specialized programs to support young carers (Aldridge & Becker, 1993a; Becker & Aldridge, 1995; Becker, Aldridge, & Dearden, 1998; Dearden & Becker, 2004). However, these efforts were not without controversy. Partly as a means to secure funding and supports and partly as a consequence of their focus on children with main caregiver responsibilities, these studies tended to emphasize negative outcomes. Critics raised questions about the ubiquitous negative consequences of child caregiving and the implied blame put on young carers' parents (Aldridge & Becker, 1999; Newman, 2002; Olsen, 1996). One key issue of this debate is whether supports should be targeted at young carers, their parents, or families. In response to these critiques, advocates of the young carer programs recently shifted their emphasis from the children to the family as a whole:

> Promoting a family approach to serve the best interests of young carers and their families emphasizes the importance of family autonomy and family rights. It shifts the focus away from children's and disabled people's rights and towards the interactive needs and rights of the whole family. (Aldridge & Becker, 1999, p. 315)

This approach recognizes that support services targeting disabled parents (or other care recipients) can lighten the burden of young carers as long as their needs are considered as well. In other countries, including the United States, programs addressing caregiving children and their families are still in their beginnings. Supports are either geared toward care recipients as individuals or at the main caregiver with little consideration for the needs of other family members. For example, the Alzheimer's Association's Web site (www.alz.org) provides a fact sheet for children and teens that describes characteristics of the disease but provides no information on how to best deal with relatives who have dementia or the main caregiver parent. It also offers no information on available supports for children.

There is also considerable need for more research on children involved in caregiving (Olsen, 1996). Our knowledge basis to date is restricted to the insights that children are involved in care for older adults (although that involvement may vary considerably), that care-giving can have numerous influences on their lives, and that it results in both positive and negative outcomes. What is not known is how prevalent different types of children's involvement in caregiving (as shown in Table 8.1) are, which conditions impinge on the extent of children's involvement, and what characteristics moderate or mediate the outcomes of children's caregiving. One of the limitations of existing studies is their nearly exclusive emphasis on care work by the children. However, indirect or passive involvement (see Table 8.1) may be at least as common as direct and active involvement and, under some circum-stances, just as stressful. For example, is it more stressful for the child to experience the care situation firsthand and thus understand the care-giving parent's stresses and anger, or is it more difficult to deal with the stressed-out and angry parent without exposure to the care situation itself (e.g., when the parent provides extensive care outside the family's home)? Similarly, we may ask whether children resent additional chores more if they involve direct care activities or if they solely relieve the caregiving parent's stress without exposure to the care recipient. Thus, more attention needs to be directed toward the different ways in which children become involved in caregiving.

Another caveat of current research is its neglect of the family environ-ment. Both family systems and life course theories stress the interlinking of family members' experiences. Such linkages are particularly relevant for research on child caregivers because it is typically a parent who is the main caregiver. As some of the illustrations from qualitative studies indicate, how well children adapt to caregiving will depend to a large extent on how well their parents cope and to what extent family dynamics are disrupted by caregiving responsibilities. To fully understand children's caregiving ex-periences, it is thus necessary to focus on the entire family unit.

Importantly, research needs to shift from small-scale qualitative stud-ies to large-scale and representative investigations that are generalizable to the population of caregiving children and address the complexity of fac-tors that may impinge on children's caregiving experiences and outcomes. In addition, there is need for prospective longitudinal research that can address well-being over time among children who are not in caregiving situations and those that encounter diverse care scenarios. Even when careful matching of groups is applied (National Alliance for Caregiving, 2005), cross-sectional studies comparing caregiving and noncaregiving children are insufficient because of nonresponse and selection bias and the problems associated with causal attributions in cross-sectional designs.

In an aging society that faces a growing number of care recipients and a shrinking of the potential traditional family caregiver population (adult children and spouses—see the chapter by Uhlenberg & Cheuk in this volume) we can expect increasing reliance on or at least participation of nontraditional family caregivers, including children. Especially in the case of children, such participation must be weighed against potential costs in terms of long-term developmental, educational, or psychological problems that may evolve from heavy care responsibilities or exposure to particularly difficult care situations such as those involving mental illness or dementia. Child caregiving also has to be assessed in regard to various cultural and subcultural contexts that may differ in terms of the normative foundations of family care obligations in general (see the chapters by Lowenstein, Katz, & Gur-Yaish and by Silverstein, Conroy, & Gans in this volume) and children's care obligations in particular. Such assessments, based on carefully designed research, can help in identifying those conditions rendering child caregiving detrimental to children and their families and in devising support strategies that reduce the vulnerabilities of caregiving children and their families.

NOTE

1. The adolescents ranged in age from 12 to 19 years and were predominantly girls (73%). All but two adolescents cared for a grandparent. Coresidence with the care recipient was an eligibility criterion. Most parents (the primary caregivers) were married and middle class. About one-quarter were African Americans. A full report of the study is available from the author. Only findings pertaining to adolescents' relationship with the caregiver and family dynamics were previously published in Szinovacz (2003), which also contains a detailed description of the study and the adolescents.

REFERENCES

Aldridge, J., & Becker, S. (1993a). Children as carers. *Archives of Disease in Childhood, 69*, 459–462.

Aldridge, J., & Becker, S. (1993b). Punishing children for caring: The hidden cost of young carers. *Children and Society, 7*(4), 277–288.

Aldridge, J., & Becker, S. (1999). Children as carers: The impact of parental illness and disability on children's caring roles. *Journal of Family Therapy, 21*, 303–320.

Ariès, P. (1962). *Centuries of childhood. A social history of family life.* New York: Vintage Books.

Beach, D. L. (1994). Family care of Alzheimer victims: An analysis of the adolescent experience. *American Journal of Alzheimer's Disease and Related Disorders, 9*, 12–19.

Beach, D. L. (1997). Family caregiving: The positive impact on adolescent relationships. *The Gerontologist, 37*, 233–238.

Becker, S. (1995). *Young carers in Europe: An exploratory cross-national study in Britain, France, Sweden and Germany.* Leicestershire, England: Loughborough University, Young Carers Research Group.

Becker, S., & Aldridge, J. (1995). Young carers in Great Britain. In S. Becker (Ed.), *Young carers in Europe: An exploratory cross-national study in Britain, France, Sweden and Germany* (pp. 1–26). Leicestershire, England: Loughborough University, Young Carers Research Group.

Becker, S., Aldridge, J., & Dearden, C. (1998). *Young carers and their families.* Oxford, England: Blackwell Science.

Bengtson, V. L., & Allen, K. R. (1993). The life course perspective applied to families over time. In P. G. Boss, W. J. Doherty, R. LaRossa, W. R. Schumm, & S. K. Steinmetz (Eds.), *Sourcebook of family theories and methods* (pp. 469–498). New York: Plenum.

Carers Australia. (2001). *Young carers research project. Final report.* Canberra: Carers Australia.

Chase, N. D. (1999). *Burdened children: Theory, research, and treatment of parentification.* Thousand Oaks, CA: Sage.

Dearden, C., & Becker, S. (1995). *Young carers: The facts.* Sutton Surrey, England: Reed Business.

Dearden, C., & Becker, S. (1997). Protecting young carers: Legislative tensions and opportunities in Britain. *Journal of Social Welfare and Family Law, 19*(2), 123–138.

Dearden, C., & Becker, S. (1998). *Young carers in the United Kingdom.* London: Carers National Association.

Dearden, C., & Becker, S. (2000). *Growing up caring: Vulnerability and transition to adulthood—Young carers' experiences.* Leicestershire, England: Loughborough University, National Youth Agency.

Dearden, C., & Becker, S. (2004). *Young carers in the United Kingdom: The 2004 report.* Leicestershire, England: Loughborough University.

Dellmann-Jenkins, M., Blankmeyer, M., & Pinkard, O. (2001). Incorporating the elder caregiving role into the developmental tasks of young adulthood. *International Journal of Aging & Human Development, 52*(1), 1–18.

Dietz, B., & Clasen, J. (1995). Young carers in Germany. In S. Becker (Ed.), *Young carers in Europe: An exploratory cross-national study in Britain, France, Sweden and Germany* (pp. 65–76). Leicestershire, England: Loughborough University, Young Carers Research Group.

Elder, G., Jr. (1995). The life course paradigm: Social change and individual development. In P. Moen, J. G. Elder, & K. Lüscher (Eds.), *Examining lives in context: Perspectives on the ecology of human development* (pp. 101–140). Washington, DC: American Psychological Association.

Gallagher, S. K., & Gerstel, N. (2001). Connections and constraints: The effects of children on caregiving. *Journal of Marriage and the Family, 63,* 265–275.

Gates, M. F., & Lackey, N. R. (1998). Youngsters caring for adults with cancer. *Journal of Nursing Scholarship, 30*(1), 11–15.

Hamill, S. B. (1994). Parent-adolescent communication in sandwich generation families. *Journal of Adolescent Research, 9,* 459–482.

Henz, U. (2006). Informal caregiving at working age: Effects of job characteristics and family configuration. *Journal of Marriage and the Family, 68,* 411–429.

Jacobson, S., & Wood, F. G. (2004). Contributions of children to the care of adults with diabetes. *Diabetes Educator, 30*(5), 820–826.

Johnson, R. W., & Lo Sasso, A. T. (2000). *The trade-off between hours of paid employment and time assistance to elderly parents at midlife.* Washington, DC: Urban Institute.

Jurkovic, G. J. (1997). *Lost childhoods: The plight of the parentified child.* New York: Brunner/Mazel.

Kreider, R. M., & Fields, J. (2001). *Living arrangements of children: 2001.* Washington, DC: U.S. Census Bureau.

Lackey, N. R., & Gates, M. F. (2001). Adults' recollections of their experiences as young caregivers of family members with chronic physical illnesses. *Journal of Advanced Nursing, 34*(3), 320–328.

MaloneBeach, E. E., Degenova, M. K., & Otani, H. (1998). Conflict, well-being, and depression: Young adults in intergenerational caregiving and noncaregiving families. *Korean Journal of Research in Gerontology, 7,* 5–16.

MaloneBeach, E. E., Otani, H., & Degenova, M. K. (1999). Intergenerational solidarity: Norms, affection, and association in caregiving and noncaregiving families. *Korean Journal of Research in Gerontology, 8,* 5–16.

National Alliance for Caregiving. (2004). *Caregiving in the U.S.* Bethesda, MD: Author.

National Alliance for Caregiving. (2005). *Young caregivers in the U.S: Report of findings.* Bethesda, MD: Author.

Newman, T. (2002). "Young carers" and disabled parents: Time for a change of direction? *Disability & Society, 17*(6), 613–625.

Olsen, R. (1996). Challenging the facts and politics of research into children and caring. *Disability & Society, 11*(1), 41–54.

Orel, N. A., & Dupuy, P. (2002). Grandchildren as auxiliary caregivers for grandparents with cognitive and/or physical limitations: Coping strategies and ramifications. *Child Study Journal, 32*(4), 192–213.

Orel, N. A., Dupuy, P., & Wright, J. (2004). Auxiliary caregivers: The perceptions of grandchildren within multigenerational caregiving environments. *Journal of Intergenerational Relationships, 2*(2), 67–92.

Ory, M., Hoffman, R., 3rd, Yee, J., Tennstedt, S., & Schulz, R. (1999). Prevalence and impact of caregiving: A detailed comparison between dementia and nondementia caregivers. *The Gerontologist, 39*(2), 177–185.

Pearlin, L. I., Aneshensel, C. S., Mullan, J. T., & Whitlatch, C. J. (1996). Caregiving and its social support. In R. H. Binstock & L. K. George (Eds.), *Handbook of aging and the social sciences* (4th ed., pp. 283–302). San Diego, CA: Academic Press.

Pezzin, L. E., & Schone, B. S. (1999). Intergenerational household formation, female labor supply and informal caregiving: A bargaining approach. *Journal of Human Resources, 34*(3), 475–489.

Piercy, K. W., & Chapman, J. G. (2001). Adopting the caregiver role: A family legacy. *Family Relations, 50,* 386–393.

Pruchno, R. A., Burant, C. J., & Peters, N. D. (1997). Typologies of caregiving families: Family congruence and individual well-being. *The Gerontologist, 37,* 157–167.

Pruchno, R. A., Peters, N. D., & Burant, C. J. (1995). Mental health of coresident family caregivers: Examination of a two-factor model. *Journals of Gerontology: Psychological Sciences, 50B,* P247–P256.

Sarkisian, N., & Gerstel, N. (2004). Explaining the gender gap in help to parents: The importance of employment. *Journal of Marriage and the Family, 66*(2), 431–451.

Shifren, K., & Kachorek, L. (2003). Does early caregiving matter? The effects on young caregivers' adult mental health. *International Journal of Behavioral Development, 27*(4), 338–346.

Stephens, M. A., & Townsend, A. L. (1997). Stress of parent care: Positive and negative effects of women's other roles. *Psychology of Aging, 12,* 376–386.

Szinovacz, M. E. (2003). Caring for a demented relative at home: Effects on parent-adolescent relationships and family dynamics. *Journal of Aging Studies, 17,* 445–472.

Szinovacz, M. E. (in press). Commentary: The future of intergenerational relationships—Variability and vulnerabilities. In K. W. Schaie & P. Uhlenberg (Eds.), *Social structures: The impact of demographic changes on the well-being of older persons.* New York: Springer.

Thomas, N., Stainton, T., Jackson, S., Cheung, W. Y., Doubtfire, S., & Webb, A. (2003). Your friends don't understand: Invisibility and unmet need in the lives of "young carers." *Child and Family Social Work, 8,* 35–46.

Wolf, D. A., Freedman, V., & Soldo, B. J. (1997). The division of family labor: Care for elderly parents. *Journals of Gerontology: Social Sciences, 52B,* S102–S109.

Wolff, J. L., & Kasper, J. D. (2006). Caregivers of the frail elderly: Updating a national profile. *The Gerontologist, 46*(3), 344–356.

SECTION III

Sociopolitical Contexts

CHAPTER NINE

Workplace Policies and Caregiving[1]

Eliza K. Pavalko, Kathryn A. Henderson, and Amanda Cott

The rise in women's labor force participation over the past half century has transformed the workplace as well as the lives of workers. Much of the focus of this transformation has been on balancing employment and the care of young children, as new cohorts of dual-career and single parents challenged the old workplace model that most workers had a source of unpaid labor to care for growing families. As the workforce ages, employers and workers will continue to face new challenges. While the demands of caring for young children will decrease, the risk that a worker will have a parent, spouse, or sibling who needs care will increase. The intersection of women's increased labor force participation and an aging workforce thus means that caregivers are increasingly likely to be employed and that workers are increasingly likely to be faced with periods of time when they are balancing caregiving with their job. Recent estimates suggest that more than half of caregivers are employed full time and that, at any given time, between 6% and 13% of employees are providing care for an ill or disabled family member (Fredriksen & Scharlach, 1999; Gorey, Rice, & Brice, 1992; National Alliance for Caregiving and American Association of Retired Persons, 1997; Pavalko & Henderson, 2006).

How many workers have access to workplace policies that may help them balance the demands of their job with this care work, and has this access increased in recent years? In the United States, solutions to work-family conflict have largely fallen on the shoulders of individual families, and, unlike workers in other industrialized countries, workers have few state protections of family time (Glass & Estes, 1997; Wisensale, 2003). However, in recent years, there has been growing public and research interest in "family-friendly" policies and increasing evidence of the benefits of some of these policies for labor force absenteeism, retention, and the well-being of adults and children (Baum, 2003; Chesley & Moen, 2006; Glass & Estes, 1997; Kossek, 2005; Pavalko & Henderson, 2006; Ruhm, 2005).

In this chapter, we review recent research on workplace policies thought to be most relevant for caregivers, including policies providing paid or unpaid time off from work, flexible hours, and health insurance. We assess some of the difficulties of determining how many workers have access to these policies and use several national data sources to examine the range of estimates for current access among U.S. workers. We then examine variation in access to workplace policies across jobs and evaluate change in access over the decade following the passage of the Family Medical Leave Act (FMLA). In these later analyses, we focus on a national sample of middle-aged women (the National Longitudinal Survey [NLS] of Young Women) because it provides one of the best sources of longitudinal data on access to workplace polices and because it targets a group of workers at greatest risk of caregiving. We conclude the chapter with a discussion of the implications of our findings for caregivers.

WHAT DO WE KNOW ABOUT WORKPLACE POLICIES AND CAREGIVING?

Attention to the impact of workplace family policies, particularly family leave, has increased in recent years (e.g., Baum, 2003; Chesley & Moen, 2006; Henderson, 2005; Kossek & Ozeki, 1999; Pavalko & Henderson, 2006; Ruhm, 1998, 2005; Schaie & Schooler, 1998). Many (but not all) of these studies have shown that policies such as family leave and flextime are associated with better labor market outcomes, work commitment, and other employment outcomes (Baum, 2003; Chesley & Moen, 2006; Henderson, 2005; Kossek & Ozeki, 1999; Pavalko & Henderson, 2006; Ruhm, 1998, 2005). For example, Pavalko and Henderson (2006) found that women working on jobs where they had access to flexible hours, unpaid family leave, and paid sick or vacation days were more likely to remain employed and maintain work hours. Women who began caregiving and had access to unpaid family leave were far more likely to remain employed than caregivers without family leave. Similarly, a study of dual-earner couples reports that women caregivers with flexible work arrangements report higher levels of well-being (Chesley & Moen, 2006).

Much of the research on family-friendly policies has focused on policies related to the care of young children, with considerably less attention to workers managing the care of an ill or disabled family member (but see Chesley & Moen, 2006; Pavalko & Henderson, 2006; Scharlach, 1994). Although there are many similarities in the needs of parents caring for young children and those caring for an ill or disabled family member, there are also differences in these two types of care work that have policy implications. Unlike the care of children—which follows a fairly predictable time schedule (i.e., heaviest during infancy and the preschool period and lighter when children enter the formal schooling period)—care for an ill or disabled spouse or parent is unpredictable and may take place over a short or long period of time. It is difficult to predict when a family member may have a health crisis that requires care, and the course, nature, and length of the caregiving career may vary widely depending on the type of health problem, the relationship of the caregiver and care recipient, and the availability of other family members to share in the care work. The need for care may be sporadic or sustained; it may involve daily contact and personal care, or it may involve long-distance management of health care and other support. Unlike caring for children, in many cases of care for those who are ill, the amount and intensity of care work increases over the course of the care episode.

This variation means that, within any given workplace, workers are likely to have a diverse and changing set of needs for policies that help them minimize work-family conflict as they traverse the life course (Glass & Estes, 1997). This diversity in needs suggests that more general policies that can be applied broadly to all employees, rather than those targeting specific demographics, may be the most effective. In a recent study assessing the impact of policies on the retention of workers in the labor force, Pavalko and Henderson (2006) found that employed middle-aged women with access to policies providing flexible hours were more likely to still be employed 2 years later, regardless of their caregiving responsibilities. Provisions in the 1993 FMLA that provide job protection for men and women needing to take family leave and that provide protection for persons needing leave for personal care, care for an ill family member, or care for a young child are consistent with this broad-based approach to family policies.

Although the FMLA is an important first step toward protecting working families, its scope and use remain limited. Under the FMLA, one may have job protection to care for an ill parent but not a parent-in-law or grandparent. Also, the FMLA is typically viewed as providing protection for parental care, but 55% of those using the leave in 2000 did so to care for their own health or disability needs, 27% to care for an ill or disabled family member, and 18% for care for a newly born or adopted child (Waldfogel, 2001). Although both men and women take family leaves, when men do so, it is almost always to care for their own health rather than that of another family member. Use of the

FMLA is limited because it only provides unpaid leave, but several states have adopted paid maternity leave. In all cases except California, these paid leave policies are limited to time off to care for newborn children (Wisensale, 2003).

Given the nature of the caregiving experience, what types of policies are most likely to be most valuable for workers who are providing care? In general, policies that provide flexibility in work schedules or opportunities to take time off to provide care while remaining employed are found to be the most valuable (Chesley & Moen, 2006; Fredriksen & Scharlach, 1999; Pavalko & Henderson, 2006; Scharlach, 1994). These policies generally include paid and unpaid family leave, paid leave for shorter periods of time (such as that provided by paid sick and vacation time), and the availability of policies allowing flexible hours. Although not typically defined specifically as a family-friendly policy, there is strong evidence that health insurance is highly salient for workers and their families and may be a deciding factor in how families manage work-family conflicts. Workers cite medical insurance as one of the most important factors in choosing jobs, and they will change jobs to obtain medical insurance even if the new job pays less (Monheit & Vistnes, 1999; Olson, 2002). In a recent study examining the impact of a wide range of workplace policies on maternal employment, access to medical insurance was found to be the most important fringe benefit for ensuring new mothers' continued employment following childbirth (Henderson, 2005). The following sections review research on each of these workplace policies.

FAMILY LEAVE AND PAID TIME OFF

The United States stands out among industrialized countries for its limited protection of new parents (Gornick & Meyers, 2003; Wisensale, 2001). The United States is the only industrialized country that does not assure some period of paid family leave for new parents, and the limits on eligibility for unpaid leave in the current FMLA mean that even unpaid leave is assured for about 47% of private-sector employees (Waldfogel, 2001). Unlike some other industrialized countries, the United States also lacks any policies specifically designed to protect workers caring for ill or disabled parents or other adult family members. However, the FMLA is unique because it does provide some protection of workers who need time off for care of an ill or disabled family member as well as those needing time off to care for a newborn child (Wisensale, 2003). The FMLA requires businesses with 50 or more workers to provide up to 12 weeks of unpaid leave without loss of one's job if the worker has worked at the establishment for at least 12 months and at least 1,250 hours in the year prior to the leave. Beyond what is required by law, Waldfogel (2001) reports that 20% to 30% of firms offering unpaid leave go beyond what is required, either by offering leaves longer than 12 weeks or by covering workers who have not met the exclusion criteria. Indeed, by the time of the FMLA passage in 1993, most states had already adopted some type of leave policy and many provided comparable or stronger laws than those approved with the FMLA (Wisensale, 2001).

Assessment of the effectiveness of the FMLA is mixed. On the one hand, the majority of firms have reported that it is somewhat or very easy to comply with the law and that implementation of the leave policy did not adversely affect their productivity or profitability (Waldfogel, 2001). While 16.5% of employees take a family or medical leave, those leaves remain relatively short. In both the 1995 and the 2000 surveys conducted by the Department of Labor to assess the FMLA (Waldfogel, 2001), the median length of employee leave was 10 days, and 90% of leaves lasted 12 weeks or less. As previously mentioned, more than half of those leaves were to deal with one's own illness or disability, and another 27% were to care for an ill or disabled family member. Although the coverage offered by the FMLA is limited, there is evidence that the small percentage of workers who do use it find it valuable. Waldfogel (2001) reports that workers were generally satisfied with their ability to take a leave, and Pavalko and Henderson (2006) find that employed caregivers who have access to family leave are more likely to be employed 2 years later than caregivers who do not have such access.

On the other hand, it is clear that many workers do not use family leave, and it is questionable whether use of family leave, at least for care of young children, has increased with the passage of the FMLA. Legislation did not increase men's use of family leave and only increased women's use of leave under certain circumstances (Han & Waldfogel, 2003). The passage of the FMLA also did not increase women's returns to their employers after the birth of a child (Klerman & Leibowitz, 1999). Besides the fact that FMLA only assures unpaid leave, an additional reason for the limited impact of FMLA legislation is that, even when legally protected, informal workplace cultures may discourage its use. A study of policy use in a financial services corporation found that use of these policies varied depending on the social context of the work group and that employees were more likely to use these policies if they were in more powerful work groups that could buffer them from the perceived negative effects on their careers (Blair-Loy & Wharton, 2002).

The mixed evidence on the effectiveness of unpaid family leave suggests that, while access to unpaid leave is helpful for a small fraction of employees, its value is limited by its narrow scope and informal sanctions in some workplace cultures. These limitations make another, more common workplace benefit a potentially valuable—albeit limited—tool for employees: paid sick time and paid vacation days. Paid sick or vacation days are the most commonly available benefit with workers in private industry, averaging 8 days of paid leave per year (United States Department of Labor, 2004). Access to this form of short-term leave may be particularly valuable for workers dealing with the sudden illness or health decline of a family member. Indeed, several studies have found that women, and particularly caregivers, in jobs offering paid sick or vacation days were less likely to leave the labor force than those whose jobs did not provide this benefit (Pavalko & Henderson, 2006; Pavalko & Woodbury, 2000).

FLEXIBLE HOURS

Access to flexible work schedules is also often mentioned as a policy that is helpful for workers managing the demands of work and family care, and there is some evidence that workers with access to flexible scheduling have reduced absenteeism and turnover (Kossek & Ozeki, 1999), that caregivers with flexible work arrangements report higher levels of well-being than caregivers without these policies (Chesley & Moen, 2006), and that the majority of employed caregivers feel that these policies are or would be useful for helping them manage their caregiving and work responsibilities (Scharlach, 1994).

Understanding the impact of flexible hours is complicated by wide variation in the meaning of this policy. A study of Chicago firms found that firms with flextime policies did not necessarily have a formal policy, but rather they tended to be individualized to particular employees or times of the year and required employees to make special arrangements or requests (Kush & Stroh, 1994). As Glass and Estes (1997) note in their review of these policies, the advantage of a systematic policy is that it does not require employees to make special deals for flexible arrangements. Flexible work arrangements may take many different forms, with some of the most common being taking time off for school or child care functions, to periodically change starting and quitting times, or to return to work gradually after birth or adoption of a child (Bond, Galinsky, Kim, & Brownfield, 2005). Far less common are policies allowing employees to change starting and stopping times on a daily basis, job sharing, or work at home or off-site on a regular basis (Bond et al., 2005; Bond, Thompson, Galinsky, & Prottas, 2002). Estimates of the percentage of workers who have access to flexible schedules reflect this variation in the definition of a flexible workplace. Data from the 1997 Current Population Surveys suggest that 27% of workers report that they can make changes in the time that they begin or end work, and that these percentages are highest among part-time workers and those who work more than 50 hours per week (Golden, 2001). However, this greater flexibility coincides with an increase in unpredictable work hours and average hours worked per week (Golden, 2001). A more limited definition of a flexible workplace in the 2000 National Compensation Survey estimates that only 5% of private industry workers have access to a flexible workplace as a specific employee benefit (United States Bureau of Labor Statistics, 2002). Variation in definitions and implementation of flextime policies make it especially difficult to assess whether these policies have an impact on employee well-being or turnover. Although some studies have found that flexible workplaces do impact employee outcomes (Chesley & Moen, 2006; Dalton & Mesch, 1990; Pavalko & Henderson, 2006), these effects are often weak (Chesley & Moen, 2006) or do not apply specifically to caregivers (Pavalko & Henderson, 2006).

HEALTH INSURANCE

Although health insurance is not typically included in the list of family workplace policies, we include it in our review because of the primary importance of health insurance to most families. Access to medical insurance is more important for new mothers' continued employment following childbirth than is access to a wide range of other workplace policies (Henderson, 2005). However, it is likely that health insurance is a fundamentally different type of family-friendly policy than those that provide time away from the job or that increase job flexibility. Whereas time and flexibility policies are designed to keep workers in the labor force by making the demands of work and family more compatible with one another, health insurance is more likely to keep workers in the labor force because it is a protection that they simply are unable to do without, particularly if a family member is ill or disabled.

TRENDS IN WORKPLACE POLICIES

The passage of the FMLA marked one of the most significant changes in workplace policies in recent decades, and, not surprisingly, access to family leave has increased since the late 1980s. However, there is some evidence that there has been a gradual erosion in access to other benefits, including health insurance, retirement coverage, and paid leave of various types (sick days, vacation time, and holidays) (Wiatrowski, 2004). Indeed, the proportion of employer compensation dollars spent on benefits has remained stable over the past 25 years despite a number of changes in benefits and despite increases in health care costs (Wiatrowski, 2004). One of the strongest overall trends in workplace policies over the past 25 years has been a shift to greater employee responsibility for benefits, including more choice among health care plans and required employee contributions to health insurance and retirement plans (Wiatrowski, 2004). We will explore these temporal changes further in this chapter.

DATA ON WORKPLACE POLICIES IN THE UNITED STATES

Although several national surveys include information on the availability of workplace benefits, there is no single data source that provides estimates of benefits for all U.S. workers. The National Compensation Survey (NCS), conducted annually by the Bureau of Labor Statistics, provides some of the most comprehensive data on worker coverage but is limited to workers in private industries.[2] The NCS is a survey of establishments, and the 2004 NCS surveyed 4,703 private establishments covering 102.3 million workers. The Current Population Survey (CPS) provides an alternative source of information on selected benefits, particularly flexible hours. The CPS is a monthly household survey that provides data on employment and unemployment among U.S. adults age 18 and older. Questions on flexible hours and shift work are included in the CPS approximately every 5 years, but information on a broader set of benefits is not provided by the CPS.

The NLS, also conducted by the Bureau of Labor Statistics, provide an alternative set of estimates on workplace benefits. The NLS provides a series of longitudinal surveys that follow national samples of U.S. adults in specified birth cohorts. These surveys include a wide range of questions on labor market experience and benefit coverage and allow estimates of coverage for all working adults in the specified age range. The original surveys include two nationally representative surveys of U.S. women that have collected data approximately every 2 years from 1967 to 2003 (United States Department of Labor, 2005). The NLS-Mature Women's cohort sampled women who were between the ages of 30 and 45 in 1967, and thus most of the women in this cohort were retired by 2003. The NLS-Young Women's cohort sampled women who were between the ages of 14 and 24 in 1967. These women provide an ideal cohort for estimating the availability of work-place benefits among employees at highest risk of caregiving—women between the ages of 49 and 60 in 2003. The NLS-79 cohort provides national estimates for a slightly younger cohort—those between the ages of 39 and 47 in 2004. Although this age group is just moving into the peak caregiving years in 2004, one advantage of this data source is that it reflects both men and women workers.

The remainder of this chapter uses these data sources to address three research questions about workers' access to workplace policies. First, how many workers have access to various workplace policies? While policies such as the FMLA are mandated by law, many employers are exempt from the law because they employ fewer than 50 employees. For example, shortly after passage of the FMLA, only 59.5% of private-sector employees worked for companies covered by the law, and only 46.5% were both covered and eligible (Waldfogel, 2001). We draw from recent data from the NCS, CPS, the NLS-Young Women, and the NLS-79 to provide a range of estimates of workers with access to various poli-cies. Our analyses focus on policies that are most relevant to caregivers, including family leave, paid sick or vacation days, flexible work hours or flexible workplace, and health insurance. Although we are primarily interested in estimates for the population of workers most at risk of care-giving (middle-aged women), by using these three data resources, we are able to assess how their coverage may differ from broader populations of U.S. workers.

A second question to be addressed is how workplace benefits vary across job and worker characteristics. For these analyses, we focus spe-cifically on the NLS-Young Women's survey because of their relevance to caregiving populations. We compare percentages of employed women who have access to family-friendly policies across job sector (comparing private and government jobs), occupational category, job tenure, firm size, and usual hours worked per week.

The final question assesses the extent of change in family-friendly benefits among employed women from 1993 to 2003. This is a particu-larly salient decade to assess change because it spans the period just prior to the passage of the FMLA to nearly a decade after passage. In addition to the overall change in coverage, we also assess this change across job and worker characteristics. These subgroup comparisons are particu-larly important because we use longitudinal data from the NLS-Young Women. Even with no policy change, we would expect the percentage of women working in jobs that provide benefits to increase because the women's job tenure and occupational position is likely to have improved as they have aged.

RESULTS

How Many Workers Have Access to Family-Friendly Policies?

Table 9.1 shows the percentage of workers with access to workplace policies that may be helpful if they need to begin caring for an ill or disabled family member. Estimates from all three surveys indicate that roughly 68% to 80% of workers report access to family leave, paid sick and vacation days, and health insurance from their jobs. The one exception is the much lower percentage of men in the NLS-79 reporting access to family leave; but given their more comparable or greater access on other benefits, we suspect that the gender difference for family leave reflects women's greater awareness of family leave policies in their workplace (Waldfogel, 1999). Flexible hours are less common for all workers, with half or fewer workers reporting they have access to flexible hours and only a handful of workers (4%) reporting that they have the option of a flexible workplace—which is defined by the CPS as a workplace that allows them to work from home at least several days a week.

Despite the many differences in the NCS, NLS-YW and NLS-79 sample designs, estimates of the percentage of workers with access to family leave, paid sick and vacation time, and health insurance are fairly consistent across these different surveys. In contrast, estimates for flexible hours and workplaces vary widely across surveys. Only 4%

TABLE 9.1 Percent of Workers With Access to Family-Friendly Workplace Policies, National Compensation Survey, National Longitudinal Surveys, and Current Population Surveys

	NCS[a]	NLS-YW[b]	NLSY-79[c]		CPS[d]
			Men	Women	
Family leave	—	72	52	68	—
Paid sick or vacation time	77	71	75	75	—
Long-term care insurance	11	—	—	—	—
Flexible workplace	4	—	—	—	—
Flexible hours		40	47	54	28
Health insurance	69	80	76	73	—

[a] National Compensation Survey, workers in private industry, 2004.
[b] National Longitudinal Survey, Young Women's Cohort, 2003, women aged 50 to 60 working in wage and salary jobs, weighted data.
[c] National Longitudinal Survey of Youth, 1979 Cohort, 2004, men and women aged 39 to 46 working in wage and salary jobs, weighted data.
[d] Current Population Survey, 2004, workers age 18 and older.

of establishments report that they offer workers a flexible workplace (defined by the NCS as allowing workers to work some days at home), and between 28% and 54% of workers report that they have access to flexible hours on their jobs. We suspect that this wide variation in estimates of flexible hours reflects the often informal nature of many flextime policies. For example, data from the CPS indicates that, while 28% of workers report that they have access to flexible hours at their workplace, only 10.7% report having a formal flextime program at their workplace (Bureau of Labor Statistics, 2004). Instead, many workers continue to rely on informal arrangements with their managers (Glass & Estes, 1997). In these cases, access is likely to vary widely in the workplace and is less likely to be available to workers in entry-level positions who are least able to afford to take unpaid family leave or to hire someone to help with caregiving tasks.

We also note that women in their 50s, represented by the NLS-YW survey, are slightly less likely than women workers in their 40s (NLS-79) to have access to paid sick or vacation days or to have flexible hours, but they have more access to family leave and health insurance. While these may reflect sampling differences, our use of weighted data and parallel samples should minimize these differences. These findings suggest that it may be important to further explore cohort differences in access to benefits in future research.

Variation in Family-Friendly Policies

Table 9.2 shows the percentage of middle-aged women workers with access to family-friendly policies across job and worker characteristics. In addition to the policies shown in Table 9.1, Table 9.2 also shows percentages of women who have more substantial sick and vacation coverage and those who have at least one of the following benefits: health insurance, flexible hours, unpaid family leave, company child care, paid sick or vacation days, profit sharing, stock options, retirement pension, life insurance, and training or educational benefits. The most common benefit available is health insurance, followed closely by family leave and paid sick and vacation time. Half of employed middle-aged women receive more than 1 work week of sick or vacation days per year, while 21% have between 1 and 5 days of paid sick or vacation time available each year. While most workers have at least one benefit available to them, 15% of middle-aged women workers report that they do not have access to any workplace benefits.

Not surprisingly, access to benefits varies across job and worker characteristics. Part-time workers are the most vulnerable, because they are least likely to have any paid sick or vacation days available to them,

TABLE 9.2 Percent of Women Wage and Salary Workers With Access to Family-Friendly Policies by Job Characteristics, National Longitudinal Survey of Young Women, 2003 (Weighted Data)

	Family leave	Any paid sick or vacation days	Six or more paid sick or vacation days	Flexible hours	Health insurance	Any benefits (from list of 10)
All workers (N = 1,446)	72	71	50	40	80	85
Job sector (N = 1,446)						
Government	79	71	52	38	86	90
Private	67	71	49	42	76	80
Occupation (N = 1,446)						
Professional/managerial	81	72	55	43	86	90
Technical/clerical	73	78	56	45	83	89
Sales/service	50	55	32	32	61	66
Manual	67	73	46	15	78	79
Job tenure (N = 1,447)						
Less than 2 years	58	62	44	33	67	73
2 years or more	78	75	53	43	85	90
Firm size (N = 1,236)						
Small	55	64	43	40	65	74
Medium	84	74	54	37	90	92
Large	80	78	57	46	87	91
Hours per week (N = 1,450)						
Less than 35	38	39	23	28	44	55
35 or more	81	79	57	43	89	92

and nearly half of part-time workers do not have access to any benefits. Ironically, many women view part-time work as a strategy for balancing work and family demands, but part-time jobs are the least likely to provide protections that allow workers to successfully combine work and family.

In addition to the limited access to family-friendly benefits among part-time workers, those working in sales or service jobs, those in small firms, and those who have been at their current job for less than 2 years also have less access to fringe benefits. There is slightly less variation in access to flexible hours across job characteristics than for more traditional benefits. For example, 37% to 40% of women working in small and medium-sized firms have access to flexible hours, while 46% of women working in large firms report access to this benefit. For family leave, the difference in coverage between workers in small and large firms is 25% (55% vs. 80%, respectively).

Change in Access to Workplace Policies 1993–2003

In the decade since the FMLA was passed, are workers increasing or losing their access to workplace policies that might help them balance caregiving and work? As shown in Table 9.3, the answer to this question is mixed. Workers have made significant gains in access to family leave, and slightly more workers have access to health insurance, but the percentage of workers who have paid sick or vacation time dropped from 83% to 71%, and the percentage of workers with 6 or more days of paid sick or vacation days dropped even more—from 73% to 50%. There is a slight decline in the percentage of workers who have access to any benefits but no significant change in the percentage who have flexible hours. In other words, while family leave is becoming more common, access to many other benefits that may be as important for short-term caregiving crises are slowly eroding (see also Wiatrowski, 2004).

These percentages are based on longitudinal data that follow the same women over time, and, thus, these estimates of declines in benefits are conservative. As workers age from their 30s to their 40s and 50s, they tend to accumulate more job experience and job tenure and move into more secure jobs. Declines in benefits are particularly pronounced among women working in more secure jobs. For example, access to paid sick or vacation days decreases 19 percentage points (from 91% to 72%) among women in professional and managerial jobs, but by less than 10 percentage points among women in sales, service, or manual labor jobs. Likewise, access to paid sick and vacation days declines among women working in large firms from 90% of workers in 1993 to 78% in 2003,

TABLE 9.3   Change in Percent of Women Wage and Salary Workers With Access to Family-Friendly Policies by Job Characteristics, National Longitudinal Survey of Young Women, 1993–2003 (Weighted Data)

	Family leave		Any paid sick or vacation days		Six or more paid sick or vacation days		Flexible hours		Health insurance		Any benefits (from list of 10)	
	1993	2003	1993	2003	1993	2003	1993	2003	1993	2003	1993	2003
All workers	55	72	83	71	73	50	38	40	75	80	89	85
Job sector												
Government	65	79	92	71	82	52	29	38	86	86	95	90
Private	51	67	80	71	69	49	42	42	71	76	87	80
Occupation												
Professional/ managerial	65	81	91	72	81	55	42	43	84	86	94	90
Technical/clerical	56	73	86	78	77	56	40	45	78	83	92	89
Sales/service	34	50	64	55	51	32	36	32	54	61	76	66
Manual	53	66	81	73	69	46	22	15	78	78	85	79
Job tenure												
Less than 2 years	38	58	69	62	56	44	38	33	62	67	79	73
2 years or more	62	78	89	74	80	53	38	43	81	85	94	90

Firm size (number of employees)											
Less than 50	25	55	64	64	51	43	37	40	44	65	76	74
50 to 500	61	84	91	74	80	54	42	37	87	90	94	92
501 or more	66	80	90	78	82	57	40	46	85	87	94	91
Hours per week												
Less than 35	25	38	51	39	37	23	36	28	36	44	65	55
35 or more	62	81	92	79	82	57	38	43	86	89	95	92

Note. Cells in bold type indicate significant change over time, as measured by comparisons between the 95% confidence intervals and corresponding point estimates.

but coverage remains stable at 64% among women working in small firms. The picture that emerges is that, at least for access to paid sick and vacation days, the variation across jobs is narrowing.

DISCUSSION

In contrast to the political rhetoric about the importance of family in the United States, U.S. workers have fewer public protections of family time in place than workers in any other industrialized country (Gornick & Meyers, 2003). Virtually all industrialized countries provide some type of maternity leave, and most provide 2 to 3 months of paid leave after childbirth (Ruhm, 2005). In contrast, most of the protections that are available to workers in the United States are from employer policies, and only one state (California) provides paid family leave to workers, which is particularly valuable for caregivers of adult family members. Because these policies vary from one workplace to another and eligibility varies both within and across workplaces, even minimal protection of working families is far from universal.

How many workers have access to family-friendly policies in the workplace? Our examination of several national data sets suggests three levels of access to these basic workplace policies. The most vulnerable are workers who have virtually no protection, receiving none of the major family-related benefits, including access to employer health insurance or any paid sick leave. Our analyses indicate that 15% of middle-aged women in wage and salary jobs fall into this category, and 45% of those working part-time lack access to even the most basic benefits. A middle group of workers has limited protection, with at least a week of paid sick and vacation days, unpaid family leave, and some form of health insurance. The most protected group of women, comprising approximately 40% of middle-aged employed women, have access to a more comprehensive set of basic benefits, such as flexible hours and 6 or more days of paid sick or vacation time. We note, however, that the package of benefits that defines this latter group of workers is fairly basic. While national data on more comprehensive benefits, such as paid family leave and job-subsidized child or elder care, is more limited, the data that are available suggest that these types of policies that provide workers with real choices are limited to a small set of the most privileged workers (Bond et al., 2005).

Of even greater concern are the indications of change in access to workplace benefits between 1993 and 2003. The passage of the FMLA did increase the percentage of middle-aged women who had access to unpaid family leave, and percentages of women with access to health insurance also increased slightly over this period. However, the percentage of employed women who have any paid sick and vacation days declined significantly over this period, and those who have 6 or more paid days declined even more sharply. One possible explanation for this change is that, over this decade, women moved into jobs where their benefits were more vulnerable. However, this appears unlikely because the drop in sick and vacation coverage occurred across a wide range of jobs. The availability of paid sick and vacation days dropped 19% among women in professional and managerial positions, 14% among women who had worked at their current job for 2 years or more, and 12% among women working in firms with over 500 employees. It appears that the increase in protections offered by family leave has come at the cost of paid sick and vacation leave (Wiatrowski, 2004).

Coinciding with this decline in the availability of paid sick and vacation days has been a slight (but statistically significant) increase in the percentage of middle-aged women workers who lack access to any workplace benefits. In 1993, 11% of workers had no benefits, increasing to 15% by 2003. These changes are particularly notable because they are taking place across a decade in women's lives when they should be moving into a peak period of job stability and earning potential.

This picture of limited—and declining—access to even minimal workplace protections of family time coincides with demographic and social trends suggesting that workers will increasingly have one or more spells during their work lives when they need to provide care for an ill or disabled family member. Between 1987 and 1997, the population aged 65 and older increased from approximately 28 million to 34 million, and the number of individuals providing care rose from 7.8% to 22% of adults, representing more than 21 million households (Wagner, 1997). At the same time, increases in women's labor force participation left fewer nonworking adults to provide this care. Exacerbating these demographic shifts is a greater reliance of the health care system on informal care, including reductions in average length of hospital stays, greater reliance on outpatient treatment, and more use of informal caregivers to perform even skilled nursing tasks such as changing IVs and catheters (Glazer, 1990; National Center for Health Statistics, 2005). These coinciding trends suggest that we are moving toward a caregiving squeeze, with greater reliance on informal care but few (and declining) protections in the workplace to allow workers to manage these needs along with their work commitments. Previous research has found that, at least for recent cohorts of women, employment is not preventing women from providing care, but that doing so does put them at greater risk of labor force exit (Pavalko & Artis, 1997; Pavalko & Henderson, 2006).

Given the prevalence and trends in workplace policies and the growing need for workers to provide informal care to an ill or disabled family member, we conclude this chapter with two recommendations. The first is that current workplace policies such as paid vacation or sick days, unpaid leave, and flexible hours be maintained and extended because they provide important, but different, stop-gaps for caregiving emergencies. Policies such as unpaid family leave should not replace paid sick and vacation time and other policies, particularly because a growing body of research indicates that many of these policies improve labor market retention, thus reducing employer costs of hiring and training new workers (Pavalko & Henderson, 2006; Ruhm, 2005).

More broadly, the workplace response to the FMLA, particularly the reduction in some benefits as others are increased, reinforces the need for broader public protections of working families. All workers, both men and women, will face greater demands to provide informal care, and for all except the most privileged, the range of choices available for providing that care are severely limited. Given the current policies, most workers are left with a choice between not providing care or leaving their job to do so. While family decisions such as these are usually framed in the United States as a private issue, the choices have implications for public health and income security in mid-life and old age.

NOTES

1. This research is supported by grant R01-AG11564 from the National Institute on Aging, Eliza K. Pavalko, P.I.
2. A separate survey on state and local government jobs was conducted through the 1990s but was discontinued in 1999.

REFERENCES

Baum, C. L. (2003). The effects of maternity leave legislation on mothers' labor supply after childbirth. *Southern Economic Journal, 69*(4), 772–799.

Blair-Loy, M., & Wharton, A. S. (2002). Employees' use of work-family policies and the workplace social context. *Social Forces, 80*(3), 813–845.

Bond, J. T., Galinsky, E., Kim, S. S., & Brownfield, E. (2005). *2005 national study of employers.* New York: Families and Work Institute.

Bond, J. T., Thompson, C., Galinsky, E., & Prottas, D. (2002). *Highlights of the 2002 national study of the changing workforce.* New York: Families and Work Institute.

Bureau of Labor Statistics. (2004). *National Compensation Survey: Employee benefits in private industry in the United States, March 2004* (Vol. Summary 04–04). Washington, DC: United States Department of Labor.

Chesley, N., & Moen, P. (2006). When workers care: Dual-earner couples' caregiving strategies, benefit use, and psychological well-being. *American Behavioral Scientist, 49*(9), 1248–1269.

Dalton, D. R., & Mesch, D. J. (1990). The impact of flexible scheduling on employee attendance and turnover. *Administrative Science Quarterly, 35,* 370–387.

Fredriksen, K. I., & Scharlach, A. E. (1999). Employee family care responsibilities. *Family Relations, 48*(2), 189–196.

Glass, J., & Estes, S. B. (1997). The family responsive workplace. *Annual Review of Sociology, 23,* 289–313.

Glazer, N. Y. (1990). The home as a workshop: Women as amateur nurses and medical care providers. *Gender & Society, 4,* 479–499.

Golden, L. (2001). Flexible work schedules: What are we trading off to get them? *Monthly Labor Review, 124*(3), 50–67.

Gorey, K. M., Rice, R. W., & Brice, G. C. (1992). The prevalence of elder care responsibilities among the work force population: Response bias among a group of cross-sectional surveys. *Research on Aging, 14,* 399–418.

Gornick, J. C., & Meyers, M. K. (2003). *Families that work: Policies for reconciling parenthood and employment.* New York: Russell Sage.

Han, W.-J., & Waldfogel, J. (2003). Parental leave: The impact of recent legislation on parents' leave taking. *Demography, 40*(1), 191–200.

Henderson, K. A. (2005). *Do workplace structures matter? A cross-cohort analysis of mothers' labor market participation and choice of child care arrangements.* Unpublished doctoral dissertation. Bloomington, IN: Indiana University.

Klerman, J. A., & Leibowitz, A. (1999). Job continuity among new mothers. *Demography, 36*(2), 145–155.

Kossek, E. E. (2005). Workplace policies and practices to support work and families. In S. Bianchi, L. Casper, & R. King (Eds.), *Work, family, health, and well-being* (pp. 97–116). Mahwah, NJ: Lawrence Erlbaum.

Kossek, E. E., & Ozeki, C. (1999). Bridging the work-family policy and productivity gap: A literature review. *Community, Work, and Family, 2,* 7–32.

Kush, K. S., & Stroh, L. K. (1994). Flextime: Myth or reality? *Business Horizons, 37*(5), 51–55.

Monheit, A. C., & Vistnes, J. P. (1999). Health insurance availability at the workplace: How important are worker preferences? *Journal of Human Resources, 34,* 770–785.

National Alliance for Caregiving and American Association of Retired Persons. (1997). *Family caregiving in the U.S.—Findings from a national survey.* Bethesda, MD: Author.

National Center for Health Statistics. (2005). *Health, United States, 2005.* Hyattsville, MD: Center for Disease Control.

Olson, C. A. (2002). Do workers accept lower wages in exchange for health benefits? *Journal of Labor Economics, 20,* S91–S115.

Pavalko, E. K., & Artis, J. E. (1997). Women's caregiving and paid work: Causal relationships in late midlife. *Journals of Gerontology: Social Sciences, 52,* S170–S179.

Pavalko, E. K., & Henderson, K. A. (2006). Combining care work and paid work: Do workplace policies make a difference? *Research on Aging, 28,* 359–374.

Pavalko, E. K., & Woodbury, S. (2000). Social roles as process: Caregiving careers and women's health. *Journal of Health and Social Behavior, 41*(1), 91–105.

Ruhm, C. J. (1998). The economic consequences of parental leave mandates: Lessons from Europe. *Quarterly Journal of Economics, 113*(1), 285–317.

Ruhm, C. J. (2005). How well do government and employer policies support working parents? In S. Bianchi, L. Casper, & R. King (Eds.), *Work, family, health, and well-being* (pp. 313–328). Mahwah, NJ: Lawrence Erlbaum.

Schaie, K. W., & Schooler, C. (1998). *The impact of work on older workers.* New York: Springer.

Scharlach, A. E. (1994). Caregiving and employment: Competing or complementary roles? *The Gerontologist, 34*(3), 378–385.

United States Bureau of Labor Statistics. (2002). *Employee benefits in private industry, 2000.* Washington, DC: United States Department of Labor.

United States Department of Labor. (2004). *National Compensation Survey: Employee benefits in private industry in the United States, March 2004.* Washington, DC: Bureau of Labor Statistics.

United States Department of Labor. (2005). *NLS handbook.* Washington, DC: Bureau of Labor Statistics.

Wagner, D. L. (1997). Comparative analysis of caregiver data for caregivers to the elderly 1987 and 1997. Bethesda, MD: National Alliance for Caregiving.

Waldfogel, J. (1999). Family leave coverage in the 1990s. *Monthly Labor Review, 122*(10), 13–21.

Waldfogel, J. (2001). Family and medical leave: Evidence from the 2000 surveys. *Monthly Labor Review, 124*(9), 17–23.

Wiatrowski, W. J. (2004). *Documenting benefits coverage for all workers.* Washington, DC: U.S. Bureau of Labor Statistics.

Wisensale, S. K. (2001). Family leave policy: The political economy of work and family in America. Armonk, NY: M. E. Sharpe.

Wisensale, S. K. (2003). Two steps forward, one step back: The Family and Medical Leave Act as retrenchment policy. *Review of Policy Research, 20*(1), 135–151.

CHAPTER TEN

Caregiving Policies in the United States: Framing a National Agenda

Steven K. Wisensale

Demographic concerns in the previous century focused primarily on the population explosion and various problems associated with migration from rural to urban areas. The 21st century, in contrast, is providing an entirely new challenge: world population aging. Longer life expectancies, combined with lower fertility rates, have produced a demographic profile in which developed nations have about the same number of children under age 15 as they have adults over 55. Consequently, we are members of a global society that is the oldest in the history of the world and we are getting older. In 2000, for example, the world's elderly population (aged 65 and older) grew by more than 795,000 a month. By 2010, the projected net gain will be 847,000 older people per month (U.S. Bureau of the Census, 2000). Put another way, the world population of those 65 and older was around 435 million in 2002, an increase of 15 million elderly since 2000.

But there is much more to say. According to Bengtson and Lowenstein (2003), there are at least three facts associated with world population aging that we need to bear in mind as we study this emerging challenge and address its potential ramifications. First, population aging is occurring in both developed and developing nations. Today, more than half the world's elderly (those 65 years and older) reside in developing nations (59%, or 249 million people). By 2030, it is expected that this will increase to 71%, or 689 million people (United Nations 1999, 2001; U.S. Bureau of the Census, 2000).

Second, Western European nations and Japan have the oldest populations in the world. It is expected that, by 2030, most European nations will have elderly populations that constitute about 25% of the total. In Japan, the elderly are expected to make up nearly 30% of the nation's population by 2030 and one-third of the population by 2050 (Kojima, 2000).

Third, the aged are aging. That is, in most industrialized countries, the fastest growing group of elderly residents is 80 years old or older. In 1996–1997, the growth rate of the world's oldest old was a relatively small 1.3%. However, by 1999–2000, it had increased to 3.5% (Bengtson & Lowenstein, 2003). By 2030 in Europe, almost 12% of all Europeans are projected to be over 75, and 7% are expected to be over 80 (U.S. Bureau of the Census, 2000). In Japan, the percentages will be 17% and 12%, respectively, for those over 70 and 80 years of age.

However, the problem does not end there. Individual nations are experiencing shifts in their particular age structures that, ultimately, will affect their respective dependency:support ratios. This ratio represents the number of people under age 15 and over age 64 who are dependent on those who are usually participating in the work force (people between ages 15 and 64) and paying taxes to support them. Typically, and not surprisingly, most debates in aging societies focus on financial issues. That is, how much should the young be taxed to support the old? Should privatized individual retirement plans replace traditional pay-as-you-go models such as Social Security? In short, how should resources be allocated across different age groups? And who should pay how much, for what programs, to serve which populations within a given society?

But another development lurks just over the horizon that extends beyond the question of who will pay for the elderly. That is, who will *care* for the elderly? Not only will there be major debates over the dependency ratio from a financial perspective (such as how much to tax the young to support the old), but there is growing concern about the availability of informal caregivers to assist the elderly as their health declines in their later years. Complicating matters further, most informal caregivers tend to be women, and many women in industrialized societies—particularly in the United States—have opted to enter the job market and, therefore, have less time for their families. What, then, is the future for industrialized societies as they struggle to not only allocate resources fairly across generations but also balance caregiving responsibilities between the family and the state?

The purpose of this chapter is fourfold. First, it provides a general overview of family care in the United States, including its role in addressing future long-term care demands. Second, it discusses family care within the context of public policy by focusing on two examples: the (FMLA) of 1993 and the adoption of the National Family Caregiver Support program (NFCSP) in 2000. Third, it discusses family care from an international perspective with a primary focus on three industrialized nations: France, Germany, and Italy. And, fourth, it proposes a framework for debating various policy initiatives related to family caregiving. Argued will be a need for key decision makers to pay closer attention to intergenerational policies that respect the demands and needs of old and young alike.

THE CHALLENGES FACING FAMILY CARE IN THE UNITED STATES

As the baby boom population ages, the demand for family care will increase and companies will be pressured by employees for release time to assist aging parents. Signs of this conflict became visible in the 1990s. A 1997 study of 1,509 people conducted for Metropolitan Life by the National Alliance for Caregivers and the American Association for Retired Persons (AARP) found that one in four families had at least one adult who had provided care for an elderly relative or friend in the previous 12 months. On average, the caregivers surveyed were 45 years of age or older and provided about 8 years of care (National Alliance for Caregiving and AARP, 1997).

In a follow-up study 2 years later, it was learned that 62% of 55 individuals surveyed indicated that they had asked supervisors, coworkers, or management for some kind of help or support with their caregiving responsibilities at home (MetLife, 1999). However, only 23% of companies with 100 or more employees have programs in place to support elder care (Families and Work Institute, 1997). "Elder care is to the twenty-first century what child care has been for the last few decades," contends Joyce Ruddock, head of the Long-Term Care Group at Metropolitan Life ("What's the Problem?" 1999, 1). Indeed, a more recent study funded by MetLife Foundation concluded that 44.4 million Americans serve as caregivers, a service valued at $257 billion a year (National Alliance for Caregiving and AARP, 2005).

Today, nearly 70% of women work full-time in the United States, and most of them assume a variety of caregiving responsibilities that are in direct conflict with their work schedules. Whether working women will be able and willing to provide informal care as they have been expected to do in the past remains an unknown (see the chapter by Johnson in this volume), as does the role that government will play in addressing both the current and future needs of family caregivers. How the government responds to this challenge may ultimately depend on the particular perspectives of those in power. But regardless of what the private or public sector does in the future to address the challenge of family care, we may still be haunted by two challenging questions posed by Shirley Burggraf in *The Feminine Economy and Economic Man*. First, "How can society get women's work done when women no longer volunteer for the traditional jobs?" And, second, "Now that the opportunity cost of women's productivity in alternative tasks is becoming increasingly and explicitly expensive, who is going to pay the costs?" (Burggraf, 1997, p. 26).

Such questions become particularly acute when viewed from the perspective of long-term health care. It is extremely expensive for the elderly, their families, and U.S. taxpayers. To understand this complex issue in the context of family care, at least four points should be emphasized. First, Medicare does not cover long-term care (other than for a short transition period), either in nursing homes or at home (Binstock, Cluff, & Von Mering, 1996). Medicaid, on the other hand, is available for such coverage, but it is means-tested and, therefore, limited to low-income elderly. Still, between 60% and 80% of Medicaid funds are consumed by the elderly for long-term care services—either for institutional or home care (Weiner 1996; Weiner, Tilly, & Alecxih, 2002).

Second, long-term care insurance, once viewed as a potential cure-all for the long-term care crisis, is not only expensive but limited in scope. At least two studies report that only 20% of the aged population can afford private long-term care insurance, and far fewer elect to purchase it (Crown, Capitman, & Leutz, 1992; Weiner, Illston, & Hanley, 1994).

Third, long-term care spending is still biased toward institutional care, with only six states spending less than half their total long-term care expenditures on institutional care (MEDSTAT Group Inc., 2002). Still, there is much variation among states. For example, in 2002, Louisiana devoted 90% of its long-term care expenditures to institutional care and 10% to home care. Oregon, on the other hand, spent 27% on institutional care compared to 73% on home care (MEDSTAT Group Inc., 2002). And, fourth, out-of-pocket expenses are high. It is estimated that about 44% of the total costs of long-term care is covered by families (Weiner, et al., 1994). Similarly, out-of-pocket payments cover 51% of nursing home costs and 26% of home care expenditures (Feinberg, 1997).

According to the National Academy on Aging (2000), uncompensated care provided by family members and friends was estimated to have an economic value of $196 billion in 1997. This amount far exceeds the total spent that year on nursing home care ($83 billion) and home health care ($32 billion) (Levine & Memmott 1999). Unpaid family care saves taxpayers billions of dollars annually. For those who are paid, however, 43% receive payments from Medicaid, and about 37% of paid caregivers receive out-of-pocket payments from the elderly who employ them (National Academy on Aging, 2000).

But the money saved for taxpayers by the efforts of family caregivers does not come without cost to someone. Nor should it be assumed that such care will continue without disruption. According to the MetLife Juggling Act Study, caregiving costs individuals as much as $659,000 over their life times in wages lost and Social Security and pension contributions not being made because they "take time off, leave their job entirely, or experience compromised opportunities for training, promotions, and 'plum assignments'" (MetLife, 1999, p. 1).

Broken down further, the caregivers studied reported $566,500 in lost wages, $67,000 in lost retirement contributions, and $25,500 in lost Social Security benefits. Added to these figures was $19,500 in food costs, transportation expenses, assistance with rents and mortgages, and the cost to retain home care professionals. Furthermore, nearly 30% stated that they had passed on promotions, training opportunities, and new assignments. About 84% of the caregivers made adjustments to their work schedules by taking sick leave or vacation time if available, decreasing work hours and thus reducing their income, taking an unpaid leave of absence, switching from full-time to part-time work, and resigning or retiring. Equally important, it was learned that few of the respondents' employers offered programs, resources, or services to assist their employees in meeting their caregiving obligations (MetLife, 1999; see also the chapter by Pavalko, Henderson, & Cott in this volume).

Not oblivious to the toll caretaking responsibilities were taking on America's families, legislators in Washington, DC, adopted two policies in an effort to address caregivers' needs and better balance work and family: the FMLA of 1993 and the National Family Caregivers Support Program of 2000.

THE FAMILY AND MEDICAL LEAVE
ACT OF 1993

The FMLA was the first bill signed by newly elected President Bill Clinton. Its adoption marked the end of 8 years of congressional debate and two vetoes by his predecessor, George Bush. It allows a worker to take up to 12 weeks of unpaid leave in any 12-month period for the birth or adoption of a child; to care for a sick child, spouse, or parent with a serious health condition; or for the worker's own health condition. The law further guarantees job security in that an employee is entitled to return to the same or comparable job and requires the employer to maintain health benefits as if the employee never took leave. The law applies only to companies with 50 or more employees and to workers who have been employed for at least 1 year or 1,250 hours. It also allows a company to deny leave to a salaried employee who falls within the highest 10% of the company's payroll if the worker's leave would create "substantial and grievous injury" to the business operations. It requires employees to notify their employers prior to taking leave and permits the employer to request medical opinions to justify the employee's absence. And, in the event a worker elects not to return to work after the leave expires, the employer may require the employee to repay all health care premiums that were paid during his or her absence.

By the time Bill Clinton signed the FMLA into law in 1993, about 34 states had already adopted some form of leave policy, with several producing comparable or stronger legislation than the federal version (Wisensale, 2001). Twenty-three states covered both private and state employees; 11 states applied their policies to state employees only. Nineteen states gave time off for pregnancy and childbirth, while 15 states had adopted broader types of legislation, permitting leave for more general family matters. There was also much variation among the states in duration of leave allowed and the size of companies to which the law applied.

With respect to structure, the FMLA has three major characteristics that place it in sharp contrast to typical models in other industrialized nations. One, the leave is unpaid. All industrialized countries except Australia and the United States provide some form of wage replacement for those taking leave. Two, the U.S. model has a family focus. That is, unlike its European counterparts that are designed for new parents, the U.S. law is intergenerational in structure, thus allowing time off from work for the birth or care of a child as well as care for an elderly parent. And, three, unlike other industrialized countries, the United States links eligibility for leave to company size (50 or more employees). Consequently, the FMLA applies to about 6% of the corporations and 60% of the labor force.

Because the FMLA is often discussed in terms of child care, little attention has been devoted to its potential for addressing major long-term care demands. However, as the baby boom generation retires and is afflicted with multiple chronic illnesses 15 to 20 years later, more families will be called upon to address the personal health care needs of elderly relatives. Between 2000 and 2002, more than 25 states introduced legislation to provide paid leave to family caregivers through the use of state unemployment insurance trust funds. However, almost all of the state initiatives limited the coverage to "baby care." That is, in pushing for paid leave, only 5 of 26 states included care of an elderly parent in their proposals. The other states, none of which succeeded, opted to limit their initiatives to baby care (National Partnership for Women and Families, 2004). In short, the original intergenerational structure of the FMLA was slowly being dismantled by well-intentioned state legislators who were seeking to provide paid leave. This can be particularly problematic in light of future projections of the long-term care needs of an aging population.

However, one success story for paid-leave advocates took place in 2002. California, by expanding its state disability insurance program from maternal to family care, became the first state to adopt a comprehensive paid family and medical leave insurance policy. Workers can receive a partial wage replacement (55% to 60% of wages) with a cap during 6 weeks of leave per year to care for a newborn or newly adopted or foster child or to care for a seriously ill family member, including an elderly parent and a domestic partner. Funded solely by employee contributions, the average annual cost per worker is about $27.

Meanwhile, in the summer of 2004, Senator Edward M. Kennedy (D-MA) and Representative Rosa L. DeLauro (D-CT) introduced the Healthy Families Act, which would guarantee 7 paid sick days a year to full-time workers. Workers in any private company or governmental unit with at least 15 employees would be covered and, therefore, eligible to take time off for their own illness or to care for a family member, including an elderly parent. However, there has been relatively little movement on the proposed bill so far.

THE NATIONAL FAMILY CAREGIVERS SUPPORT PROGRAM

In 2000, the passage of several Older American Act Amendments (Public Law 106-501) included the adoption of a new and important program for family caregivers. The NFCSP was developed by the Administration on Aging within the U.S. Department of Health and Human Services. The NFCSP represented "the first federally-funded program implemented at the state level designed specifically to support the needs of family caregivers of older people," according to Feinberg and Newman (2004, p. 760).

With initial funding of $125 million in fiscal year 2001, about $113 million was allocated to states through a congressionally mandated formula based on a proportionate share of the population aged 70 years and older. Under the program, all states are responsible for working closely with area agencies on aging as well as local community service providers to offer five basic services designed to support family caregivers. These include the following:

- information to caregivers about available services in their community;
- assistance to caregivers in gaining access to supportive services;
- individual counseling, organization of support groups, and caregiver training to caregivers to assist them in making decisions and solving problems related to their caregiving roles;
- respite care to allow caregivers to receive temporary relief from their caregiving obligations; and
- supplemental services, on a limited basis, to complement the care provided by family caregivers.

Under the law, three types of caregivers are eligible to receive assistance: family caregivers of older adults; grandparents; and other family caregivers, such as aunts, uncles, and cousins. Priority is given to those in greatest social and economic need, such as poor minorities and older individuals who are providing care and support to those with developmental disabilities.

In 2004, the Family Caregiver Alliance, in cooperation with the National Conference of State Legislatures, completed a major study on the implementation of the NFCSP (Family Care Alliance and the National Conference of State Legislatures, 2004). Four major conclusions were drawn. First, in all 50 states, key program administrators identified the lack of resources to meet caregiver needs in general, and limited respite care in particular, as the top unmet needs confronting family caregivers. Even if respite care is available in all 50 states, there is much unevenness in both the quantity and quality of this service, leaving some families very vulnerable.

Second, although the NFCSP is emerging as a key program in supporting caregivers and is inspiring much program innovation in the states, it is sorely underfunded. New models of caregiver education, family counseling, support groups, and care management are not only evolving rapidly, but states are learning from each other as they move forward under the NFCSP. However, states' abilities to replicate successful programs are often hindered by funding limitations. Complicating matters further, most states experienced economic downturns during the first 4 years of the NFCSP's existence.

Third, there is little if any consensus among the 50 states on approaches to program development, the importance of caregiver support services, and the integration of family care programs with traditional home care and community services for the aged. Although the NFCSP represented a paradigm shift with respect to providing services to family caregivers of the elderly, there is still much confusion within states as to how family care is to be an important component in the restructuring of long-term care policy in the United States (Family Care Alliance and the National Conference of State Legislatures, 2004).

Fourth, greater emphasis needs to be placed on caregiver needs and their access and utilization of various support services. If policymakers are interested in replacing fragmented care with integrated care, then it is imperative that they put in place an ongoing program that assesses the continuing challenges and conflicts confronting family caregivers.

Other shortcomings that were identified in the 2004 study include a lack of information and outreach to the public. That is, nearly half (46%) of the service providers feel that many families who might benefit from their services do not know where to go for help. Also, it was learned that there is a growing shortage of professional service providers, such as social workers and nurses aides, who play an important role in supporting family caregivers. Another problem is that caregivers seldom self-identify. In other words, instead of viewing themselves as informal service providers who need support, many caregivers tend to view themselves as husband, wife, and daughter doing what family members are expected to do. Finally, there is concern that certain caregivers—such as those who are racially and ethnically diverse, working full-time, or at a distance—may fall through the cracks of most caregiver support programs (Family Care Alliance and the National Conference of State Legislatures, 2004).

That said, the 2004 report concluded by offering five major recommendations for improving the NFCSP. One, funding levels need to be raised and existing gaps in caregiver support services, such as those mentioned in the previous paragraph, need to be filled. In the long run, such actions will prevent higher Medicaid costs and reduce community-based expenditures.

Two, improve data collection and reporting procedures under the NFCSP so that uniform requirements produce more useful data that can be shared by the states and used by the federal government to better target funds. A national clearinghouse that not only collects data, but shares it with the states, will create more economically efficient programs that serve family caregivers better.

Three, strengthen and expand uniform assessment tools to measure caregiver contributions and identify their specific needs. Currently, no consensus exists on how to assess family care or what an effective assessment tool should look like. More consistency in caregiver assessment should ultimately assist both the caregiver and the care recipient while simultaneously containing or reducing long-term care costs.

Four, conduct a national public awareness campaign on family caregiving. Outreach is crucial, particularly when so many caregivers do not self-identify and thus fail to view themselves as true caregivers who could benefit from appropriate community-based services and other support mechanisms.

Finally, invest in more innovation, recognized best practices, and technical assistance. Specifically, respondents in the survey listed training and technical support, a knowledge base of best practices, culturally and ethnically appropriate services, reliable assessment tools, and outreach strategies as the most important things that can be done to harvest the potential benefits of the NFCSP.

Other studies of the NFCSP, including work by Feinberg and Newman (2004), Dal Santo, Scharlach, and Fox (2005), and Giunta (2007), focused on implementation, program design, and service utilization. In a statement before the U.S. Senate Health, Education, Labor and Pension Committee, Suzanne Mintz, President of the National Family Caregiver Association, testified that the NFCSP helped over 2.5 million people in the first 3 years of its existence. For example, over 1.5 million caregivers have received help in accessing services; nearly a half million caregivers got respite care under the NFCSP; and more than 814,00 received counseling, joined support groups, or learned new caregiving skills (Mintz, 2005).

Despite their weaknesses, the adoption of the FMLA and the NFCSP represent the recognition of a problem (pressures of family care) and a commitment on the part of government to address it. While the former policy is geared primarily to balancing work and family and the latter policy serves as a major component of an emerging long-term health care strategy, both are interconnected. Even though the FMLA is typically thought of in terms of baby care and the NFCSP is usually associated with elder care, both are intergenerational in structure, meaning that caregivers of the young and old are both acknowledged and supported.

FAMILY CARE FROM AN INTERNATIONAL PERSPECTIVE

To analyze recent policy initiatives directed at family caregivers is one thing; to put such an analysis in broader perspective is quite another matter. In short, the question that needs to be asked is this: Compared to what? That is, how does U.S. policy on family care differ from similar policies in other industrialized countries? More specifically, are the issues, concerns, and proposed solutions regarding family care substantially different in European nations? Because an overview of caregiving policies in all 25 European Union countries is beyond the constraints of this chapter (but see chapters by Lowenstein, Katz, & Gur-Yaish and by Sundström et al. in this volume), three countries (France, Germany, and Italy) have been selected for comparative purposes.

These countries were chosen for two reasons. First, they were in the news frequently for having extremely low fertility rates, growing aging populations, and major street demonstrations that protested government cutbacks and/or proposed tax increases to cover a variety of social policies, including pensions and long-term health care. For example, on April 3, 2004, hundreds of thousands of people in Rome, Berlin, and Paris marched in a coordinated protest against proposed welfare reforms in their respective countries. Second, compared to other nations in Europe and North America, these three countries spend the greatest percentage of their gross domestic product on their elderly citizens.

Family Care in France

With respect to family care of the elderly in France, the problem is embedded in a history of gender inequality that has manifested in two significant events that occurred within the last 2 years. Today women make up 57% of the French workforce, compared with 30% in the 1960s. However, more than 75% of part-time workers are women, and they earn on average 25% less than men. They are more likely to be concentrated in particular job categories (71% in the service sector), are more likely to be unemployed compared to men, and are far less likely to assume top executive (less than 14%) or managerial (under 35%) positions (Meda, 2004).

But even more pertinent to this discussion is the relatively heavy burden of family and household tasks assumed by women, as they perform 80% of the hardcore domestic chores. That is, while the husband spends an average of an hour and a quarter on domestic work per day, the wife spends an average of four and a half hours performing such tasks. This division of household labor, which has remained fairly stable over the last two decades, widens upon the arrival of a child, with women investing twice as much time as men (25 hours to 12 hours) on average per week. Clearly, this gap is likely to widen further if the family is required to assume the responsibility of elder care ("France Tries Again," 2005).

Two events within a 2-year span have changed the French political landscape with respect to family care, focusing more attention on the well-being of the elderly. In August 2003, nearly 15,000 people, mostly elderly, died during a summer heat wave. Occurring during the nation's traditional vacation month, many bodies remained unclaimed in morgues for weeks. This, coupled with a government study that reported that one-third of French suicides each year, (3,232 of 10,000, or 62 a week) are committed by people over age 65, produced two policy reforms designed to affect society at large and, on a micro level, family caregivers as well.

First, to cultivate national solidarity between generations, the French government converted a long-treasured holiday (Pentecostal Monday) to a "free labor" day in an effort to raise 2 billion euros ($2.6 billion) for a fund for the elderly and disabled. The primary purpose of the fund is to assure that basic services and care not available during the 2003 heat wave will be guaranteed in the future under similar emergency circumstances. However, in polls prior to the scheduled holiday, three out of four French opposed the elimination of the holiday and more than two-thirds ultimately refused to go to work on May 16.

Second, in February 2004, the government announced that it will punish families that do not keep in touch with elderly relatives regularly. Under existing French law, adult offspring are required to provide for aging parents who do not have the means to look after themselves. Article 207 of the Civil Code states that children are obligated to honor and respect their parents, pay them an allowance, and provide a fund or a home for them if necessary. But the February 2004 initiative tightens the code further, declaring it a crime for descendants of people living alone to fail to keep themselves regularly informed of their state of health or not to intervene should they suddenly be taken ill. According to a special government report, relatives' checkbooks had replaced their passion. More was expected from families.

The implications of such a policy for caregivers in general and women in particular are clear. In light of the fact that most women work part-time and are available for variety of caregiving tasks, it is likely that informal care responsibilities will fall on them. And, with major disparities already existing between men and women in completing housework chores and raising children, one may safely conclude that the future demands on women produced by an ever-growing aging population will exacerbate the large rift that currently exists between men and women with respect to caregiving responsibilities.

Family Care in Germany

Of the three countries discussed here, Germany presents perhaps the most unique case study, primarily because for 45 years it was two countries with each creating its own history. But German reunification in 1990 resulted in two ideologically divergent states being merged into one. With respect to attitudes about family caregiving and the role of women in the workforce and at home, the two states could hardly be more different. Women in the former East Germany were not only encouraged to work but were also expected to assume the role of mother and wife, often supported by comprehensive child care and parental leave policies. Consequently, 91% of East German women worked before the Berlin Wall came down. This is in sharp contrast to women's status in the former West Germany, where the male breadwinner model was dominant and women who remained home to keep the house and raise children were viewed as important as men who were employed in factories. Therefore, only 58% of women worked and that figure has not changed much for all German women since 1990 (Adler & Brayfield, 1997).

An equally significant event occurred just 5 years later, when Germany began implementing new provisions in its national health insurance law to provide for long-term care assistance. With the passage of the Social Dependency Insurance Program, payments are available for family caregivers, community-based services and nursing homes, and other facilities for the disabled. Funded by eliminating the Pentecostal Monday vacation, the same policy that would throw France into a political tailspin 9 years later, the heart and soul of the program is the compensation of family members for caring for their loved ones (Wagner, 2001). Depending on the level of disability, the amount paid to a family caregiver may range from $250 to $450 a month in U.S. dollars. According to a study funded by the Robert Wood Johnson Foundation, "there has been nearly unanimous agreement that Germany's Social Dependency Insurance Program is a public policy success" (Polivka, 2001, p. 6).

However, while Germany should be applauded for its success in designing effective programs to address the challenges of an aging population, one cannot overlook the fact that in a traditionally patriarchal society in which many women continue to stay home to care for children, it is highly likely that it will be women who will assume this role in caring for the nation's ill elderly as well. When the new insurance system was introduced in 1995, 750,000 people over 65 years of age utilized it. In 2002, the number of recipients in this age group had practically doubled to 1.43 million. This is already occurring when the population aged 65 years and older in Germany is expected to rise from 13.4% in 2000 to about 23% in 2040 and while the number of future contributors to the program and potential caregivers is expected to decline continuously due to lower birth rates (International Labor Organization, 2004).

Family Care in Italy

As Italian women's educational attainment rose, beginning in the 1970s, their entry into the job market increased, marriage was delayed, and the national birth rate plummeted. Within two decades, between 1972 and 1993, the fertility rate dropped from 2.4 to 1.2 and has continued downward ever since. But despite these developments, only 38% of Italian women work outside the home (University of Southern California, 2004).

As is the case with the United States, France, and Germany, Italy not only faces a financial challenge that is produced by a distorted dependency ratio, it must also be concerned about the availability and support of potential caregivers of the elderly. Although Maroni (2002) reports that 78% of women over the age of 75 identify themselves as care providers for relatives, one cannot conclude that this pattern will hold for younger generations. For example, with one-fifth of the population over 65, many Italians are addressing the caregiving issue by outsourcing home care for the elderly to immigrants—a recent development that is distinct from what has occurred in the other three countries discussed in this chapter. It is also a far cry from traditional Italian society, in which the elderly and disabled lived with their families and were cared for by their female relatives (Screti, 2005). As society has changed, so too has the rate of immigration in Italy.

According to statistics provided by the National Social Security Institute, 51,110 immigrants worked as domestics in Italy in 1994 (or nearly 27% of all domestic workers), compared to nearly 500,000 domestic workers (or 83%) in 2003. Today, foreign caregivers total more than 600,000, with most coming from the Ukraine (21%), Romania (16.4%), the Philippines (9.5%), Poland (7.0%), Ecuador (6.4%), Moldova (5.7%), and Peru (5.0%). Not surprisingly, almost all of these immigrant caregivers are women who work at relatively low wages ($900 to $1,200 a month) and often leave behind their husbands and children in their home countries (Smith, 2005).

With a government either unable or unwilling to address long-term care of the elderly straight on, families face a difficult situation in Italy. They are confronted with expensive private services and lengthy waiting lists produced by underfunded and inadequate public programs. At the same time, they see a cheap domestic labor pool consisting of inexpensive workers from abroad. Not surprisingly, a fairly large number of Italians have opted for immigrant domestic workers to address their caregiving needs. This approach is not necessarily unsatisfactory for the government. If institutionalized, the elderly would be extremely costly for the government and, therefore, a private system costs taxpayers much less. And it is even cheaper if foreign labor, rather than Italian labor, is employed.

So, unlike the United States—which has tinkered at the margins in supporting caregivers of the elderly with programs such as the FMLA and the NFCSP—and France and Germany—which have adopted specific policies to address the problem of long-term care—Italy appears content in outsourcing its problem by welcoming more immigrants. Though controversial perhaps, such an approach may solve two problems at once: increasing the population while simultaneously addressing the nation's long-term care needs. In fact, to maintain its working age population at 1995 levels, Italy will require approximately 350,000 immigrants each year. It is estimated that Germany will require 500,000 per year.

CREATING A FRAMEWORK FOR ANALYZING AND DEBATING FAMILY CAREGIVING

In 1999, the theme for the United Nations International Year of Older Persons was "Towards a Society for All Ages." Recognizing that the globe is graying rapidly; that this process is not confined to just the wealthier Western industrialized societies; that there is great potential for conflict between generations over limited resources; and that greater, not lesser, demands will fall on family caregivers in the future, the United Nations encouraged countries to address these challenges and share with each other their solutions to problems.

With respect to the United States, future aging policy in general and caregiving policies in particular should be debated within a framework that requires accuracy in gathering data and demands balance in formulating policies. In the process, not only should we fortify existing policies, such as the FMLA and the NFCSP, we should also strive to create new ones, such as expanding access to respite care services. Five recommendations regarding the future debate over the direction of U.S. caregiving policies follow:

1. *Avoid misunderstandings about the implications of population aging.* An aging society can create much anxiety. This anxiety, sometimes referred to as "apocalyptic demographics," often revolves around the dependency ratio—the number in the labor force compared to those younger than age 16 and those older than age 64. However, two points should be emphasized. First, this ratio is questionable because it fails to take into account the constantly changing labor force participation of women, the potential for the elderly to postpone retirement and work longer, and the possibility of economic growth. Second, this ratio tends to ignore the fact that policymakers can make a difference. Adjustments in monetary and fiscal policies, a shift in education policy that can affect worker productivity, and a different focus on research can all help shape a different future than that projected. Demography need not be destiny.

2. *Recognize the diversity of the elderly population.* The elderly population in the United States is heterogeneous. They are rich

and poor, strong and weak, "young old" and "old old," conservative and liberal, and at times burdens and contributors. Failure to recognize the heterogeneity among the elderly may affect how social problems are defined and, therefore, ultimately determine how they are addressed. Stereotyping—particularly that which furthers certain political ends, such as a reduction of social programs—should be challenged.

3. *Be prepared to correct misunderstandings about relations between generations.* Although examples of conflict between age groups can be found on occasion in the United States, such conflict is more the exception than the rule. In short, while there will always be some tension between various groups in any society, the bonds between generations remain strong. People understand that successive birth cohorts and generations (particularly within families) are interdependent. If the young generation chooses to dismantle social programs for the old, it is also dismantling social programs for itself. For example, Social Security could offer "care credits" so that those who must leave the labor force to care for children, the elderly, or others will not be penalized financially when their Social Security benefits are calculated.

4. *Avoid using narrow and misleading definitions of fairness.* Although it may be desirable to achieve equity between generations, such an outcome would be fairly narrow in that it would not necessarily address other questions of social justice in a given society. For example, the idea that per capita public expenditures on children and the elderly ought to be equal sounds good, but it is probably not realistic. As Norm Daniels (1988) has argued, we all have different needs at different stages of our lives. Thus, to pit one age group against the other is not only unfair but it diverts attention away from other societal inequities. Therefore, policy initiatives that are intergenerational in structure, such as the FMLA and the NFCSP, should be encouraged and adopted.

5. *Address the issue of gender equity aggressively, particularly with respect to family caregivers.* Currently, women provide a disproportional amount of care, be it child care or elder care. More efforts need to be put forth that are designed to balance caregiving responsibilities between men and women. To some extent, this is a problem that needs to be addressed in the privacy of the family home. However, policymakers should not ignore their responsibility in this matter. For example, in an effort to create a state of equality between parents of newborns, the Swedish

government introduced "the father's month." Under this provision, Swedish couples are granted longer leaves from work for child care, provided the father uses at least 1 month of leave to care for the child. The United States could adopt a similar policy but not necessarily confine it to baby care. Why not extend it to care of the elderly?

These are just a few examples of key items on a checklist for policymakers that should be considered as they attempt to formulate an effective integrated system of care for our most vulnerable citizens. Clearly, family caregivers will be expected to play a major role in this endeavor and, therefore, should expect to receive the support they deserve. To do otherwise is to abandon two generations in need simultaneously. We can do better by fortifying existing policies, such as the FMLA and the NFCSP.

REFERENCES

Adler, M., & Brayfield, A. (1997). Women's work values in unified Germany: Regional differences as remnants of the past. *Work and Occupations, 24*, 245–266.

Bengtson, V., & Lowenstein, A. (2003). *Global aging and challenges to families.* Hawthorne, NY: Aldine de Gruyter.

Binstock, R., Cluff, L., & Von Mering, O. (1996). Issues affecting the future of long-term care. In R. Binstock, L. Cluff, & O. von Mering (Eds.), *The future of long-term care: Social and policy issues.* Baltimore, MD: Johns Hopkins University Press.

Burggraf, S. (1997). *The feminine economy and economic man.* Reading, MA: Addison-Wesley.

Crown, W., Capitman, J., & Leutz, W. (1992). Economic rationality, the affordability of long-term care insurance, and the role for public policy. *The Gerontologist, 32*, 478–485.

Dal Santo, T., Scharlach, A., & Fox, P. (2005). *Implementation of the National Family Caregiver Support program: How has caregiver service use changed in California?* Paper presented at the 58th annual meeting of the Gerontological Society of America, Washington, DC.

Daniels, N. (1988). Justice between age groups: Am I my parents' keeper? *Millbank Memorial Fund Quarterly*, Summer, 489–522.

Families and Work Institute. (1997). *National study of the changing workforce.* New York: Author.

Family Care Alliance and the National Conference of State Legislatures. (2004). *The state of the states in family caregiver support: A 50-state study.* San Francisco: Family Care Alliance.

Feinberg, L. (1997). *Options for supporting informal and family caregiving: A policy paper.* San Francisco: American Society on Aging.

Feinberg, L., & Newman, S. (2004). A study of 10 states since passage of the National Family Caregiver Support program: Policies, perceptions, and program development. *The Gerontologist, 44*(6), 760–769.

France tries again to give women equal pay. (2005, May 11). *Mail & Guardian* (London), p. 18.

Giunta, N. (2007). *Examining the implementation of the National Family Caregiver Support program: A mixed-methods analysis of efforts in 50 states.* Paper presented at the 11th annual conference of the Society for Social Work and Research, San Francisco, CA.

International Labor Organization. (2004). *Frail older people—The long-term care challenge.* Washington, DC: Author.

Kojima, H. (2000). Japan: Hyper-aging and its policy implications. In V. L. Bengtson, K.-D. Kim, G. C. Myers, & K. S. Eun (Eds.), *Aging in East and West: Families, states and the elderly.* New York: Springer.

Levine, A., & Memmott, M. (1999). The economic value of informal caregiving. *Health Affairs, 18*(2), 182–188.

Maroni, R. (2002). *Statement by the Honorable Roberto Maroni, Italian Minister of Labor and Social Policies.* Madrid, Spain: Second World Assembly on Aging.

Meda, D. (2004). *Women and work.* Briefing paper. Washington, DC: Embassy of France in the U.S.

MEDSTAT Group Inc. (2002). *The long-term care tab.* Ann Arbor, MI: Author.

MetLife. (1999). *MetLife juggling act study.* Westport, CT: MetLife Mature Market Institute.

Mintz, S. (2005). *Statement of Suzanne Mintz before the Senate Health, Education, Labor, and Pension Committee.* United States Senate. Washington, DC, February 14, 2005.

National Academy on Aging. (2000). *Caregiving: Helping the elderly with activity limitations.* Washington, DC: Author.

National Alliance for Caregiving and American Association for Retired Persons (AARP). (1997). *Family caregiving in the U.S.* Washington, DC: National Alliance for Caregiving.

National Alliance for Caregiving and American Association for Retired Persons (AARP). (2005). *Family caregiving in the U.S.* Washington, DC: National Alliance for Caregiving.

National Partnership for Women and Families. (2004). *Get well soon: Americans can't afford to be sick.* Washington, DC: Author.

Polivka, L. (2001). *Paying family members to provide care: Policy considerations for the states.* Policy Brief no. 7. Princeton, NJ: Robert Wood Johnson Foundation.

Screti, F. (2005). *Elderly depend on immigrant women for caregiving.* Briefing paper. New York: Global Action on Aging.

Smith, T. (2005). *Aging Italy leans on immigrants.* Briefing paper. New York: Global Action on Aging.

United Nations. (1999). *The sex and age distribution of the world populations* (1998 revisions). New York: Author.

United Nations. (2001). *World population prospects.* New York: Author.

University of Southern California. (2004). *Inclusion/exclusion in the workplace.* Briefing paper. Los Angeles: University of Southern California School of Social Work, Center for the Inclusive Workplace.

U.S. Bureau of the Census. (2000). *International data base.* Washington, DC: Author.

Wagner, E. (2001). Restructuring care for the elderly in Germany. *Current Sociology, 49*(3), 175–188.

Weiner, J. (1996). *Can Medicaid long-term care expenditures for the elderly be reduced?* New York: Commonwealth Fund.

Weiner, J., Illston, L., & Hanley, R. (1994). *Sharing the burden: Strategies for public and private long-term care insurance.* Washington, DC: Brookings Institution.

Weiner, J., Tilly, J., & Alecxih, L. (2002). Home-and community-based services in seven states. *Health Care Financing Review, 23*(2), 90–114.

What's the problem? (1999, August 9). *New York Times,* p. A14.

Wisensale, S. (2001). *Family leave policy: The political economy of work and family in America.* Armonk, NY: M. E. Sharpe.

CHAPTER ELEVEN

Family Care for Elders in Europe: Policies and Practices[1]

Gerdt Sundström, Bo Malmberg,
Mayte Sancho Castiello, Élena del Barrio,
Penélope Castejon, Maria Angeles Tortosa,
and Lennarth Johansson

INTRODUCTION

Many preconceptions exist about how European countries differ in terms of policies and practices affecting older adults. For example, many assume greater autonomy but also more loneliness and lack of family care for elderly people in the north, while elders in the south bask in the warm but controlling care of their family network. Social life and social services in Portugal, Spain, Italy, and Greece are, by northern Europeans, perceived as similar; and, likewise, welfare states in the north are seen by southerners as being similar. Although differences between countries tend to be homogenized, there is, in fact, much more variation than commonly thought in elder care (and in many other respects) between countries in the south and countries in the north, and within each country.

Some signs of convergence also can be identified, but not to the extent that there is a European perspective despite official expectations by the European Union (EU) that member countries improve services for elderly people. Care in the community is in all of Europe official policy, which often implies that elders will be cared for by their families, with or without public support. Assessing family care and the policies affecting them in European countries is beyond the scope of this chapter. Fortunately, a few recent research projects by the Organisation for Economic Co-operation and Development (OECD) and one funded by the EU describe some of these aspects.

Country-specific reports are available for most European countries in the EUROFAMCARE (2006) project, our source when no reference is given. The Survey of Health, Ageing, and Retirement in Europe (SHARE) project, with national population sample surveys of middle-aged and older persons, covers several European countries and has some information on care, and EUROSTAT (the European Union statistical agency) publishes useful information on social life in Europe. We will draw on these and other sources to clarify explicit and implicit policies on family care for elders and their rationales. In this chapter, we begin by considering the most relevant dimensions along which old age policies and practices vary across European countries. In this context, we consider two contrasting nations—Spain and Sweden—in greater depth. Because care is a function of policies, demographics, and family values, these countries demonstrate that there can be considerable change over even short periods of time.

FAMILY CARE: POLITICAL AND CULTURAL ASPECTS

Family policies are politically sensitive and were even more so in the turbulent 20th century of European history. When Spain became a republic in 1931, one of its first acts was to legalize divorces. In occupied France, the collaborationist Vichy regime immediately appointed a family minister who set out to promote fertility. The family in the "new order" was to be "honored, protected and supported." The provocative motto about *liberté* on French currency was shifted to *travail-famille-patrie* on coins made from a worthless light alloy. Earlier pronatalist policies in France paid child allowances to the father, an unwed mother received nothing. When universal child allowances were introduced in Sweden in 1948, payable to mothers regardless of marital status, there was a debate about whether this might further "immorality," and popular weeklies ran reports about teenage mothers.

Sweden had a bachelor tax (higher tax rates for single men) in the 1930s and 1940s, later followed by joint taxes for married persons and family deductions that made it unprofitable for women to work; these taxes were abolished in 1971. France introduced a similar bachelor tax in 1920 (25% higher tax for bachelors older than age 30 who did not support a family). Mussolini did likewise in Italy in 1927 for men older than age 25. Many countries still have marriage subsidies, nearly always as tax concessions (Montanari, 2000). States have, in various ways, tried to monitor and influence family life, and this appears to have been more acceptable in the Nordic countries with their traditionally more state-friendly culture. Until recently, explicit family policies were directed almost entirely toward young families and children. Because policies affecting elders and their care are still developing, we also consider living arrangements and help patterns of the elderly in a number of countries, as well as availability of public services and their allocation.

We will cover themes of responsibility for care (public and family based) and policies and various models of support for caring families. It is common to distinguish between the state and the private sphere (that is, the family), the market, and nonprofit organizations as alternative or supplementary providers of care. Market in the wider meaning as financial incentives will be touched upon, as they are important in many countries in continental Europe and in the Nordic countries, as the state sometimes has difficulty financing constant service coverage. With the term *state*, we mean public bodies: municipal, regional, and national. In the Nordic countries, municipalities have near monopoly in formal elder care.

POLICIES OF SUPPORT FOR ELDERS AND THEIR CARERS IN CONTEMPORARY EUROPE AND THE ADMINISTRATIVE CONTEXT

Esping-Andersen (1990) suggested one way to group European countries along ideological-political categories, but following Iacovou (2002) we simply refer to countries as Nordic, northern, and southern, which roughly corresponds to the Esping-Andersen taxonomy. This also happens to make reasonable sense for elder care, because countries in these categories tend to differ visibly in how common it is for elders to live alone, to live with offspring, to have access to public services, and also in regard to the legal framework of care.

The Nordic countries are Denmark, Finland, Iceland, Norway, and Sweden; northern Europe includes Belgium, France, Germany, Luxemburg, The Netherlands, and the United Kingdom; southern Europe consists of Spain, Greece, Italy, and includes Austria and Ireland, mostly for religious reasons (Iacovou 2002), as elaborated below. Switzerland and Israel stand on their own. Alternatively, countries could be grouped according to tax levels and expenditures on social protection, both as proportions of the gross domestic product, which would provide a similar ordering. This is a useful heuristic framework to summarize the situation for elders and their carers. Statistical analyses of demographic aspects, patterns of care, public expenditures on the elderly, and service levels disclose a rather more complex pattern (Glaser, Tomassini, & Grundy, 2004). Some countries are also changing their whole concept of care, which may eventually invalidate these categories. The Netherlands is now "municipalizing" services, and Spain differs in some important regards from the other southern countries. Table 11.1 illustrates differences in family care policy characteristics as a function of these country groups.

Drawing on country reports in the EUROFAMCARE (2006) project, we may distinguish countries with an official policy on family care from those without. There may still be an implicit policy, which can be deduced from administrative documents and routines. The Nordic countries and Britain have had a decentralized, local-level approach to poor relief and welfare since medieval times. There is a trend in many European countries to decentralize programs that used to be organized at the national or regional level. Now all countries except Greece,

TABLE 11.1 Variations in Dimensions of Family Care Policies and Obligations

Country group	Family care policy	Level of responsibility	Official responsibility	Financing
Nordic	Yes, explicit	Municipality	State	Local tax
Northern	Yes, implicit	National	Shared	Insurance
Southern	No, implicit	Individual	Family	Individual
	Variation in responsibility **Legal obligation for family**			
	Extended family	Offspring only		No obligation
	Bulgaria	Austria		Denmark
	Greece	Belgium		Finland
	Hungary	France[a,b]		Iceland, Ireland
	Italy	Germany[b]		Luxembourg
	Portugal	Israel[a]		The Netherlands
	Spain	Slovenia		Norway
				Sweden
				United Kingdom

Note. Most countries also require a user copayment. Spouses seem everywhere to be responsible, although adjustments may be made when a spouse is institutionalized. From Millar and Warman (1996), adapted and expanded.

[a] May apply only when institutional care is the option.
[b] Both family obligations and clear state obligation.

Luxembourg, and Portugal have locally organized services for the elderly. They tend to be strictly regulated at the national level in the Nordic countries and in The Netherlands. Decentralization sometimes occurs when central authorities wish to save money, but it may also reflect attempts to make service provision more efficient. A valuable analysis of these issues was done in the OASIS project (Lowenstein & Ogg, 2003).

Yet, there are also cases of the opposite movement for the very same reason. Denmark recently collapsed small municipalities into bigger ones, and Norway nationalized hospital care, previously financed and run regionally. Some countries, like the United Kingdom, have a confusing mix of local and regional bodies, and the sheer number of local authorities (36,000 municipalities in France and 8,000 in Spain) can cause difficulties. In the latter case, a national plan (Plan Gerontologico) and an energetic national drive to improve service coverage in collaboration with regional authorities runs parallel with decentralization to regions and municipalities, which can be improved by using national assessment schemes (e.g., France, Germany, Israel, and Spain).

Some countries with many small municipalities and/or in the absence of an independent municipal tax base and income equalization schemes, often cannot muster resources for costly elder care. In federal countries (Germany and Austria), other problems of coordination and implementation may plague attempts to formulate national policies. Clearly, almost everywhere, large differences in service coverage and quality prevail. Although user copayment is the rule in most countries, it is frequently waived for low-income users, and fees typically cover only a fraction of the costs of public elder care. British, French, and Swedish studies indicate that informal care and/or services vary substantially between regions—variation can be explained partly by varying levels of need among the elderly (Davey, Johansson, Malmberg, & Sundström, 2006; Jeger, 2005; Wheller, 2006; Young, Grundy, & Kalogirou, 2005). A British study found that service coverage was due more to local authority discretions and fees than to needs of elders (Evandrou, Falkingham, Le Grand, & Winter, 1992), whereas a recent Swedish analysis found Home Help services to be quite equitable (Davey et al., 2006).

Some countries have no family policy; one or two even had trouble identifying an indigenous word for the concept of family care in the EUROFAMCARE project. Even once the concept is named, the choice of words can present difficulties. In France, the legislation on a dependency allowance (*prestation spécifique dépendence,* or PSD) introduced in 1997 chose to use the concept *natural carer* instead of *family carer.* Spain uses the term *cuidadores familiares* (family carers) in a law of dependency to be phased in from 2007 with financial provisions for nonprofessional carers—usually, although not necessarily, family.

Public awareness concerning family care issues also varies considerably, from the rather intense discussion and extensive research underpinned by statistics and census data in Britain and Germany to a near-total lack of a public agenda in Bulgaria, Poland, and Slovenia. (The Bulgarian country report appears to misunderstand the concept and confuses it with public home help services.) Some countries may lack policy but have very active carers' associations and other lobbying groups which keep the issue on the agenda (notably Ireland). At the time of this writing, initiatives are trying to establish a pan-European organization Eurocarers. These issues emerged later and more hesitantly in the Nordic countries—with the exception of Finland, which in 2006 introduced a law that addresses the issue of support for family carers. Typical from an expansionist public welfare perspective, a Swedish government commission in 1987 stated that "family may supplement public services." In 1998, the Swedish social service act added a nonbinding clause that municipalities ought to support family carers.

There is considerable variability in how well European countries have prepared for the projected radical increases in age-related expenditures, with public debt a serious issue for many countries if unchecked (European Union, 2006). Family policies and practices are not static, with expectations that families will shoulder more of the care in future. A 1998 Council of Europe survey about elder care to the national ministries of social affairs referred to the need for increased reliance on family care to reduce government spending (Council of Europe, 1998). A year later, the parliament of Europe reaffirmed "the importance of the family—and argues in favour of it being restored to its rightful place" (Recommendation 1428, 1999). A Norwegian econometric study shows the vast impact on finances of varying assumptions about how much informal care is provided to the elderly (Statistics Norway, 2006). The problem is aggravated by the official wish in the European Union to reconcile informal care with higher rates of employment (among women) and gender equality, often captured in statements about a "proper balance" between work and family life.

In Britain, carers in the 1990s were granted the right to have their needs assessed when the person cared for was assessed for public services, and, recently, a government "green paper" proposed choice and prevention in future elder care but also stated repeatedly with varying formulations that "when support from family and friends is not enough, it is supplemented by more formal models" (Department of Health, 2005, p. 99). (Scotland deviates slightly, for example, with free Home Help services.) Similarly, a large part of continental Europe subscribes to *subsidiarity*, a concept established by the Roman Catholic church and used to describe a desirable social order: interventions shall be done where they "belong." Private family tasks and problems are not to be solved by the state or other higher entities. (Other denominations may endorse similar principles.) This should be seen in perspective. When pronounced by Pope Pius XI in an encyclical in 1931, his statement of the "natural" rights of the family was directed against the strivings of expanding fascism to put individuals and families in service of the state. Without formally endorsing subsidiarity, similar results may emerge in the United Kingdom and the Nordic countries when the state primarily targets elders who need help with health care and personal care, whereas the family is expected to help the many more persons who primarily need help with household tasks of various kinds.

INFORMAL CARE AND LEGAL
FILIAL DUTIES

Family and household patterns of elders have implications for who may provide care or whom they may have to give it to. If old people live alone, with just their spouse (partner) and/or with others, this may also affect their likelihood of using public services—for example, Home Help and institutional care. Therefore, an overview of these living arrangements is given in Table 11.2 for some European countries. Although policies are often considered to be responsible for specific living arrangements, they are, of course, in response to them as well.

Nordic countries are characterized by their long-standing and far-reaching household separation—with many elders living alone, comprehensive services, and no legal responsibility of the family, except spouses ("individualism"). In the northern countries, solitary living is nearly as common, living with offspring has declined, but public services (especially community-based) usually have lower coverage, and filial obligations mostly apply. In the southern countries, solitary living is on the rise among the elderly but is relatively uncommon. Joint households are still typical and have, for example, in Italy not declined at all. Legal family obligations, often elaborate, still apply.

Living alone is much more common in the Nordic countries than in the southern region; the northern countries are more similar to the Nordic countries. The trend in need for care is the same for men and women, but levels of public services are everywhere much higher for women, roughly corresponding to the two to three times greater risk for a marriage to end with the death of the husband than that of the wife. A widely preferred living arrangement, living only with one's partner, is also more common

TABLE 11.2   Household Structure in Selected European Countries (ca. 2004) for People Age 65 and Older Living in the Community

Country	Living alone	Partner only	Other (%)
Nordic			
Denmark	41	55	4
Sweden	39	59	2
Northern			
Belgium/Flanders	27	63	10
Britain	36	51	13
France	36	55	10
Germany	39	53	8
The Netherlands	42	54	5
Southern			
Austria	43	43	14
Greece	38	44	19
Italy	32	42	26
Spain	27	38	35
Switzerland	35	57	8
Israel	25	45	30

Note. Other living arrangement includes any other type of living arrangement (with partner and child, with child(ren), etc.). Percentages reported here may differ from those in other sources. From our own computations on SHARE. Data for Denmark and Sweden were corrected for institutional population (8% and 7%, respectively); in the other European countries, samples are of persons living in the community. Belgium data are calculated from the LOVO-survey (2001), courtesy Benedicte de Koker. Data for Israel are from Brodsky, Shnoor, & Be'er (2005). Information kindly provided by Ariela Lowenstein. Data for Britain are from our own calculations on Glaser and Tomassini (2003).

in the Nordic countries and is everywhere much more common among men. Other living arrangements—with offspring, siblings, other relatives or unrelated people, live-in housekeepers, and others—is now rare in the Nordic countries but is still frequent in the south.

Increasing numbers of elders remain married into advanced age, with obvious consequences for their chances to receive—or have to provide—informal care. Also cohabitation and "living alone together" (LAT) are becoming more common among the elderly, but more so in northern Europe than in the south. For example, in Sweden, 56% of people who are age 65 and older are married, 5% live with a partner (Britain 2%, Spain 1%), and 7% are in LAT relationships (Socialstyrelsen, 2006). These are superficial indicators that family life, in some regards, has improved—for example, marriages of older people last longer than before. Other aspects may be more worrisome, such as rising divorce rates and delayed independence of younger generations, who remain unmarried and stay longer in their parents' household because of adverse housing and labor markets, particularly in southern Europe. This may be a way to economize for both generations; in Britain, nearly a million households have three generations under the same roof (Age Concern, 2005). The phenomenon has been studied among both older and younger generations in Italy. Solitary living as an important social fact is now recognized symbolically by the United Nations' demographic fact chart on aging, which provides data on solitary living for men and for women (United Nations, 2006). The reason is said to be elders' greater risk of social isolation and vulnerability in case of illness or disability.

Do differences in living arrangements translate to variations in caregiving in European countries? It is well known that old persons all over Europe depend primarily on their families, but this does not necessarily imply that care is similar, seen from the providers' perspective. This aspect is assessed with recent data shown in Table 11.3. Because women are often assumed to be the primary caregivers, their data are displayed separately.

Unexpectedly, caregiving in total—inside and outside of one's household—is more common among people who are age 50 and older in central Europe and in the Nordic countries of Denmark and Sweden, with their extensive welfare programs, than in southern countries such as Spain and Italy, with their strong family traditions. Yet, external caregiving frequently may be help with less demanding tasks than the heavier personal care tasks inside the household. Higher rates of male helpgiving to other households in the Nordic countries probably reflect greater male involvement in maintenance and other practical tasks, also probed in this question. Care for someone in one's own household is two to three times more common in the southern than in the northern and Nordic countries—for example, 10% in Spain and 4% in Denmark and Sweden. In the Nordic countries, in-household care is mostly spouse care, because it is rare for old persons to live with anyone else other than their spouse. In the continental and southern countries, this will often be care for parents (or parents-in-law). When Danes and Swedes help their parents, it is typically help to another household, because coresidence with parents is very rare for this age group in these countries (near zero), compared to 4.1% in Italy and 5.6% in Spain (Attias-Donfut, Ogg, & Wolff, 2005). Needy Nordic elders mostly received help from outside; southern elderly received help mostly from people in their households, but in total they received help about equally as often. The same pattern held for the giving of help and support by elders themselves (Socialstyrelsen, 2006). It is also possible that *help* is interpreted differently in northern and southern Europe (Ogg & Renault, 2006). Cross-sectional rates of caregiving greatly underestimate the lifelong risk of ever being a caregiver, which is roughly two to three times greater. Many stop, and many begin, a caregiving episode

TABLE 11.3 Prevalence of Care and Employment in Selected European Countries for People Age 50 and Older by Gender, 2004 (%)

	Gives care in household[a]		Gives help outside household[b]		Employed		Employed among household carers	
	All	Women	All	Women	All	Women	All	Women
Nordic								
Denmark	4	4	47	37	52	47	35	25
Sweden	4	4	41	39	52	51	38	30
The Netherlands	5	5	41	38	40	32	27	15
Northern								
Germany	6	7	32	29	46	33	18	15
France	6	8	31	31	33	30	17	16
Southern								
Austria	8	9	25	24	32	26	21	18
Greece	6	7	20	21	35	24	22	19
Italy	8	9	23	22	25	18	16	10
Spain	10	12	14	15	27	20	17	12
Switzerland	6	8	36	37	54	48	36	27

[a] Regular care for sick or disabled adult in household last year.
[b] Help to family, friend or neighbor in other household. Help can be with personal care, household, and/or paperwork.
Source: Authors' computations using SHARE data.

every year (Aeldre Sagen, 2005; Hirst, 2002). Data on elders as caregivers are scarce, but, in Sweden, roughly 40% of elderly women and 20% of elderly men report having ever been carers, mostly for parents or spouses (Socialstyrelsen, 2006). Who becomes a caregiver and who does not is likely influenced by the density of one's social network, among other things (Amirkhanyan & Wolf, 2003; Socialstyrelsen, 2006). For international comparisons of caregiving, we have to make do with available time-point estimates.

Interestingly, there are few gender differences among who provides care inside the household in Denmark, Sweden, and The Netherlands, but differences are more evident in the southern countries. These patterns are seen, for example, in national surveys of informal care in Spain and Sweden (IMSERSO 2005a, 2005b; Socialstyrelsen, 2006), in part possibly due to gender differences in care to parents-in-law. Evidence for partner care indicates small differences between men caring for their wives and women caring for their husbands, in absolute and relative terms. The differences are smaller than expected in northern European countries, with about equal numbers of husband and wife carers in Sweden, England, and Wales (Socialstyrelsen, 2006; Young, Grundy, & Jitlal, 2006). Husbands less often care for their wives in Ireland and in Spain, even in spouse-only household constellations (National Council for the Aged, 1988, and our own calculations on Spanish survey data).

The SHARE study asks whether one has helped someone in the household "daily or almost daily during at least three months—during the last twelve months with personal care, such as washing, getting out of bed, or dressing." In the total population sample of people age 50 and older, this is affirmed by 2% to 3% of European men and by 4% to 6% of the women. The rates are naturally higher for married persons who live with their partner only. In this group, men provide care only slightly less often than women (5% and 6%, respectively, European average). For both men and women, this is more common in southern countries, possibly due to less adequate housing and/or poorer health (for example, 3% and 4%, respectively, for married men and women in Denmark and Sweden and 7% and 8% to 9%, respectively, in Italy and Spain).

Differences between men and women in the help they give to persons in other households are small, but less is known about the nature of this help: it may frequently concern practical tasks such as house repairs and car maintenance that typically involve men. In general, then, informal care is common, and when time series exist (Norway, The Netherlands, Spain, Sweden, United Kingdom), there is no indication that informal care is on the decrease. It is, for example, estimated that, in Sweden, about 60% of all elder care, including institutional care, is provided informally (Szebehely, 2005).

German studies hint at weakening support for family care, suppos-
edly due to the new care insurance, but Swedish studies indicate a remarkable growth in informal care (EUROFAMCARE, 2006; Sundström,
Johansson, & Hassing, 2002). Research in Norway, The Netherlands,
Poland, Spain, Sweden, and the United Kingdom indicates that about
60% to 70% or more of informal care is directed from a younger generation to older persons, typically parents or parents-in-law. Also, as
mentioned, care between aging spouses is not negligible.

As shown in Table 11.3, employment rates are remarkably high
in the northern and Nordic countries, for both men and women age
50 years and older (Sweden, Denmark, The Netherlands, Germany,
and Switzerland) and very low for men and women in Italy and Spain.
Among women, employment (especially part-time employment) has
been on the rise for a long time in most countries. (Finland is an exception, with high rates of women in full-time positions.) Do care commitments, then, generally prevent carers from gainful work, as evidenced
by Spanish surveys of informal carers (IMSERSO, 2005a)? Evidence of
this is ambiguous. An overview of the situation in Europe was cautious
in its conclusions, because it is difficult to disentangle cause and effect
of working and caring and the effects of care allowances on caregiving
(Jenson & Jacobzone, 2000). A major European survey also found little
effect on the labor supply of help provision to persons in other households, for men and for women ages 50 and older (analyses on SHARE,
not shown here). Those who give more demanding help inside their own
households are everywhere less often employed, although this tendency
is more pronounced in the southern countries.

A Swedish overview of population-based data on care concluded
that carers were mostly in better health than the general population,
and there were no major effects on employment (Socialstyrelsen, 2006).
Yet the British census of 2001 that included two questions on health
and two on caregiving found that carers both suffer poorer health in
general and are financially disadvantaged (Young et al., 2006), again
hitting on the question of cause and effect. Importantly, many people
both work and provide care. Thus, in Switzerland, it is estimated that
12% of women aged 50 to 54 are in paid work and have dependent
parents; rates are lower before and after this age range. In Sweden, the
figure approaches 20% (Perrig-Chiello & Höpflinger, 2005; Socialstyrelsen 2006).

In 2000, 21% of the adult population (16 years and older) in the
United Kingdom were carers, and 5% gave heavy care (at least 20 hours
of care per week)—proportions that have remained stable since the first
General Household Survey probing this topic in 1985 (Office for National
Statistics, 2002). As indicated, British carers often suffer from poor health

and are outside of the labor market, with heavy care frequently being a working-class prerogative (Young et al., 2006).

Heavy care commitments may be less common in the Nordic countries and mostly established rather late in life, when people may have stopped working for other reasons. Importantly, many dependent persons in the northern countries receive both public services and family help, which may facilitate carers remaining in the labor market or other life roles. Informal caregiving seems to be expanding in Sweden in response to stagnating public services (Sundström et al., 2002). In all European countries, most elders have children living in relative proximity, as evidenced in SHARE. In Sweden, over half of elders have at least some adult child in the same municipality (Socialstyrelsen, 2006).

It is possible that patterns of care partly reflect the demographics of a country. For example, there are more middle-aged men and women per thousand old people in Spain than there are in Sweden. Old Swedes hypothetically, then, have fewer family ties (children) to rely on, and the children may thus feel more committed to being caregivers. This has been conceptualized as the caretaker pool, following seminal work by Moroney (1976), defined as the ratio of the number of women ages 45 to 69 to the number of persons age 65 and older. In 1991, the caregiver pool ratio was 1.01 in Spain and 0.88 in Sweden, reflecting higher fertility rates in the 1920s and 1930s in Spain, when Sweden experienced extremely low fertility. This is likely to change, because later cohorts in Spain had low fertility, when it was high in Sweden, but still in 2004 the average number of children was higher in Spain. (In both countries, the majority of people age 50 and older had no, one, or two children.) Given the smaller caregiver pool, one would expect informal caregiving to be more common among middle-aged adults in Sweden than in Spain (see the chapter by Uhlenberg & Cheuk in this volume for the comparable perspective in the United States). This may be reflected in generally more frequent help provided to persons in other households in Sweden than in Spain, but an analysis that pinpoints time transfers (help) to parents finds them to be more frequent in Spain—where 35% of people who are 50 years and older give such help, compared to 27% in Sweden (Attias-Donfut et al., 2005). We suspect that it is problematic to substitute demographical arithmetics for the complex dynamics of informal and formal care.

Legal responsibility for financial support and/or hands-on care is an obvious clue to care policy. Countries vary in the extent to which they enforce these obligations. Sometimes they do so only when costly institutional care is the alternative. Denmark never had any legally prescribed family obligations for elders, whether in poor law or in the family code, yet there is nothing to indicate that Danish family care was any worse—or better—than elsewhere. Other Nordic countries had these obligations but abolished them in the 1950s or somewhat later (Iceland last, in 1991). On the continent, most countries retain prescribed family obligations, except Ireland, Luxembourg, the United Kingdom, and The Netherlands. Examining this issue in a larger context, the Nordic countries jointly liberalized marriage clauses of their family laws in the 1920s, with, for example, no-fault divorce, which most continental countries did not accept until the 1970s. One interesting case is Israel, which applies both family obligations and clear state obligations—under specified conditions—in its care insurance law (Lowenstein, 2006). Refer to Table 11.1 for an overview of who bears legal responsibility for care across selected countries.

Spanish civil law clearly prescribes these obligations, corresponding to the order of inheritance. Italy has similar prescriptions, but with the amendment that family must either pay for care or provide care of dependent persons. (Families in Spain also have this choice.) The EUROFAM-CARE country report for Italy remarks that this law is sometimes used by authorities to blackmail families into providing care. Laws may also prescribe responsibility for stepparents (Slovenia) and aunts and uncles and nieces and nephews (Portugal). Italy and Spain include half-siblings among the legally responsible, but Spain also makes a distinction between the extent of support by which spouses, children, and grandchildren carry a heavier commitment than siblings and their ascendants and descendants. Obligations extend to grandparents in France and some other countries, and sometimes the locus of responsibility in the family is not exactly defined (Bulgaria, Greece, Hungary). Services may be restricted to "persons who have no relatives to take care of them" (Bulgaria).

One may speculate that these obligations tend to correspond with legal prescriptions to keep inheritance within the family. Lack of obligations and testamentary freedom are "natural" partners, as demonstrated in a comparison of France and England (Twigg & Grand, 1998). In a traditional society, aging parents may more often negotiate inheritance against provision of care, as shown in a comparison of inheritance patterns in Japan and England (Izuhara, 2002).

In countries with filial obligations, the state may reclaim some of its costs for care from the old person's legacy, as was the case in Nordic countries in the poor-law era. For example, in France, it was applied with the PSD but so far *allocation personnalisée d'autonomie à domicile* (APA) compensation is exempt from filial obligations, although this has been considered as a means to save costs. In the PSD, this discouraged elders from seeking this assistance (Morel, in press).

In practice, access to close family may determine patterns of care at large, including use of public support. For example, in contemporary Spain, only 17% of institutionalized elders have children, and 61% report that they have no one to support them outside of their residence. The most common motive given for entering an institution was to avoid solitude. In France, 40% of residents have children. In general, their networks are small and many are socially isolated (Cribier, 1998; Desesquelles & Brouard, 2003). Obviously, then, children have rarely "dumped" their parents in these countries. Institutional care in the Nordic countries is more "democratic." In Sweden, 19% of elders in institutions are childless, compared with 14% in the community.

Never-marrieds are over-represented in all institutional care. These patterns gradually change when institutional care shifts from being a place to live for the socially underprivileged to being a residence for the very old and frail at the end of life—as seen, for example, in repeated French surveys (Tugores, 2006). This explains the higher proportions of very old and frail who eventually enter an institution, but for a shorter period of time. For example, in Sweden in 1950, most institutionalized elders were never married and childless, but frequently not frail at all. Some 15% spent the rest of their lives there. Today, more residents are much frailer and less socially underprivileged than in the past, but they also stay a shorter time in institutional care. Yet residents with few family ties are likely to always be over-represented in institutions, because the most important support is the partner, and married persons rarely are institutionalized. Men are no more likely than women to place their partner in an institution in Britain and Sweden; in France, more married men than married women are institutionalized (Tugores, 2006). Family responsibility is sometimes stipulated only for financial maintenance of dependents, but in practice this tends to include care, because institutional care is usually scarce and expensive in countries with this type of legislation. Even in countries with many community services, a tendency of rationing makes itself felt in The Netherlands, for example, through long waiting times (Social and Cultural Planning Office, 2001). In Sweden, access to family networks is increasingly considered in needs assessments, although doing so lacks legal underpinning (Johansson, Sundström, & Hassing, 2003).

State responsibility for care may or may not coexist with family obligations. Thus, France has both state responsibility and family obligations and Ireland has neither state responsibility nor family obligations. Some countries, such as Austria, have a clear state responsibility only in the realm of health care, whereas cases of primarily social needs may be ambiguous. Sometimes the degree of responsibility of the state is unclear or extended only to financial maintenance of elders. Countries also may be in transition, as are Spain and The Netherlands. Officially, Norway guarantees care in the community for elders regardless of how large their needs, whereas Sweden recently had a case in the administrative appeal courts that overturned this official cornerstone of elder care (the municipality refused to provide unlimited Home Help and instead offered a room in a retirement or nursing home, accepted by the court). How far state responsibility extends may, in practice, depend on resources and political will, as it does in any other domain of public affairs.

Norms on responsibility for the elderly have been probed in a few international studies. In the OASIS project, representative samples of elders in Norway, Germany, Britain, Spain, and Israel varied somewhat in their definition of responsibility, but everywhere most wanted responsibility to be shared between family and state, or what has been termed *partnership* (Nolan, 2001). Preferences vary, as may be expected, by actual availability of government support. More than half of those sampled in Israel and Norway were for "mainly state" responsibility for financial support, domestic help, and personal care (see the chapter by Lowenstein, Katz, & Gur-Yaish in this volume). Similar opinions were held about who should be responsible for increasing, future needs (Daatland & Herlofson, 2004). Another international study found similar patterns, shown in Table 11.4.

In Sweden, one-quarter of carers endorse main responsibility for family, compared to three-quarters or more in the other countries. Only in Poland does a large fraction (36%) accept total family responsibility. (A couple of national studies confirm the pattern; see the concluding comparison of Spain and Sweden.) The OASIS study is exceptional in that it considers family and state support simultaneously (Daatland & Lowenstein, 2005). It is unusual to find a discourse on this topic in official publications. A rare exception is a French analysis of the APA that contains a systematic consideration of network configurations of elders at different levels of need and the interaction of family and public

TABLE 11.4   Desired Division of Responsibility Between Family and State Among Carers of the Elderly in Selected European Countries, 2005

Desired responsibility (%)	Sweden	United Kingdom	Poland	Germany	Italy	Greece
Family all	3	3	36	4	12	15
Mainly family, state contributes	22	65	57	71	77	78
Mainly state, family contributes	57	12	5	11	6	3
State all	6	2	1	0	1	0
Don't know or no answer	12	18	1	14	4	4
N	581	320	875	451	863	290

Source: Calculations derived from EUROFAMCARE (2006).

support (Campéon & Le Bihan, 2006). These aspects are likely to be more important in coming years. A survey in Flanders (Belgium) found that most people age 55 and older oppose legal filial responsibility for residential care (Vanden Boer & Vanderleyden, 2003). Still, we rarely encounter discussions of the ambivalence and conflicts that may be inherent for both sides in obligatory care for a dependent older relative.

MODELS OF SUPPORT TO CARING FAMILIES: PAYMENTS OR SERVICES?

Some countries primarily support dependent elderly persons, and others primarily support (caring) family members. The former are the Nordic countries, Britain, and The Netherlands, although the distinction is not always clear-cut and tends to change. Extensive public support to dependent elders is also indirect support to caring families. Direct support to carers includes respite care, day care, and financial support including cash allowances and tax rebates. Countries with relatively high levels of community services have often thought less about informal care and provided rather little direct support to family carers. In Sweden, an aging parent housed by a relative may have to pay more taxes for benefits in kind. In France and in Spain, the same family can take a tax deduction. Payments made under these obligations are tax deductible, for example, in France and Israel. In France, the care recipient has to report the payments as income. If housing is provided, any rent forgone is also tax deductible (Jacobs, 2003).

Germany may be the best example of a country where service levels are rather low, but where persons in need of care are recognized by a care insurance (introduced in 1995, for both institutional and community care), and many family carers are financially compensated. Austria, with comparatively high service levels, only provides cash, but in Germany the person cared for can choose to receive cash or have services paid for. Luxembourg and The Netherlands also have programs akin to a care insurance, Spain introduces one in 2007, some countries (parts of Belgium, Hungary) will introduce them, while others (Ireland, Italy, Slovenia) consider them. A new Finnish program to contract family care also may be considered in this context. Care insurances have mostly been considered in countries with less extensive public elder care and weak local responsibility for services to the elderly. Care insurance typically uses standardized needs assessments, with simple and uniform criteria that provide rights and some choice to persons who are dependent on care, usually fixed in steps with corresponding compensations or services. The Netherlands lets clients decide whom they will hire to provide the care but covers very few elderly people. The Austrian insurance scheme covers 15% of the elderly population, the German one 6% of those age 65 and older, and the Israeli 16%. Countries vary considerably in the level of services provided and distinctions made among levels of need.

France, with its 2002 APA, covers nearly 900,000 beneficiaries, or 5% of the population aged 60 years and older. Dependency is assessed by teams of social workers and health care professionals and is graded on a scale, with ensuing compensations (minus copayments) similar to Austria and Germany. The French APA pays for a needs-assessed care plan, and money can also be used to pay a carer chosen by the client, for home adaptations, and for institutional care (about 40% of the beneficiaries). Frequently, the beneficiaries live with their families, but spouses are not eligible. No compensation is paid when needs are only for household help, which has led to a decrease in public Home Help. With APA, 93% of the users report that they are now able to use professional services, compared with 65% under PSD (Petite & Weber, 2006). Coverage rates of APA vary locally; they are highest in rural regions with higher rates of poverty and working-class and farmer dominance (Jeger, 2005), where many old people suffer health problems. Similar patterns are found for Swedish municipal Home Help (Davey et al., 2006). Large local variations in frailty among old people also emerge in Britain from an analysis of its 2001 census (Young et al., 2006).

Financial compensations to carers may be a mixed blessing. In many countries—less clear in the Nordic ones—family carers are often underprivileged and poor and women. A compensation may improve their situation but may also trap them in the situation. Outcomes should be assessed individually to make sure that the dependent person receives adequate care and the carer is not overtaxed. There may also be consequences of these financial compensations, such as an underdeveloped service sector: it is reported that the attendance allowance in Austria led to a price increase for social services (Evers, Leichsenring, & Pruckner, 1994). The notion of trapping (especially women) carers in the home should be considered and is indeed discussed by professionals in the field (e.g., IMSERSO, 2005a, 2005b). One review concluded that payments that coexist with reasonable coverage of other services may be the best solution, because they provide some measure of choice to both the giver and receiver of care (Millar & Warman, 1996).

INDIRECT SUPPORT TO CARERS

Home Help in some countries covers only housekeeping-type help (such as in Denmark and Norway and several other countries), and some countries have a home care program that provides personal care. In Finland and Sweden, public Home Help is an integrated service that officially does everything except purely medical treatments (but frequently also that); in other countries, the service may provide very limited help with household chores. These and other administrative distinctions complicate any comparison, further worsened by a plethora of providers in some countries, where people may use more than one. Fewer elders in Britain have Home Help than do elders in the Nordic countries.

Statistics on these forms of support are mostly scarce and flawed, but levels of public services are generally higher in the northern parts of Europe, where many countries provide public Home Help to 5% to 10% or more of people age 65 and older; Denmark provides the service to 15% of its elderly population, and Iceland provides Home Help to 20% of its elderly. Many countries in southern Europe report rates around 1% or less, and some lack these services altogether; Spain is an exception with 4% of elderly people using Home Help and another 2% or more using other community services (for example, 3% have *teleasistencia* and 0.5% use day care centers) but not Home Help. Other significant services that may relieve carers are often unreported in the statistics; these include intermediate services such as day care and day centers for dementia sufferers.

Simple coverage rates for individual countries are presented in Table 11.5. Targeting of Home Help and other services differs. In some countries, these services are means-tested; in others, they are for anyone in need. In the Nordic countries, for example, fees are graded by income, and in Denmark the services are free. Users are often elders who live alone (80% to 90% of the users in Nordic countries), and it is not uncommon to focus services on people with low incomes and those who do not have a family to care for them. In southern Europe, users sometimes live with or near family who are typically busy in the daytime (Slovenia expressly mentions this). A criterion of severe dependence may also apply. To disentangle the degree of overlap between various forms of services is statistically tricky, and is reported systematically only in Britain, where, in 2001, 5% reported using Home Help, and 5% reported using some other service but not Home Help. We estimate from 2000 survey data that these proportions are 9% and 8%, respectively, in Sweden.

Coverage rates of community services are generally higher than institutional care in northern Europe, though not uniformly so. In southern Europe, institutional care often has higher coverage rates than community care, in a way mirroring the situation in northern Europe some decades ago. It seems to take longer for community care to develop and receive sustained financing. In Bulgaria, Italy, Poland, and Greece, about 1% or

TABLE 11.5 Home Help Use and Institutionalization Rates of People Age 65 and Older in Selected European Countries, ca. 2000 (%)

Country	Home help coverage rates	Institutiona- lization rates	Year of data
Nordic			
Denmark	15	8	2005
Finland	11	4	2002
Iceland	20	9	2001
Norway	13	6	2004
Sweden	9	6	2005
Northern			
Belgium/Flanders	10	6	2004
Britain	5	5	2003
France	5	7	1998, 1996
Germany	7	4	2003
Luxembourg	5	7	2003
The Netherlands	14	7	1999
Southern			
Austria	15	4	2000
Greece	<1	<1	present
Ireland	5	5	2000
Italy	~1	~1	present
Portugal	n.a. but low	4	2001
Spain	4	4	2005
Not categorized			
Bulgaria	n.a. but low	n.a.	no information
Chechnya	n.a. but low	n.a.	no information
Estonia	~3	~2	2005
Hungary	~5	n.a.	2000
Israel	16	4	2004
Poland	<1	n.a. but low	present
Slovenia	~1	4	present
Switzerland	5	7	2000

Note. Despite our attempt to cover the panorama of care and services in the community, variations may reflect organizational as much as substantial differences. For example, Norwegian Home Help mostly provides household help and an independent organization helps with personal care (and also more or less regular home health care, etc.). This is likely to inflate public services for the elderly in Norway compared to Sweden, where a single organization provides both household help and personal care. On the other hand, many old people in Sweden only use transportation services or some other service, but not Home Help. In Denmark, with more extensive Home Help, few old people rely only on these other services.

Source: EUROFAMCARE (2006).

fewer elders use residential care; in Portugal, Slovenia, and Spain, 3% or a little more use the service. Ireland has little Home Help, and about 4% of its elderly are institutionalized. The Netherlands, which used to have a vast number of various sheltered and unsheltered residences, is now at a 7% institutionalization rate. The United Kingdom is steady at 5%, and Denmark and Iceland are remarkable for their high coverage of Home Help and relatively low coverage of institutional care. As already mentioned, there are often large local variations in coverage rates for services, although regular statistics on local and regional public elder care exist, to the best of our knowledge, only in Britain, France, Spain, and the Nordic countries.

Most European countries are in a process of adaptation to the changing profile of service users, with an increasing number of elders who need much help with their ADLs. For example, both France and Spain now face the same challenge: they have to turn often large social institutions with residents who were there for socioeconomic reasons into smaller residences that provide much more care and health care. Many obstacles make the transition difficult, such as vested private interests in large-scale institutions. The countries in northern Europe have more or less successfully gone through this complicated process, which also requires a restructuring of the work force, training, and other changes.

Except in the Nordic countries, Ireland, The Netherlands, and the United Kingdom, residential care is usually very expensive for the users, although a number of residents may be on welfare. Frequently, there is a two-tiered system with public residences and private ones (for-profit and nonprofit). Many countries have programs for quality controls of Home Help and institutional care, but follow-up is sometimes inconsistent and unsatisfactory, typically varying between providers. This has been the case in the Nordic countries, with their extensive public services. Typically, Swedish authorities used to inspect only the few private nursing homes. Controls may be more systematic and thorough when private providers are publicly financed to provide a service. Where private and public services coexist, comparisons are possible. In the Nordic countries, private (very expensive and rare) institutional care may typically be of higher standing, whereas the picture is more varied in the southern countries. In Spain, public institutions for the elderly are reportedly of higher quality than many private ones.

DIRECT SUPPORT TO CARERS

Several European countries have recently undertaken systematic studies of carers for elderly people and their potential problems and needs for support. As shown in Table 11.2, the frequency of caregiving in the household varies between 4% and 10% for the population aged 50 and older. Between 13% (Norway) and 29% (The Netherlands) of the adult population report that they have care tasks, inside or outside their household. Caring is most common in the 45–64 age span, when parent care is frequent. Country differences may be due to shifting ways to probe care and what is included in the concept. For example, many people in Spain and Sweden report that they "keep an eye on someone": care can be anything—and everything—from relatively easy monitoring to intense personal care.

It is commonly thought that many women take on multiple roles: caring for frail parents, working, and providing for family and small children (Moen & Chermak, 2005). Slovenia reports that this is common, but data in SHARE indicate that this type of situation is (on average) unusual, affecting only about 2% of adult subjects in the multicountry study. Similar results emerge from analysis of German studies (Künemund, 2006), although this situation may become somewhat more common, with delayed "launching" of the younger generation, as previously mentioned (Attias-Donfut et al., 2005). For Britain, evidence indicates that women performing multiple roles is relatively rare, but increasingly common (Evandrou & Glaser, 2004); many women have competing obligations to parents and children, but most manage to fulfill both commitments (Grundy & Henretta, 2006).

Work and care was explored in the EUROFAMCARE project. In Sweden, with high employment rates for both men and women well into their late 50s, it is estimated that one employee in five is also a carer (Socialstyrelsen, 2006). British studies report that between 14% and 19% of the work force have caring duties (Rands, 1997), and German estimates indicate that about one-third of employees are also carers. Several countries have programs meant to soften this predicament, and variations are impressive. In Austria, a maximum of 1 week per year can be used for care, but there are many restrictions and compensation is low. Belgium allows a maximum of 10 days unpaid leave; the Czech Republic allows 9 paid days per diagnosis; Denmark, Norway, and Germany have a certain right to paid leave at serious illness or death in the family. This also appears to be the case in Greece, but only for public employees and for a maximum of 6 days, whereas Italians can use 3 paid days per month for their entire life. Israeli carers have the right to 6 days of paid leave a year (deducted from their allotted sick days) to care for completely dependent parents or parents-in-law. If they have to resign from their job, they are entitled to all dismissal benefits. Luxemburgians can use 3 weeks per year, paid by the national health insurance, and Ireland has a little-used program that offers up to 65 unpaid weeks leave per care recipient, with a prescribed minimum of 13 weeks. In The Netherlands, some unpaid leave is available in central labor agreements, but the program Career Break also theoretically could be used. In Portugal, public employees can have up to 15 unpaid days off per year to care for a sick family member over 10 years old who lives in the same household. In Slovenia, leave is granted for care of a spouse up to 7 paid days per year and up to 30 unpaid days. Spain has a program whereby workers receive 3 to 5 days of unpaid leave when a family member has a disease, accident, or is hospitalized, and public employees in 2005 reached an agreement of up to 1 month of paid, reduced working hours to care for an immediate relative who is seriously ill, with full salary. Swedish employees have a right to take a leave only when someone "near" is fatally ill or dying from an accident, providing up to 60 paid days per person cared for. In the United Kingdom, employers are required to give employees "reasonable" time off under two different programs (Carers Leave and Compassionate Leave). From 2007, carers can request flexible working arrangements under the new Carers' Equal Opportunities Act. Care leave is unheard of in Finland, France, Hungary, Malta, and Poland. These examples illustrate the confusing variation and the limited attempts to facilitate caring and paid work.

Programs in many countries directly or indirectly remunerate carers for their efforts. The largest in scope is undoubtedly the Austrian and German care insurance. The German program gives the user a choice between cash and services, and the monetarized alternative is frequently used to remunerate the carer. Norway and Sweden remunerate a small and shrinking number of carers. The Swedish program was introduced in the 1960s, when a government commission found that many women— mostly never-married—in their 50s and 60s were on welfare after caring for their elderly parents for a long time. Finland has recently (in 2006) formalized an experimental program to reimburse carers on a larger scale; in 2004, about 28,000 persons were reimbursed, and this number is expected to grow. Carers, who must be family or "close," conclude a contract with their municipality that regulates the compensation (from 300 to 600 euros per month), provides 2 days of relief per month, social security, and insurance. The program is tailored for heavy care and persons with smaller needs for care and their carers are said to be better helped in other ways. Municipalities can reclaim 33% of their expenses from the state.

The British special program called Direct Payment covers about 1 in 10,000 of the over-65 population, corresponding to about 1% of service users in this age group. The vision is to expand this considerably (Department of Health, 2005; Fernandez, Kendall, Davey, & Knapp, 2005). The Swedish program covers 0.1%, and the Netherland's personal budget program covers 0.8%—these programs are all quite restrictive. Importantly, a thorough analysis of carers in England and Wales found that carers with heavy commitments are frequently over-represented in disadvantaged segments of the population; providing financial (or other) support for them may be a way to address social inequalities (Young et al., 2006).

A COMPARISON OF SPAIN AND SWEDEN: CARERS AND CARED-FOR ELDERS

Community care is generally agreed to be the most important resource in an era when official policy is that old people are expected to remain at home as long as possible. To learn something about the forces that shape formal and informal care, we compare Spain and Sweden, two European countries that are geographically distant and can be seen as opposites in most regards. They differ in terms of religion and tradition, family and household structures, in their social services and naturally also in their social policy, which is family-oriented in Spain and individualistic in Sweden.

Spain has found services to be unsatisfactory and launched ambitious investigations to assess the situation of elders and their carers. A comprehensive Plan Gerontologico set out in 1993 to reform elder care, and some notable progress has been achieved (see Table 11.5). Sweden, on the other hand, seems to have reached the ceiling of its public service capacity. The implications for the Home Help services and their clients in Spain and Sweden have been studied (Sundström & Tortosa, 1999). Recent data show that coverage rates increase rapidly in Spain but with lower intensity of care, while Sweden has had shrinking coverage rates but higher intensity of help.

Relevant for this comparison is the fact that older people increasingly live alone in Spain (21% in 2006); in Sweden this peaked at about 40% in the 1980s (refer to Table 11.2). A large number of old Swedes are married or partnered only, a life-style that is increasing in Spain but is still less common. As shown in Table 11.6, it is noteworthy that old Swedes who live alone on average need help much more often (28%) than coresident elders (17%), while this is not the case in Spain (21% vs. 19%). In Spain, elders who live with others are on average the frailest group (analysis not shown here). This group is nearly nonexistent in Sweden.

Given these sociodemographic differences, elders who need help often live with family (or others) in Spain, but frequently live alone in Sweden. It is estimated that 5% of Spanish households house one or more dependent elder. Earlier research has shown that older Swedes who live with family (for 96%, this is a spouse) rarely use Home Help. The bulk of Swedish services goes to persons who live alone, and indeed the

TABLE 11.6   Use of Public Services (Home Help) and Source of Help Among People Age 65 and Older Living in the Community in Spain (2004) and Sweden (2002–2003) by Household Structure

	Use of Home Help					
	Living alone		Coresident[a]		All	
	Spain	Sweden	Spain	Sweden	Spain	Sweden
All	22	39	78	61	100	100
Percentage using home help	7	15	2	3	3	8
Percentage needing help with activities of daily living	19	28	21	17	20	21
Percentage of above using Home Help	18	54	6	19	9	37

	Source of Help					
	Spain	Sweden	Spain	Sweden	Spain	Sweden
Percentage who need help	19	28	21	17	20	21
Family only	65	38	76	78	73	58
Home help only	5	24	0	5	1	15
Both	6	30	3	15	4	23
Neither or no help	24	8	21	2	22	5
N	83	392	323	349	406	741

Note. Ns refer to those who need help with one or more of the following activities of daily living: Spain—shopping, cooking, bathing and showering, outdoor mobility, (un)dressing, indoor mobility. Sweden—shopping, cooking, cleaning, laundry, bathing and showering, (un)dressing, getting into and out of bed. From our own computations on Encuesta de condiciones de vida de los mayores 2004 for Spain, and on Statistics Sweden Level of Living Surveys 2002–2003 for Sweden.

[a] Any relationship.

Social Service Act states that municipalities have to provide help when someone "has a need that can not be seen to otherwise." To assess how well services target old people in need, it is therefore crucial to define *need* in a reasonably comparable manner.

We consider people living alone who need help with their ADLs to compare targeting of Home Help services in Spain and Sweden (see Table 11.6). We note that 3% of all elders in Spain use public Home Help compared to 8% in Sweden. In both countries, those who live alone are more likely to use services—7% and 15%, respectively, in Spain and Sweden. Among coresident elders, 2% to 3% use Home Help in either country. Needs for help with ADLs as measured here (as similarly as possible with our data) are about as common in Spain as they are in Sweden (20% and 21%, respectively). Elders who need help more often use Home Help, 9% in Spain and 37% in Sweden. Use rates among coresident persons are higher: 6% in Spain and 19% in Sweden. The service use of frail persons who live alone is, as expected, still higher: 18% of elders who need help and who live alone get Home Help in Spain, compared to 54% of a similar group in Sweden.

After adjusting for differences in living arrangements and frailty, public services target many more elders than we can deduce from the raw national averages, in both Spain and Sweden. Yet, for the most critical group—those who live alone and need help—the service still reaches out to just a minority in Spain. In Sweden, public Home Help targets a little more than half of the eligible recipients. This implies that most of them will need help from other sources in both Spain and Sweden. This takes us to the important issue of the degree of interplay and overlap between what the family and the state are doing respectively for elders in need, analyzed in the lower part of Table 11.6. These tabulations use different items, which explains some of the discrepancies between the two tabulations. This may have led to some underreporting of overlap of family help and public support in the lower part, but it will not seriously distort the major patterns.

Once again we discern national differences, but also some similarities. The family is the main resource for help in both Spain and Sweden (though somewhat less often in Sweden): 73% in Spain and 58% in Sweden of elders who need help rely on their family only. In Spain, 1% of elders rely on Home Help only; in Sweden, a substantial minority of 15% rely on Home Help alone. To get help both from family and from Home Help is more common than relying on Home Help only in both countries: 4% in Spain and 23% in Sweden benefit from overlapping care. Noteworthy is the large group (22%) in Spain who use neither family care nor Home Help. Most of them (17%) hire private help. There are an estimated 1 million caregivers for elders in Spain and at least 100,000 private helpers, often immigrants, legal and illegal (IMSERSO, 2005b). In total, help from family for older people in need is forthcoming about equally often in Spain and Sweden: 77% and 81%, respectively. (About 2% to 4% in either country report unmet needs.) The important difference is the degree of overlap with public services, which is much larger in Sweden, and the use of private help, which is much more prevalent in Spain.

Despite the substantial differences in demographic structure, household arrangements, and coverage of public services between Spain and Sweden and present patterns of care, preferences for care are largely similar in the two countries, as shown in Table 11.7. In the Swedish case, data refer to a population sample of adults age 45 and older, where 32% still had parents alive and 11% had parents who needed help. Families do not want to abandon their elders, but they desire to share the task of providing for them with the state. Table 11.7 also indicates that families bear the main responsibility in Spain (84%); in Sweden, they mostly share it with public services (in 38% of cases, the family is mainly responsible). Carers want the state to take on a larger share of responsibility: there is a marked discrepancy in both countries between actual patterns of care and how carers would prefer them but also a clear distinction between Spanish and Swedish patterns of care. They are, again, mostly family-based in Spain, though a change is underway. A national Spanish opinion survey in 2004 found that 28% wanted the state to provide all or nearly all care of the elderly, 40% were for principal responsibility of the state with the family as participant, 26% were for state support to caring families, and 5% were for total family responsibility—largely the same pattern as in a 2006 survey with older people (12%, 33%, 43%, and 6% respectively; 7% no answer). In the 2004 survey, 31% said that they wanted more community services, and 17% said they wanted more financial support to family carers. Seventy-three percent said that, in case of permanent needs for care, they wanted to remain in their own home rather than institutional care or other solutions (Centre de Investigaciones Sociológicas, 2004).

The remaining differences in preferences between Spain and Sweden probably reflect that families are carrying a larger share in Spain, but preferences also may be affected by what is available in terms of public services for elders. The international OASIS survey found that 61% of the Spanish elderly age 75 and older wanted public services to cover increasing needs of elders in the future, compared to 89% in Norway (Daatland & Herlofson, 2004). Sweden was not part of that study, but an explicit question about who should do more for aging parents confirms that Swedes aged 45 and older who have elderly parents in need of care want the state to take on more responsibility, not less (Table 11.7; Socialstyrelsen, 2004a).

TABLE 11.7 Actual and Preferred Source of Support[a] in Spain and Sweden, 2003–2004 (%)

	Spain				Sweden	
			Parents need help		Family is carer[b]	
	Carers					
Care is...	Actual	Desired	Actual	Desired	Actual	Desired
Mostly or partly public	14	83	54	80	—	70
Wholly or mostly family	84	16	38	16	100	28
Other, don't know, etc.	3	—	6	4	—	3

Note. Data for Spain are from Encuesta de apoyo informal a los mayores en Espana 2004. Data from Sweden are raw data from Socialstyrelsen (2004), a national, representative survey of the population aged 45 and older that was undertaken in 2003. Our own computations.

[a] In Spain, carers of elderly persons, any relationship; in Sweden, persons age 45 and older who have parents alive and care patterns for these parents.

[b] Any person in the family who provides care to parent(s), alone or with public services.

DISCUSSION

Family care for the elderly is the most common form of care in all European countries, despite widely varying household patterns. Rates of solitary living have leveled off in the north but are increasing in the south. Nordic and northern countries experience more overlap of family care and public services, at least when needs for care are extensive. These countries have relatively high coverage rates of Home Help (and other types of community services) and institutional care, but they struggle to maintain them, and, in some countries, these rates have begun to decline.

The introductory overview depicted the confusing and ad hoc character of programs to support dependent elders and their families that have evolved in many European countries. This was also the conclusion of an OECD study that covered several European and some non-European countries. Programs seem rarely to be the outcome of rational considerations, but rather reflect more profound distinctions, and many European countries strive to establish an ideal relation between state and family in elder care.

There are the relatively affluent and (benignly) paternalistic societies, such as the Nordic countries, The Netherlands, and the United

Kingdom, that primarily provide in-kind support to carers (services) and reasonably adequate pensions to most citizens. In other countries, support is mainly financial, be it to carers or cared-for persons, with Austria and Germany as prime examples. There are, lastly, a number of countries where many old people have very small or no (Poland) pensions. The predicament of small or no incomes frequently holds also for the carers, as borne out by the findings of several studies.

The concluding section examines specific data for Spain and Sweden, which are interesting because service provision has shrunk in Sweden in the last decade and has expanded in Spain, where it is set to continue, after a decision on new legislation for a law of dependency. There will also be financial support for about 300,000 carers. It should be noted in this context that popular support for government responsibility does not necessarily mean a desire for major state provision of defined volumes of care but an expectation of a reliable presence of services when they are needed. This is obviously most critical for frail old persons living in the community. It was very helpful that the British census in 2001 asked about caregiving, because all municipalities now can provide information on this for family carers and their support groups and often do so on their Web sites.

A sizable overlap between family care and public services seems to be a workable path toward safeguarding care, both formal and informal, and also implies support to carers. It emerges from international studies that find that sharing between families and the public services is often the preferred situation, both by the elderly and by their families. This may be especially true when needs for care are high. Yet, we may also ask whether the users of services and recipients of family care really want to be objects of planned coordination.

Even in countries with extensive community services, it is felt that targeting may be less than efficient, and unnecessary institutionalization occurs. Clearly, no European country has a perfect model of support to family carers, whether direct or indirect. This should not surprise us, because most countries still spend a small fraction of their gross domestic product on dependency. The experience of the Nordic countries indicates that there is a ceiling to how much will be used for this purpose. Except for the United Kingdom, there is little in the way of citizen rights for carers; they are, for example, not covered by appeal rights in Sweden. Another lesson is that it is not only resources that count but also how they are used. Institutional care is expensive and benefits few people (who may have little family support), while the same resources used for community care may help many dependent persons and their families.

NOTE

1. We want to thank, in no special order, Nathalie Morel, Dorly Deeg, Benedicte de Koker, Thérèse Jacobs, Edith Lodewijckx, Svein-Olav Daatland, Ariela Lowenstein, Mette Nörgaard, Anna Howe, Karin Janzon, Vanessa Davey, Cristina Goncalvez, Alexandra Lopes, Adam Davey, Steffen Hougaard, Marja Vaarama, Viveca Arrhenius, Maria Iacovou, and Anders Klevmarken for help, valuable information, and comments. We have used data from the early release 1 of SHARE 2004. This release is preliminary and may contain errors that will be corrected in later releases. The SHARE data collection has been primarily funded by the European Commission through the 5th framework program (project QLK6-CT-2001–00360 in the thematic program Quality of Life). Additional funding came from the US National Institute on Aging (U01 AG09740–13S2, P01 AG005842, P01 AG08291, P30 AG12815, Y1-AG-4553–01, and OGHA 04–064). Data collection in Austria (through the Austrian Science Fund, FWF), Belgium (through the Belgian Science Policy Office), and Switzerland (through BBW/OFES/UFES) was nationally funded. The SHARE data set is introduced in Börsch-Supan et al. (2005); methodological details are contained in Börsch-Supan and Jürges (2005). See www.share-project.org/

REFERENCES

Aeldre Sagen. (2005). Pårørende til svage aeldre i tal [Carers of frail old people in figures] (mimeo). Copenhagen, Denmark: Author.

Age Concern. (2005). *Three generation households on increase.* Retrieved May 8, 2007, from www.ageconcern.org.uk

Amirkhanyan, A., & Wolf, D. (2003). Caregiver stress and noncaregiver stress: Exploring the pathways to psychiatric morbidity. *The Gerontologist, 43,* 817–827.

Attias-Donfut, C., Ogg, J., & Wolff, F.-C. (2005). European patterns of intergenerational financial and time transfers. *European Journal of Ageing, 2,* 161–173.

Börsch-Supan, A., Jürges, M. (2005). The Survey of Health, Aging and Retirement in Europe—Methodology. Mannheim, Germany: University of Mannheim.

Brodsky, J., Shnoor, Y., & Be'er, S. (2005). *The elderly in Israel.* Statistical Abstract 2005 [in Hebrew]. Jerusalem, Israel: JDC Brookdale and ESHEL.

Campéon, A., & Le Bihan, B. (2006). Les plans d'aide associés à l'allocation personnalisée dáutonomie. Le point de vue des beneficiaires et de leurs aidants. *Études et Résultats No. 461.* Paris: Direction de la Recherche des Études de l'Évaluation et des Statistiques, Ministère de la Santé et des Solidarités.

Centro de Investigaciones Sociológicas. (2004). *Estudio 2.581 Barómetro Nov. (2004).* Observatorio de Personas Mayores, IMSERSO.

Council of Europe. (1998). *Elderly people within their family—Legal and social responsibilities.* Questionnaire for Research Programme, Coord/Elderly (98) 3 Def.

Cribier, F. (1998). La vie au grand age d'une génération de Parisiens (des retraités nés en 1906–1912). *Revue Prevenir, 35,* 99–106.

Daatland, S. O., & Herlofson, K. (2004). Familie, velferdsstat og aldring. Familiesolidaritet i et europeisk perspektiv [Family, welfare state and ageing. Family solidarity in a European perspective]. Rapport 7/04. Oslo: NOVA.

Daatland, S. O., & Lowenstein, A. (2005). Intergenerational solidarity and the family-welfare state balance. *European Journal of Gerontology, 2,* 174–182.

Davey, A., Johansson, L., Malmberg, B., & Sundström, G. (2006). Unequal but equitable: An analysis of variations in old-age care in Sweden. *European Journal of Ageing, 3,* 34–40.

Department of Health. (2005). *Independence, well-being and choice: Our vision for the future of social care for adults in England*. London: Author.

Desesquelles, A., & Brouard, N. (2003). Le réseau familial des personnes agées de 60 ans ou plus vivant à domicile ou en institution. *Population-F, 58*(2), 201–228.

Esping-Andersen, G. (1990). *The three worlds of welfare capitalism*. Princeton, NJ: Princeton University Press.

EUROFAMCARE. (2006). Retrieved September 4, 2006, from www.uke.uni-hamburg.de/extern/eurofamcare/presentations.html

European Union. (2006). *European economy. Special Report No. 1, 2006. 2004 Living conditions in Europe. Statistical pocketbook. Data 1998–2002*. Luxembourg: European Communities.

Evandrou, M., Falkingham, J., Le Grand, J., & Winter, D. (1992). Equity in health and social care. *Journal of Social Policy, 21*, 489–523.

Evandrou, M.,& Glaser, K. (2004). Family, work and quality of life: Changing economic and social roles through the lifecourse. *Ageing and Society, 24*, 771–791.

Evers, A., Leichsenring, K., & Pruckner, B. (1994). Austria. In A. Evers, M. Pijl, & C. Ungerson (Eds.), *Payments for care: A comparative overview* (pp. 191–214). Aldershot, England: Avebury.

Fernández, J. L., Kendall, J., Davey, V., & Knapp, M. (2005). *Direct payments in England: An analytical first cut at the evidence on variation*. Manuscript submitted for publication.

Glaser, K., & Tomassini, C. (2003). Demography: Living arrangements, receipt of care, residential proximity and housing preferences among older people in Britain and Italy in the 1990s: An overview of trends. In K. Sumner (Ed.), *Our homes, our lives: Choice in later life living arrangements*. London: Centre for Policy on Ageing.

Glaser, K., Tomassini, C., & Grundy, E. (2004). Revisiting convergence and divergence: Support for older people in Europe. *European Journal of Ageing, 1*, 64–72.

Grundy, E., & Henretta, J. (2006). Between elderly parents and adult children: A new look at the intergenerational care provided by the "sandwich generation." *Ageing and Society, 26*, 707–722.

Hirst, M. A. (2002). Transitions to informal care in Great Britain during the 1990s. *Journal of Epidemiology and Community Health, 56*, 579–587.

Iacovou, M. (2002). Sharing and caring: Older Europeans' living arrangements. *Schmollers Jahrbuch, 122*, 111–142.

IMSERSO. (2005a). *Cuidados a las personas mayores en los hogares Españoles. El entorno familiar*. Madrid: Ministerio de Trabajo y Asuntos Sociales.

IMSERSO. (2005b). *Cuidado a la dependencia e inmigración. Informe de resultados*. Madrid: Ministerio de Trabajo y Asuntos Sociales.

Izuhara, M. (2002). Care and inheritance: Japanese and English perspectives on the "generational contract." *Ageing and Society, 22*, 61–77.

Jacobs, T. (2003). Paying for informal care: A contradictio in terminis? *European Societies, 5*, 397–417.

Jeger, F. (2005). L'allocation personnalisée d'autonomie: Une analyse des disparités départementales en 2003. *Études et Résultats No. 372*. Paris: Direction de la Recherche des Études de l'Évaluation et des Statistiques, Ministère de la Santé et des Solidarités.

Jenson, J., & Jacobzone, J. (2000). *Care allowances for the frail elderly and their impact on women care-givers*. Labour Market and Social Policy Occasional Papers, No. 41. Paris: Organisation for Economic Co-operation and Development.

Johansson, L., Sundström, G., & Hassing, L. (2003). State provision down, offspring's up: The reverse substitution of old-age care in Sweden. *Ageing and Society, 23*, 269–280.

Künemund, H. (2006). Changing welfare states and the "sandwich generation": Increasing burden for the next generation? *International Journal of Ageing and Later Life, 1*, 11–30.

Lowenstein, A. (2006, December). *Care networks for the elderly in Israel: The community long term care insurance law.* Paper presented at the seminar on Process of Home Care Management in Long Term Care Insurance Systems, Daegu Haany University, South Korea.

Lowenstein, A., & Ogg, J. (2003). *OASIS—Old age and autonomy: The role of service systems and intergenerational family solidarity.* Final Report. Haifa, Israel: Center for Research and Study of Aging.

Millar, J., & Warman, A. (1996). *Family obligations in Europe.* London: Family Policy Studies Centre.

Moen, P., & Chermak, K. (2005). Gender disparities in health: Strategic selection, careers, and cycles of control. *Journals of Gerontology: Social Sciences, 60B*, 99–108.

Montanari, I. (2000). From family wage to marriage subsidy and child benefits: Controversy and consensus in the development of family support. *Journal of European Social Policy, 10*, 307–333.

Morel, N. (in press). Providing coverage against new social risks in Bismarckian welfare states: The case of long-term care. In K. Armingeon & G. Bonoli (Eds.), *The politics of postindustrial welfare states: Adapting postwar social policies to new social risks.* London: Routledge.

Moroney, R. M. (1976). *The family and the state.* London: Longmans.

National Council for the Aged. (1988). *The caring process: A study of carers in the home.* Dublin, Ireland: Author.

Nolan, M. (2001). Working with family carers: Towards a partnership approach. *Reviews in Clinical Gerontology, 11*, 91–97.

Office for National Statistics. (2002). *Carers 2000.* London: Author.

Ogg, J., & Renault, S. (2006). The support of parents in old age by those born during 1945–1954: A European perspective. *Ageing and Society, 26*, 723–742.

Perrig-Chiello, P., & Höpflinger, F. (2005). Aging parents and their middle-aged children: Demographic and psychosocial challenges. *European Journal of Ageing, 2*, 183–191.

Petite, S., & Weber, A. (2006). Les effets de l'allocation personnalisée sur l'aide dispensée aux personnes agées. *Études et Résultats No. 459.* Paris: Direction de la Recherche des Études de l'Évaluation et des Statistiques, Ministère de la Santé et des Solidarités.

Rands, G. (1997). Working people who also care for the elderly. *International Journal of Geriatric Psychiatry, 12*, 39–44.

Recommendation 1428. (1999). Parliament of Europe.

Social and Cultural Planning Office. (2001). *Report on the elderly 2001.* The Hague, The Netherlands: Author.

Socialstyrelsen. (1999). Hur gick det sen? [What happened afterward?]. *Äldreuppdraget 99*, 3.

Socialstyrelsen. (2004a). *Framtidens anhörigomsorg* [Family care in the future]. Retrieved September 4, 2006, from www.sos.se

Socialstyrelsen. (2004b). *Äldres levnadsförhållanden 1988–2002* [Living conditions of old people 1988–2002]. Retrieved September 4, 2006, from www.sos.se

Socialstyrelsen. (2006). *Omsorg människor emellan* [Care between people]. Retrieved September 4, 2006, from www.sos.se

Statistics Norway. (2006). Et grånende Norge [A graying Norway]. Rapporter 21.

Sundström, G., Johansson, L., & Hassing, L. (2002). The shifting balance of long-term care in Sweden. *The Gerontologist, 42*, 350–355.

Sundström, G., & Tortosa, M. A. (1999). The effects of rationing home help services in Spain and Sweden: A comparative analysis. *Ageing and Society, 19*, 343-361.

Szebehely, M. (2005). *Anhörigas betalda och obetalda äldreomsorgsinsatser*. Forskarrapport till Jämställdhetspolitiska utredningen SOU 2005:6 Makt att forma samhället och sitt eget liv [Unpaid and paid old-age care. Research report to the government commission on gender equality SOU 2005:6].

Tugores, F. (2006). La clientèle des établissements d'hébergement pour personnes agées. *Études et Résultats No. 485*. Paris: Direction de la Recherche des Études de l'Évaluation et des Statistiques, Ministère de la Santé et des Solidarités.

Twigg, J., & Grand, A. (1998). Contrasting legal conceptions of the family obligation and financial reciprocity in the support of older people: France and England. *Ageing and Society, 18*, 131-146.

United Nations. (2006). *Population ageing 2006*. New York: Author, Department of Economic and Social Affairs.

Vanden Boer, L., & Vanderleyden, L. (2003). Voor of tegen de onderhoudsplicht: Het woord aan de ouderen. *Wijs over Grijs, 7*, 25-26.

Wheller, L. (2006). *Caring and carers*. London: Office for National Statistics.

Young, H., Grundy, E., & Jitlal, M. (2006). *Care providers, care receivers: A longitudinal perspective*. London: Joseph Rowntree Foundation & London School of Hygiene and Tropical Medicine.

Young, H., Grundy, E., & Kalogirou, S. (2005) Who cares? Geographical variation in unpaid caregiving in England and Wales: Evidence from the 2001 census. *Population Trends, 120*, 23–34.

CHAPTER TWELVE

Caregiving Contexts: Implications for Research and Policy[1]

Maximiliane E. Szinovacz and Adam Davey

The perspective of caregiving guiding this volume draws attention to the various interconnected contexts that impinge on selection of care as well as on the consequences of care provision for caregivers and care recipients, their families, and society. This approach stresses the need to go beyond the predominant models used in past research. Even though the stress model of care (Aneshensel, Pearlin, Mullan, Zarit, & Whitlatch, 1995) includes contexts as moderators of caregiving stress, studies rarely considered such contexts. Similarly, the rational choice models on which much of the research on care selection is based (Henretta, Hill, Li, Soldo, & Wolf, 1997; Silverstein, Conroy, Wang, Giarrusso, & Bengtson, 2002; Wolf, Freedman, & Soldo, 1997) typically consider which specific characteristics of adult children relate to their participation in care but rarely address interrelationships among these characteristics or moderating effects of larger cultural and societal contexts. At the most basic level, viewing care from the perspective of divergent contexts (personal, familial, societal, cultural) affords a more comprehensive perspective than the predominant exclusive emphasis on caregivers or care recipients. More importantly, the contextual perspective emphasizes interconnections among divergent care contexts. Consideration of such interconnections is not only important to grasp the interplay among the diverse forces that shape care decisions and outcomes but also to overcome the static view of care that characterizes much of the care literature. Care systems are constantly in flux, and changes within each context have repercussions for the other contexts.

CONTEXTUAL PERSPECTIVES

The chapters in this volume represent each of these approaches to a contextual perspective of caregiving and care systems. First, as discussed in the introductory chapter, this volume covers divergent contexts (sociocultural, familial, and sociopolitical) and thus contributes to our knowledge base on each specific care context. Caregiving reflects the personal situation and characteristics of caregivers and care recipients. Because much of the literature has emphasized these characteristics, they were not explicitly addressed in this volume. We know from previous research (Altonji, Hayashi, & Kotlikoff, 1992; Johnson & Lo Sasso, 2000; Silverstein et al., 2002; Whitbeck, Simons, & Conger, 1991) and some of the chapters in this volume (Johnson; Lowenstein, Katz, & Gur-Yaish; Silverstein, Conroy, & Gans) that careprovision by family members, though partly driven by altruistic motives (i.e., parents' or spouses' care needs), also reflects caregivers' and care recipients' past relationship history, or the caregivers' competing obligations both within and outside the family.

Family contexts are addressed in three distinct ways. First, by juxtaposing different types of family care (spouse, adult children, young children—see chapters by Davey & Szinovacz, Stoller & Miklowski, and Szinovacz), we draw attention to the differences and similarities of care by different family members. For example, spouse care distinguishes itself from care by others through its primary and strongly obligatory character, its implications for the marital relationship, and the relative absence of competing obligations because most caregiving spouses are of retirement age and have no dependent children. In contrast, care by adult children typically involves some choice—especially if more than one child is available to provide care—and thus raises issues of bargaining among potential adult-child caregivers. Many adult-child caregivers also face competing obligations both inside and outside their families. Young children's involvement in care, on the other hand, is mainly non-normative—especially if children are primary caregivers—or serves to supplement parental caregiving. While adult caregivers can manipulate their other role obligations at least to some extent, children's school attendance is mandatory, and school attendance or performance problems can have legal repercussions. Nevertheless, there are similarities across family systems as well. For example, all pertinent chapters point to the greater involvement of women in care. Racial and ethnic or social class variations in the use of supplemental formal services also appear to permeate all types of family care.

Second, family contexts such as number of children, proximity of at least one child to the parent, or change in adult-child caregivers over time are considered as predictors of care decisions and outcomes. In this way, features of the family system can be shown to impinge on individual caregivers. For example, number of children and especially daughters increases the likelihood of reliance on unpaid help from children (Johnson; Lowenstein et al., this volume), and a sibling's leaving the care network seems to enhance remaining adult-child caregivers' depressive symptoms (Davey & Szinovacz, this volume), which is important because care is most often shared. There is also considerable change in the composition of care networks even over a fairly short time frame. Alternatively, one can focus on families as bargaining systems that distribute care among their members. Although the bargaining perspective is not new (Checkovich & Stern, 2002; Pezzin & Schone, 1997), it draws attention to the equity of care responsibilities within and across families. Some family contexts may promote under- and overproviders within the care system (Silverstein et al., this volume), whereas others may encourage a division of responsibility strictly in terms of cost-benefit calculations.

Third, while family systems shape individual caregiver decisions and outcomes, they are themselves subject to sociocultural and sociopolitical forces. Structural changes at the societal level such as those described by Uhlenberg and Cheuk (this volume) determine the availability of potential caregivers and the composition of care systems. In societies characterized by high fertility among middle-aged cohorts, most adult children will have the option to share care responsibilities and to allow overburdened caregivers to leave the care system; whereas in societies with low fertility among middle-aged cohorts, many adult children may be forced to either assume care under high costs or to rely increasingly on formal help. Whether such formal help is available will, in turn, depend on state or municipal family care policies and the development of formal care systems (Lowenstein et al.; Sundström et al.; Wisensale, this volume).

As in the case of family contexts, sociocultural contexts are addressed in multiple ways. At the macro level, the volume offers estimates on social structural changes that will have profound effects on the future availability of caregivers and the composition of care networks (Uhlenberg & Cheuk, this volume) as well as a cross-national comparative perspective of normative contexts that impinge on the interplay between informal and formal care systems (preference for state versus family responsibility for care; see Lowenstein et al.; Sundström et al., this volume). These chapters remind us that care occurs within sociostructural and cultural settings that may differ widely across countries and vary over time. These contexts constitute the parameters within which care decisions are made.

Indeed, numerous chapters in this volume demonstrate that sociocultural contexts permeate care systems at all levels. The cultural climate in different countries impinges on individuals' and families' care preferences and thus family members' inclination to assume care and to use available formal services. Consequently, even though most family members in Western nations feel some obligation to care for frail or disabled members, preferences for and the actual allocation of responsibility between state and family vary considerably across countries (Lowenstein et al., Sundström et al., this volume). Various other normative influences are also apparent, ranging from the predominant role of women as caregivers to subcultural variations (e.g., by race and ethnicity or socioeconomic status) in the acceptability of paid services and nursing home placement. Whether such preferences and norms are expressed in actual behaviors is contingent on other parameters. Silverstein et al. (this volume) show, for example, that filial responsibility attitudes matter most when the relative costs of care are low. We can speculate that other contexts such as the availability and price of formal services (Johnson, this volume), local labor markets, or workplace policies (Pavalko, Henderson, & Cott, this volume) may also moderate the impact of filial responsibility attitudes on the assumption of care and the extent of care by family members.

The last set of contexts addressed in this volume is sociopolitical—that is, policies and programs pertaining to the legal allocation of responsibility for care, the development and financing of formal care, and supports for family caregivers. We present several chapters (Lowenstein et al.; Pavalko et al; Sundström et al.; Wisensale) that show the diversity of both inter- and intranational policies for elder care. Comparison of these approaches affords a macro-level perspective on how states and municipalities attempt to deal with the growing need for elder care, on the political underpinnings of these diverse approaches, and on the effectiveness of diverse solutions.

In addition, several chapters demonstrate the interplay between cultural and political contexts. For example, the more family-oriented southern European countries tend toward implicit family policies and assignment of care responsibility to families, whereas the more welfare state–oriented Nordic nations tend to develop explicit policies and allocate more responsibility to states and municipalities (Sundström et al., this volume). It is also telling that some solutions such as long-term care insurance financed through the elimination of holidays are accepted in some cultural and political climates but not in others (Sundström et al., this volume). Similarly, the heat-wave related death toll among elderly in France was seen as an elder care and filial obligation issue and spurred the legalization for care responsibilities for families (see the chapter by Wisensale), whereas the albeit regionally confined and smaller death toll of the heat wave in Chicago in 1995 was primarily viewed as a city problem (e.g., in terms of electrical systems failures and lacking shelters) and resulted in the amelioration of city emergency response systems (Klinenberg, 2002).

Yet another way in which sociopolitical contexts are addressed is through the emphasis on the interplay between informal and formal care systems. Several chapters (Johnson; Lowenstein et al.; Sundström et al.) consider the relative reliance on informal and formal help. These chapters demonstrate the supplemental or complementary roles of paid and family care, and their relative impact on each other. For example, in the OASIS study (Lowenstein et al., this volume), use of services at home is associated with less family support, whereas use of community services seems to supplement family care. Indeed, some programs such as the NFCSP (see the chapter by Wisensale) are specifically designed to support family caregivers and to further the coordination of family and formal care.

In summary, then, the chapters in this volume describe different contexts of care, show differences and similarities between contexts at the same level (cultural, familial, political), assess linkages among contexts, and attend at least to some extent to the dynamics of social contexts and care systems. What are the implications of this approach and our findings for research and policy?

IMPLICATIONS FOR RESEARCH

The caregiving scenario awaiting baby boomers as they reach old age will differ substantially from that experienced by their parents. Fewer elderly will have spouses, and, among those who do, we will increasingly see husbands caring for wives as the gender gap in life expectancy narrows. The baby boom elderly will also have to rely on a smaller pool of adult children. Because of delays in child bearing (Szinovacz, in press), many of these children will be in the labor force, and more caregivers will still have dependent children than is typical among current generations. On average, these children will also be better educated than today's caregivers. This means that the potential costs of caregiving to family members and especially to adult children will increase substantially, both because of decreased opportunities to share care with siblings or with spouses (many middle-aged women will be divorced as well) and because of heightened opportunity costs of care (labor force participation, employment in higher-level jobs as a function of higher education). At the same time, funding for Medicare and Social Security will be stretched to its limits, and the squeeze on the labor force as the large baby boom generation retires may render low-paying home care or nursing aid jobs less attractive.

This rather gruesome scenario presents a special challenge to researchers. It clearly shifts the focus of attention from the individual care situation to the larger picture of ensuring quality care for the large number of baby boom elders. A contextual perspective is particularly suited for this endeavor. One possible line of research is the assessment of caregiving experiences for subgroups of caregivers who fit (or do not fit) the predominant demographic profile expected for caregivers of the baby boom cohorts. By contrasting care decisions and experiences among adult children with divergent marital statuses and different numbers of sisters and brothers, it will be possible to gain some insights into potential effects of expected demographic change. It is essential that such family context characteristics are used as moderators in such studies—that is, the focus would be on the interrelationship between family contexts and other predictors on care decisions and outcomes.

Because the future demographic profile of caregivers, as well as the caregiving experience, are likely to differ substantially for divergent racial and ethnic groups (Dilworth-Anderson, Williams, & Gibson, 2002) further exploration of the effects of subcultural contexts is indicated. As described by the chapters in this volume showing cross-national variations, such research should take a comparative perspective that allows for the assessment of within- and across-group differences.

Given expected demographic change, one of the potential features of future care systems will be the greater use of supplemental paid services by family caregivers. Research has only begun to explore interactions among divergent care systems. Because the type and extent of paid service use will differ among selected population subgroups (e.g., socioeconomic status groups), for divergent family care contexts (spouse, adult child, other family members), or for subgroups differentiated by divergent attitudes toward filial responsibility or toward reliance on outside supports, studies will need to investigate the interplay of paid and unpaid care among varying contexts. Results from such research could help develop paid services that better fit caregivers' needs.

One important aspect of the contextual perspective is its emphasis on the dynamics of care. We still know very little about how care experiences change over the caregiving career from a network perspective (Aneshensel et al., 1995; Lawton, Moss, Hoffman, & Perkinson, 2000), and we know even less about the circumstances under which individual caregivers drop out or enter already existing care systems or the circumstances under which they start to obtain or terminate use of paid help (Jette, Tennstedt, & Branch, 1992; Kelman, Thomas, & Tanaka, 1994; Lyons, Zarit, & Townsend, 2000; Szinovacz & Davey, 2007). By its very nature, such research must be contextual because it requires linking characteristics of the care system to individual caregiving decisions and outcomes.

As demonstrated by the cross-nationally comparative chapters in this volume, filial responsibility attitudes and care provision vary considerably across divergent welfare systems. Further exploration of such variations will be helpful to assess how state welfare and care support systems impinge on care decisions and outcomes, and which specific family caregiver problems prevail under specific systems. Because formal care systems often diverge across municipalities or other regional entities (Davey, Johansson, Malmberg, & Sundström, 2006), similar comparative analyses across such entities would be informative as well. As indicated by the chapters in this volume, several cross-national studies are currently underway in Europe. However, we lack analyses that include the United States. Given that the SHARE project was inspired by the U.S. HRS, it should be possible to conduct some cross-national comparisons including the United States by combining SHARE and HRS data.

IMPLICATIONS FOR POLICY

In recent policy debates pertaining to the aging of the baby boom cohorts, long-term care received relatively little attention except in relation to rising health care costs. However, as several chapters in this volume document, we may also face a crisis in regard to the availability of family caregivers and the need for formal help. How can a contextual perspective of caregiving inform policy?

In light of the shrinking pool of potential caregivers and little indication that public funds (especially for formal home care) will increase substantially in the foreseeable future, it will become essential to target scarce subsidized services to the most vulnerable groups. A contextual approach can help in identifying such subgroups through careful analysis of the circumstances under which care needs are not or only marginally met and by identifying those programs that function best for selected subgroups of caregivers.

In addition, the contextual perspective draws attention to the connectedness among divergent life spheres and implicitly the policies pertinent for these life spheres. Policy debates about specific concerns raised by the aging baby boomers have been largely compartmentalized. For example, the debates concerning financing of Social Security or the aging work force have been largely separated from debates about long-term care, and policy issues pertaining to the elderly are rarely tied to issues that concern younger population groups. Yet these concerns are usually intricately linked. For example, caregiver burden is likely to rise as the ratio of potential caregivers to care recipients declines, leading to greater need for caregiver supports. One such need is the expansion of workplace policies to accommodate caregiving employees; another is the expansion of formal help. Employers and employees largely bear the costs of workplace policies for caregivers, whereas costs for subsidized formal care are shared among national, state, and local entities. The costs of financing formal care will thus have to be weighed against labor market costs. On the other hand, it is conceivable that the large pool of young-old nonfrail retired baby boomers could be used to supplement formal care, especially for tasks that require little physical effort. Similarly, it is well known that caregiver stress has negative health outcomes, as evidenced in increased morbidity and mortality among caregivers (Schultz & Beach, 1999; Schulz, O'Brien, Bookwala, & Fleissner, 1995). Yet the health care costs associated with caregiving are rarely weighed against the costs of programs that may alleviate caregiver stress.

Once the relative success of the divergent strategies developed by European nations to deal with long-term care issues is better understood, the more successful programs could provide useful guidelines for policymakers in the United States. However, these strategies will have to be carefully assessed within each country's welfare system and infrastructure context. A strategy that works well in Germany may not work in France (see the chapter by Wisensale, this volume), and workplace policies that are acceptable to European employers may be opposed by those in the United States. In addition, the specific cultural climate in each country and cultural variations within each country (e.g., in regard to the preferred mix between state and family responsibility for the elderly; see chapters by Lowenstein et al. and by Sundström et al., this volume) would have to be taken into account.

In devising strategies for dealing with the increased demand for care in the future, it will also be important to consider foreseeable changes in diverse contexts such as the labor force in general or the home care industry in particular. Technological advances in the workplace are likely to increase opportunities for work at home, a trend that will aid coresident caregivers. On the other hand, the shrinking pool of workers after the retirement of the baby boom cohorts and increases in the average level of education among future workers will render lower-level and poorly paid care service jobs such as home help aids less attractive and thus more difficult to fill. More coordination and perhaps specialization of services may serve the divergent needs of caregivers and also enhance the appeal of home care jobs.

Amid generalized projections about future care needs it is essential to acknowledge the heterogeneity of family caregivers and care recipients. Selected policies are likely to benefit some groups more than others. For example, some jobs lend themselves to flexible work hours while others do not; some family caregivers require only occasional reprieve from their care responsibilities, while others need daily supports; some care recipients might prefer formal help over aid from relatives; and some will require care only at very old ages when caregiving relatives are likely to have retired but may themselves suffer from diverse ailments, whereas others will need care at relatively young ages when caregiving relatives are in the labor force and still have dependent children. Thus, any care system is only likely to work if it is sufficiently flexible to accommodate the divergent needs and preferences of caregivers and care recipients in a heterogeneous society.

The chapters presented in this volume offer a multifaceted picture of caregiving and care systems within and across sociocultural, familial, and sociopolitical contexts. The linkages among these contexts and their dynamics over time will shape the care scenario for future generations of elders. Although there is little evidence supporting the often-publicized concerns that families may abandon their needy elderly, the expected squeeze on future caregivers will require more concerted efforts on the part of formal care systems to lighten family caregivers' burden. As both the European and U.S. contributors to this volume contend, the solution to quality care for future elders lies not only in the improvement or expansion of specific care systems and supports, but also (if not foremost) in the development of collaboration between caregiving families and support systems. Research guided by a contextual perspective can help identify the complex interplay among diverse care systems and its implications for policy and practice.

NOTE

1. Preparation of this chapter was funded in part by a grant from the National Institute on Aging, R01024045, Maximiliane E. Szinovacz, P.I.

REFERENCES

Altonji, J. G., Hayashi, F., & Kotlikoff, L. (1992). Is the extended family altruistically linked? Direct evidence using micro data. *American Economic Review, 82*(5), 1199–1220.

Aneshensel, C. S., Pearlin, L. I., Mullan, J. T., Zarit, S. H., & Whitlatch, C. J. (1995). *Profiles in caregiving: The unexpected career.* San Diego, CA: Academic Press.

Checkovich, T. J., & Stern, S. (2002). Shared caregiving responsibilities of adult children with elderly parents. *Journal of Human Resources, 37*(3), 441–478.

Davey, A., Johansson, L., Malmberg, B., & Sundström, G. (2006). Unequal but equitable: An analysis of variations in old-age care in Sweden. *European Journal of Ageing, 3*, 34–40.

Dilworth-Anderson, P., Williams, I. C., & Gibson, B. E. (2002). Issues of race, ethnicity, and culture in caregiving research: A 20-year review (1980–2000). *The Gerontologist, 42*(2), 237–272.

Henretta, J. C., Hill, M. S., Li, W., Soldo, B. J., & Wolf, D. A. (1997). Selection of children to provide care: The effect of earlier parental transfers. *Journals of Gerontology: Social Sciences, 52B,* 110–119.

Jette, A. M., Tennstedt, S. L., & Branch, L. G. (1992). Stability of informal long-term care. *Journal of Aging & Health,* 4(2), 193–211.

Johnson, R. W., & Lo Sasso, A. T. (2000). *The trade-off between hours of paid employment and time assistance to elderly parents at midlife.* Washington, DC: Urban Institute.

Kelman, H. R., Thomas, C., & Tanaka, J. S. (1994). Longitudinal patterns of formal and informal social support in an urban elderly population. *Social Science Medicine,* 38(7), 905–914.

Klinenberg, E. (2002). *Heat wave: A social autopsy of disaster in Chicago.* Chicago: University of Chicago Press.

Lawton, M. P., Moss, M., Hoffman, C., & Perkinson, M. (2000). Two transitions in daughters' caregiving careers. *The Gerontologist,* 40(4), 437–448.

Lyons, K. S., Zarit, S. H., & Townsend, A. L. (2000). Families and formal service usage: Stability and change in patterns of interface. *Aging & Mental Health,* 4(3), 234–243.

Pezzin, L. E., & Schone, B. S. (1997). The allocation of resources in intergenerational household: Adult children and their elderly parents. *American Economic Review,* 87(2), 460–464.

Schultz, R., & Beach, S. (1999). Caregiving as a risk factor for mortality: The caregiver health effects study. *Journal of the American Medical Association,* 282(23), 2215–2219.

Schulz, R., O'Brien, A., Bookwala, J., & Fleissner, K. (1995). Psychiatric and physical morbidity effects of dementia caregiving: Prevalence, correlates, and causes. *The Gerontologist,* 35(6), 771–791.

Silverstein, M., Conroy, S. J., Wang, H., Giarrusso, R., & Bengtson, V. L. (2002). Reciprocity in parent-child relations over the adult life course. *Journal of Gerontology: Social Sciences,* 57(1), S3–S13.

Szinovacz, M. E. (in press). Commentary: The future of intergenerational relationships—variability and vulnerabilities. In K. W. Schaie & P. Uhlenberg (Eds.), *Social structures: The impact of demographic changes on the well-being of older persons.* New York: Springer.

Szinovacz, M. E., & Davey, A. (2007). Changes in adult-child caregiver networks. *The Gerontologist.*

Whitbeck, L. B., Simons, R. L., & Conger, R. D. (1991). The effects of early family relationships on contemporary relationships and assistance patterns between adult children and their parents. *Journal of Gerontology,* 46(6), S330–S337.

Wolf, D. A., Freedman, V., & Soldo, B. J. (1997). The division of family labor: Care for elderly parents. *Journals of Gerontology: Social Sciences, 52B,* S102–S109.

Index

AARP. *See* American Association for Retired Persons (AARP)
Absolute support, 85
Active coping, 181
Activities of daily living (ADL)
  data analysis and, 19
  defined, 11
  disability rates and, 14
  formal vs. informal care and, 21
  HRS study questions and, 43
  linked data and, 133–134
  service user changes and, 255
  technology advancements and, 15
  types of, 11, 43
ADL. *See* Activities of daily living (ADL)
Adult children caregiver
  characteristics of, 136
  constraints and, common, 135
  factors of care and, 136
  parental assistance and, 135
Affect and consensus questions, 98–99
Age (cohort) differences, 126
Aging population
  baby boom cohorts and, 9
  caregivers and, access to, 10
  elder care and, future of, 9
  formal care and, 10

  home health care and, 10
Aging process, 93
Aging workforce, 195
Albeit limited tool, 200
Allen, S. M., 121
Allocation personnalisée d'autonomie à domicile (APA), 248, 250, 252
American Association for Retired Persons (AARP), 134, 217
Amirkhanyan, A. A., 149
Analytic strategy in commitment to caring, 79–81
APA. *See* Allocation personnalisée d'autonomie à domicile (APA)
Arlinghaus, K., 119
Article 207 of the Civil Code, 225
Assistance, distribution of, 136
Assistance, multiple child
  biological vs. stepchildren care providers and, 139
  care expectations and, 139
  caregiver change and, 140
  care networks and, 138
  care tasks and, allocating, 139
  filial responsibility and, 138
  gender differences and, 138
  informal vs. formal care and, 139–140